MEDICAL TECHNOLOGY REVIEW

MEDICAL TECHNOLOGY REVIEW

Lorraine D. Doucet, CSC, PhD., Editor

Medical Technology Program Director
Professor of Biology
Notre Dame College
Manchester, New Hampshire

J. B. LIPPINCOTT COMPANY • Philadelphia • Toronto

1 3 5 6 4 2

Library of Congress Cataloging in Publication Data
Main entry under title:

Medical technology review.

   Includes bibliographies and index.
   1. Medical technology. I. Doucet, Lorraine D.
[DNLM: 1. Technology, Medical. QY 46 M4895]
RB37.5.M43   616.07'5'028   80-28781
ISBN 0-397-50459-4

The authors and publisher have exerted every effort to ensure that drug
selection and dosage set forth in this text are in accord with current
recommendations and practice at the time of publication. However, in
view of ongoing research, changes in government regulations, and the
constant flow of information relating to drug therapy and drug reactions,
the reader is urged to check the package insert for each drug for any
change in indications and dosage and for added warnings and precautions.
This is particularly important when the recommended agent is a new or
infrequently employed drug.

Cover photograph courtesy of

G. Berry Schumann, M.D.

Contributors

SHIRLEY H. BRIEN, BA, MT(ASCP)
Chief Technologist, Catholic Medical Center
Manchester, New Hampshire
Assistant to Regional Inspector for the College
  of American Pathologists' Inspection and
  Accreditation Department
Skokie, Illinois

JOYCE M. CUFF, PhD.
Assistant Professor Biology
Notre Dame College
Manchester, New Hampshire

LORRAINE D. DOUCET, CSC, PhD.
Director, Medical Technology Program
Professor of Biology
Notre Dame College
Manchester, New Hampshire

RAYMOND L. METHOT, BS, MS, MT(ASCP)
Manchester, New Hampshire

PAULA M. MILLER, MST, CLS
MLT Program Director
Assistant Professor Medical Technology
Department of Biological Science
Anna Maria College
Paxton, Massachusetts

MARGARET MUELLER-SHORE, MT(ASCP), CLS (NCA), MS
Medical Technology Program Director
Central Maine Medical Center
Lewiston, Maine

ALBERT E. PACKARD, BS, MT(ASCP)
Instructor of Biology
Natural Science Division
Notre Dame College
Manchester, New Hampshire

JAMES J. VAILLANCOURT, MT(ASCP)
Supervisor Clinical Chemistry
Concord Hospital
Concord, New Hampshire

Preface

This book has been designed for students of medical technology and practicing clinical scientists and has been written by Medical Technologists and educators involved in medical technology programs. This book attempts to bridge the gap between the classroom and the clinical laboratory; to blend theoretical scientific knowledge with clinical laboratory experience.

Since each chapter could be a separate text, this book does not intend to compete with large technical volumes in the field, but rather to serve as a broad foundation upon which technical details may be assimilated, understood and applied in a clinical setting.

Each chapter is not condensed for the sake of condensation and distillation but rather, each contributor has included only those salient theoretical and practical points believed important. Theory, and diagnostic procedures are presented in a straightforward manner.

Tables, charts, illustrations and typical laboratory profiles are used to facilitate comprehension of the most widely used clinical principles.

"Med Techs" and educators share their knowledge and clinical experience in special topics in Bacteriology, Clinical Mycology, Parasitology, Virology, Immunology/ Serology, Immunohematology, Hematology, Clinical Chemistry, Nuclear Medicine (Wet Work), Urinalysis/Body Fluid Analysis, and Quality Control/Management in the Clinical Laboratory.

Consequently, this Medical Technology Review text is intended to help the students of clinical medicine and clinical laboratory practitioners to prepare for either multidisciplinary certification, registry or proficiency examinations. Furthermore, in this age of specialization, laboratorians and educators will also find this book to be a helpful tool to refresh their memories in less familiar clinical areas.

The updated Bibliography and Recommended Readings at the end of each chapter will also aid to identify the relevant texts in several clinical areas.

Acknowledgements

A special acknowledgement is due to the contributors who realize the value of the Medical Technology profession and care and dare enough to share their knowledge with prospective and practicing "Med Techs".

The excellent work performed by Medical Technologists should be noted; work which is too frequently taken for granted and not fully appreciated and recognized.

I also wish to express my appreciation to: Juliette LeBlanc, CSC and Jeannette Vezeau, CSC for their ongoing support; my friends for their patience, endurance and loyalty; Blanche E. Duval for typing the manuscript; Cathy Morrison for finalizing the art work, and Jim Morrison for providing this opportunity.

Contents

Chapter 1

Bacteriology

LORRAINE D. DOUCET, CSC, PhD.
Medical Technology Program Director
Professor of Biology
Notre Dame College
Manchester, New Hampshire

OUTLINE

INTRODUCTION

The role of Bacteriology in the clinical laboratory cannot be overemphasized. Morphological traits, isolation, and identification procedures are routine for the experienced microbiologist. However, the student of microbiology, the prospective Medical Technologist, or the relatively inexperienced practitioner may be overwhelmed or "swamped" by the numerous diagnostic procedures and results. This could be avoided if academic courses were structured in such a way so as to bridge the gap between the classroom and the laboratory. Many educators teaching Pathogenic or Diagnostic Bacteriology courses do not have the clinical experience to help the students bridge the "college to laboratory" gap.

This section attempts to help students, prospective "med techs", and practitioners to link the theoretical and the practical by listing theory and diagnostic procedures in a straightforward and simple manner. No text can replace "hands on" experience, but hopefully this section will familiarize the reader with the frequently encountered bacterial pathogens and diagnostic procedures. Stepwise test procedures are not included in the section, but diagnostic results are included. It is suggested that the reader use procedure manuals for stepwise laboratory procedures (see Bibliography and Recommended Readings). To maintain simplicity, serological techniques are not in this section, However, several pertinent serological tests can be found in the IMMUNOLOGY/ SEROLOGY section.

BACTERIOLOGY

The Staphylococci

FAMILY: MICROCOCCACEAE
GENUS: STAPHYLOCOCCUS

Three staphylococcal species are reocgnized. These are: *Staphylococcus aureus, Staphylococcus epidermidis*, and *Staphylococcus saprophyticus*.

MORPHOLOGY/STAINING/PHYSIOLOGY

As a group, the staphylococci are non-motile, non-spore forming Gram positive cocci which measure 0.5 to 1.0 μm in diameter. Most of the staphylococci are non-encapsulated, however, a limited number of strains are encapsulated. Since encapsulation seems to impede phagocytosis of the pathogenic staphylococci, encapsulation has been associated with virulence.

When stained, the staphylococci usually appear in irregular clusters often referred to as "grape-like" clusters. Occasionally, however, the stained staphylococci may be found singly, in pairs, or in short chains.

The staphylococci are facultative anaerobes which grow well aerobically or anaerobically. An increased carbon dioxide atmosphere (5-10% CO_2) may enhance their growth aerobically. The staphylococci are not nutritionally fastidious and meat peptone containing media will serve as general purpose growth media. These bacteria grow abundantly on enriched media, such as blood agar. Trypticase soy agar is an excellent stock culture medium. For primary isolation, blood agar is the medium of choice.

Although the staphylococci demonstrate a fairly wide temperature and pH growth range, their optimum temperature range is 35-40°C and their optimum pH range is 6.8-7.3.

The staphylococci are halophilic; they can grow on media containing 7-10% to (w/v) sodium chloride. A few strains have been reported to grow on media containing as high as 15% sodium chloride. This halophilic trait is useful in differentiating and isolating staphylococci from related and morphologically similar bacteria.

Staphycococcus Aureus

Since *S. aureus* is ubiquitous, it is frequently encountered. *S. aureus* is generally considered to be the most pathogenic member of the family Micrococcaceae. *S. aureus* is isolated from diseased skin and mucous membranes. This bacterium is commonly recovered from absesses, pustules and furuncles. Furthermore, this organism is the causative agent of septicemia, pneumonia, meningitis and osteomyelitis. Certain strains of *S. aureus,* which produce a soluble, heat-stable enterotoxin, may cause food poisoning. Vomiting and intestinal disorders are experienced 24-48 hours after consuming foods contaminated with S. aureus. Creamy pastries or potato salads containing either mayonnaise or salad dressings enriched with eggs may support the growth of *S. aureus*. This type of food poisoning is categorized as an intoxication caused by the ingestition of the enterotoxin. Recovery is usually apparent within 24-48 hours. *S. aureus* organisms are not usually recovered from stool specimens therefore foods ingested by the patients, which are suspected of being contaminated with *S. aureus,* should be used to recover the agent responsible for the intoxication. The enterotoxin itself may be identified immunologically by the gel diffusion technique. Following incubation at 37°C for 24 hours, most primary isolates will demonstrate a clear zone of hemolysis on blood agar. This total dissolution of the sheep or rabbit blood cells is due to the extracellular alpha hemolysin elicited by most *S. aureus* strains. Since the *S. aureus* hemolysin is not highly effective on human red blood cells, human blood is not recommended for blood agar preparations. The more virulent the *S. aureus* strain, the greater the alpha toxin production, and consequently the broader the zone of hemolysis around the individual clones. The alpha toxin is perhaps the most dangerous toxin produced by *S. aureus* strains. In animal tests, the alpha exotoxin has been demonstrated to be hemolytic, leukocidal, dermonecrotic and lethal. Other important toxins and enzymes produced by *S. aureus* strains include: P-V leucocidin, coagulase, hyaluronidase, staphylokinase (fibrinolysin), deoxyribonuclease, lipase, phosphatase and enterotoxin. Only those *S. aureus* strains which produce enterotoxin can cause food poisoning. The enterotoxin may be identified serologically.

Leukocidin is a soluble substance which destroys leukocytes. Coagulase is a plasma chelating enzyme which forms a protective fibrin wall around lesions formed by *S. aureus* coagulase producing strains. Hyaluronidase is an enzyme which breaks down hyaluronic acid. As a result of hyaluronic acid destruction, connective tissue can be destroyed and thereby virulent staphylococci may spread throughout the host.

Staphylokinase (fibrinolysin) is an enzyme which breaks down fibrin clots and consequently allows the virulent staphylococci to invade the body.

Enterotoxin is the heat stable toxin which is responsible for gastroenteritis in *S. aureus* food poisoning.

BACTERIOLOGICAL IDENTIFICATION

PIGMENTATION

Since there are several strains of *S. aureus*, colony color may vary. Growth on agar slants may be white, creamy, yellow or orange, depending upon the strain. Primary isolates on sheep blood agar plates are usually beta hemolytic and the colonies may be white, cream, yellow or yellow-orange in color. Laboratory identifi-

TABLE 1

BACTERIOLOGICAL MEDIA AND COLONY CHARACTERISTICS

Media	Characteristics
Blood Agar	Smooth, circular, creamy or golden, beta hemolytic clones. (*S. aureus* strains are generally beta hemolytic on sheep blood agar preparations).
Staphylococcus Agar #110	Circular, creamy or golden colonies.
Chapman Stone Agar	Circular, golden, glistening colonies. Frequently, a clear ring or zone may form around the colonies.
Mannitol Salt Agar	Salt tolerant, mannitol fermenting strains grow on this medium. A yellow zone or halo around the colonies is indicative of mannitol fermentation.
Coagulase Mannitol Agar	Coagulase positive and mannitol fermenting strains form large yellow rings or zones around the colonies; coagulase negative mannitol fermenting strains may form clear yellow halos or zones in the medium; coagulase negative, mannitol negative strains do not discolor the medium and the medium remains a clear bluish-purple. The appropriate coagulase plasma is added after autoclaving the mannitol agar.
Tellurite Glycine Agar	Coagulase positive strains reduce tellurite and appear as grayish-black colonies.
Vogel and Johnson Agar	Coagulase positive, mannitol fermenting strains appear as black colonies surrounded by yellow zones.
D Nase Agar	Deoxyribonuclease producing strains, when treated with 1N HCl, demonstrate a clear ring or zone around the colonies; when treated with 0.1% toluidine, D Nase positive colonies demonstrate pink zones.

cation of *S. aureus* is dependent upon isolation of the bacterium. To screen for, and identify *S. aureus* strains, most laboratories employ a combination of the following as DIAGNOSTIC CRITERIA:

1. Gram positive cocci
2. Beta hemolysis on sheep blood agar preparations
3. Coagulase positive tube or slide test
4. D Nase positive test
5. Acid production or anaerobic fermentation of mannitol
6. Phosphatase positive test
7. Salt tolerance (up to 15% NaCl)

Although most beta hemolytic *S. aureus* strains are coagulase positive, D Nase positive and mannitol fermenters, there are exceptions to all cases. Some beta hemolytic *S. aureus* strains have been found to be coagulase negative, other strains have been reported to be D Nase negative and still others have failed to ferment mannitol. Consequently, it is recommended that all or a combination of the diagnostic tests be performed to clinically identify *S. aureus* strains.

It might also be important to note that most bacteriologists recommend the tube test which demonstrates "free" coagulase over the slide test which shows "bound" coagulase and suggest that negative coagulase slide tests be checked by the coagulase tube test. To bacteriologically screen and identify *S. aureus*, most bacteriologists use a combination of the media listed in Table 1.

Antibiotic Resistance

S. aureus strains demonstrate resistance to antibiotics. Some strains demonstrate multiple antibiotic resistance, i.e., the strains fail to be sensitive to a multiplicity of antibiotics. Consequently, antibiotic sensitivity tests should be routinely performed. Because of the general use of antibiotics in the last decade, the staphylococci are believed to have acquired new genes which are responsible for the acquired drug resistance. These "new" genes are usually present on extrachromosomal materials and replicate independently of the organisms.

To date, different *S. aureus* strains have demonstrated resistance to penicillin, erythromycin, the tetracyclines and chloramphenicol.

EPIDEMIOLOGY

Healthy carriers harbor *S. aureus* on the mucous membranes of the nose, on the skin and in the intestines. Healthy carriers are primarily responsible for the spread of *S. aureus*. The nasal carrier is believed to be responsible for the high incidence of staphylococcal infections in hospitals.

IMMUNIZATION

In the past, alpha toxoid culture filtrates, attenuated vaccines, and phage lysates were used to control and prevent chronic staphylococcal infections. Evidence does not suggest that these were highly effective in chronic and recurring infections.

TREATMENT

Sensitivity testing demonstrates whether the *S. aureus* strain in question is penicillin resistant. If it is not resistant, penicillin is the drug of choice. However, should the isolated pathogenic staphylococcus produce penicillinase, then

oxacillin, methicillin, cloxacillin, erythromycin, the tetracyclines, the sulfonamides, and chloramphenicol usually are effective against this Gram positive bacterium.

Staphylococcus Epidermidis

GENERAL CHARACTERISTICS

Staphylococcus epidermidis biotypes resemble Staphylococcus aureus strains with
regards to Gram staining characteristics; salt tolerance pH, growth and oxygen requirements, however, with regards to colony pigmentation, *S. epidermidis* clones are nearly
always white. Physiologically, *S. epidermidis* strains usually are:

1. Not beta hemolytic on blood agar
2. Coagulase negative
3. Deoxyribonuclease negative
4. Mannitol negative, and
5. Novobiocin sensitive

VIRULENCE

S. epidermidis is relatively nonpathogenic on the skin and on the mucous membranes
of the upper respiratory tract. Nevertheless, different *S. epidermidis* biotypes have
been implicated in stitch infections and subacute bacterial endocarditis.

TREATMENT

Should *S. epidermidis* be the causative agent of an infection, then the antibiotics
effective against the Gram positive bacteria could be used. However, to assure proper
antibiotic administration, antibiotic sensitivity tests should be performed in the
laboratory.

Staphylococcus Saprophyticus

S. saprophyticus strains are Gram positive cocci which occur most frequently in
irregular clusters, but may occasionally occur either as single cells, pairs or
tetrads. *S. saprophyticus* is a non-motile, facultative anaerobe which grows on
fairly complex media and requires a minimum of 5% NaCl for best growth results. Four
S. saprophyticus biotypes have been reported, based on carbohydrate utilization. Some
strains produce acid from mannitol. Hemolysis production has not been reported.

PATHOGENICITY

Generally, *S. saprophyticus* strains are considered non-pathogenic, however some
strains have been involved in urinary bladder infections.

ISOLATION

When medically or clinically significant, *S. saprophyticus* may be isolated from
the urine of infected persons. Otherwise, this organism may be recovered from dust,
soil, dairy products and from the surface of dead animal tissues.

TABLE 2

DIFFERENTIATION OF THE STAPHYLOCOCCI

Species	Gram Stain	Alpha Toxin	Coagulase	Mannitol	D Nase	Phospha- tase	Novobi- ocin	Salt Tolerant (7-10%)	Cata- lase	Gelatin Liquifaction
S. aureus	+	+	+	+*	+	+	S	+	+	+
S. epidermidis	+	-	-	-*	-	-	S	+	+	D
S. saprophyticus	+	-	-	-*	-	**+/-	R	+	- (usually)	+

+ = positive   - = negative   S = sensitive   R = resistant   D = delayed

*Most strains of *S. aureus* are mannitol positive.
Most strains of *S. epidermidis* are mannitol negative, but one strain produced acid from mannitol.
**Two of the 4 *S. saprophyticus* strains were positive and 2 were phosphatase negative.

TREATMENT

Sensitivity tests hould be performed to determine drug resistance. Penicillin, erythromycin methicillin and any other antibiotic. effective against Gram positive bacteria should be effective.

The Streptococci

FAMILY: STREPTOCOCCACEAE
GENUS: STREPTOCOCCUS

MORPHOLOGY/STAINING/PHYSIOLOGY

The streptococci are Gram positive, non-motile, non-spore forming spherical bacteria which measure approximately 0.6 to 1.0 μm in diameter. The streptococci characteristically appear in chains because the members of this genus divide in only one plane. Growth in broth cultures seems to increase the chain length. The streptococci are facultative anaerobes which are nutritionally fastidious, especially upon primary isolation. Although Gram positive, older cultures may appear Gran negative. As a group, the streptococci are catalase and oxidase negative, and do not contain heme compounds. The streptococci grow best at 35-37°C. Since some strains are microaerophilic, and do not grow best in atmospheric oxygen, an increased CO_2 atmosphere (10%) may enhance their growth. Since the streptococci are faily fastidious, enriched media are essential. Blood agar and the following broths are used to cultivate the streptococci: Todd-Hewitt, thioglycollate, brain-heart infusion, Mueller Hinton and casein digest.

Some of the clinically significant pathogenic streptococci are listed in Table 3.

TABLE 3

Species	Lancefield's Classification	*Hemolysis on Sheep Blood Agar
S. pyogenes	Group A	Beta
S. agalactiae	Group B	Usually Beta but some strains can be either Alpha or Gamma
S. faecalis	Group D	Gamma (few strains are Alpha)
S. pneumoniae	None	Alpha
S. mitis	None	Alpha
S. facium (durans)	**Group D	Alpha

*Hemolysis data from Bergey's *MANUAL OF DETERMINATIVE BACTERIOLOGY* (8th Edition).
**Listed as *S. facium* in Bergey's *MANUAL OF DETERMINATIVE BACTERIOLOGY* (8th Edition).

CLASSIFICATION OF THE STREPTOCOCCI

   Bergey's *MANUAL OF DETERMINATIVE BACTERIOLOGY* (8th Edition) groups the streptococci as: pyogenic, viridans, enterococcus and lactic. The Lancefield classification
system is based on the antigenic properties of the streptococci. Precipitin reactions
for a cell wall polysaccharide (C substance) are different for each group of streptococci and permit the formation of a number of antigenic groups. Clinically however,
the simplest classification is based upon the hemolytic action of the streptococci
grown on sheep blood agar preparations. Streptococci activity on sheep blood agar
preparations are: (1) Alpha--green or brownish zones around the clones due to the
partial dissolution of RBC's; (2) Beta--a clear zone around the clones due to the
complete breakdown of RBC's; (3) Gamma--no hemolysis or lysis of RBC's. Sheep blood
agar preparations are recommended for the cultivation of the streptococci. This will
prevent confusing the streptococci with *Haemophilus haemolyticus* which is also hemolytic, but only on rabbit or human blood agar. Furthermore, a Gram stain will readily
differentiate this Gram negative rod shaped mucous membrane commensal from the Gram
positive streptococci.

PATHOGENICITY

   Streptococcus pyogenes (Group A, beta hemolytic) may cause numerous infections or
diseases among which are: sinusitis, tonsillitis, pharyngitis, erysipelas, impetigo,
rheumatic fever, scarlet fever, puerperal fever, glomerulonephritis, bronchitis,
bronchial pneumonia and pleurisy. *Streptococcus pyogenes* is also frequently found
in wound infections and infections of burn victims.

   Streptococcus pyogenes strains (Group A) account for 90-95% of all streptoccal
infections. Group A streptococci produce extracellular enzymes and other substances
which permit them to invade their host. These are listed in Table 4.

   The toxic substances listed in Table 4 are not restricted to the Group A, *Streptococcus pyogenes* strains. Certain members of Groups C and G streptococci produce
streptokinase and streptolysin S.

LABORATORY IDENTIFICATION

1. Hemolysis

   The type of hemolytic reaction (Alpha, Beta or Gamma) on sheep blood agar preparations provides preliminary separation of streptococcal species.

2. Gram Stain

   Suspected colonies should be Gram stained for verification. Streptococci colonies
should appear Gram positive and be mostly in a chain arrangement.

3. Catalase Test

   The catalase test is useful and recommended by many as a means of separating the
beta hemolytic streptococci from the hemolytic staphylococci (*S. aureus*). The Beta
hemolytic streptococci are catalase negative while the hemolytic staphylococci are
catalase positive.

TABLE 4

GROUP A STREPTOCOCCI BODY INVASION FACTORS

Hyaluronidase	An enzyme which breaks down hyaluronic acid. Since hyaluronic acid holds cells together, its breakdown allows bacterial penetration throughout tissues.
Streptokinase (Fibrinolysin)	An enzyme which dissolves fibrin clots formed by the host in an attempt to isolate the invading bacteria or to limit the site of infection. Hemolytic streptococci elicit streptokinase.
Streptodornase (Deoxyribonuclease)	An enzyme which liquifies purulent exudates thereby allowing the spread of the pathogens into body tissues.
Hemolysins	Substances produced that, either totally or partially, lyse red blood cells. Hemolysins are responsible for alpha or beta hemolysis of sheep red blood cells. Streptolysin S and O are hemolysin components.
Streptolysin S	A non-antigenic, oxygen stable hemolysin which produces beta hemolytic reactions around surface colonies grown on sheep blood agar. Strains which become deficient or devoid of streptolysin S appear non-hemolytic (Gamma). Phospholipids inhibit streptolysin S.
Streptolysin O	An antigenic hemolysin produced by Group A, C and G streptococci. Its production induces the body to elicit antistreptolysin O. Since this hemolysin is oxygen labile, it is responsible for hemolytic reactions around subsurface colonies or colonies grown anaerobically.
M antigens	This antigen is antiphagocytic and therefore contributes to the invasiveness of the streptococci.
Erythrogenic Toxin	This toxin is responsible for the scarlet fever rash; resists heating at 60°C for several hours; is soluble and is destroyed when boiled for one hour. Only those strains or S. pyogenes which produce erythrogenic toxin can cause the scarlet fever rash. Immunity to this toxin does not provide immunity to streptococcal infections.

BETA STREPTOCOCCI

Cultural and physiological characteristics serve as a basis for the identification of the beta streptococci. Table 5 lists some biochemical tests which aid to identify the groups of streptococci which are the causative agents of many human infections.

Streptococcus Pyogenes

The isolation and identification of *Streptococcus pyogenes* is usually no problem. Sheep blood agar preparations should contain white to grayish pinpoint colonies that are surrounded by zones of beta hemolysis. Sheep blood agar plates containing *Streptococcus pyogenes* will have:

A. white to grayish colonies
B. generally small and opaque colonies
C. zones of beta hemolysis surround the colonies
D. the colonies are susceptible to bacitracin
E. smear preparations of suspected colonies demonstrate chains of Gram positive cocci

Colonies with the above characteristics may be presumed to be *Streptococcus pyogenes*. Further biochemical tests (Table 5) should be performed to clinically diagnose *Streptococcus pyogenes*. In addition, many bacteriologists employ fluorescent antibody (FA) techniques as well as antistreptolysin O, antihyaluronidase, or anti-D Nase titers for diagnostic purposes.

IDENTIFICATION OF ALPHA AND GAMMA STREPTOCOCCI

The "green" or alpha hemolytic streptococci can cause subacute bacterial endocarditis. For proper treatment, these must be isolated and identified, since the beta straphylococci, gonococci, and meningococci may also cause bacterial endocarditis. Species from both the enterococci (Group D) and veridans group have been implicated in bacterial endocarditis. The streptococci most frequently recovered from patients suffering with this disease are: *Streptococcus mitis, Streptococcus salivarius,* and *Streptococcus faecalis* (Group D). Recent reports indicate that *Streptococcus bovis* (Group D) is increasingly being recovered from patients with acute bacterial endocarditis. The alpha or "green" streptococci, on rare occasions, have been reported to be the etiological agents of pneumonia and meningitis. However, these bacteria are rarely found in wound infections. Since some streptococci produce zones of alpha (green) hemolysis after 48 or 72 hours of incubation (e. g., *S. faecalis*), one should not hastily conclude non-hemolysis. Subsurface colonies frequently give best hemolytic results.

INULIN fermentation and BILE solubility tests should be performed to distinguish the alpha hemolytic (green) streptococci from the alpha hemolytic *Streptococcus pneumoniae.*

IDENTIFICATION OF GROUP D STREPTOCOCCI, ENTEROCOCCI, AND NONENTEROCOCCI

Presumptive identification of the group D enterococci may be derived using the bile esculin test. The group D enterococci hydrolyze bile esculin to 6, 7 dehydroxy-coumarin, which forms deep brown or black agar or broth preparations. For best results, it is recommended that the cultures be incubated at 35-37°C for 48 hours. *S. faecalis* and *S faecium* constitute the group D enterococci. The group D enterococci are also salt tolerant, therefore a positive bile esculin medium (BEM) and positive salt tolerance test aid in the indentification of these bacteria. *S. bovis* is a group

D nonenterococcus. *S. faecalis* and *S. bovis* are both causative agents of bacterial endocarditis. Clinical distinction and identification are important, since *S. faecalis* is penicillin resistant and *S. bovis* is penicillin sensitive. Selected biochemical characteristics of the group D streptococci are listed in Table 5.

EPIDEMIOLOGY

The upper respiratory tract harbors *Streptococcus pyogenes*, therefore the healthy carrier is a prime source to disseminate the infection. Infected people may transmit this pathogen via aerosols, contaminated bandages, dust or by direct contact.

TREATMENT OF STREPTOCOCCI INFECTIONS

Antibiotics effective against Gram positive bacteria may be used to combat streptococcal infections. The effectiveness of different chemotherapeutic agents is dependent upon the type of streptococcal infection treated. Penicillin remains the antibiotic of choice unless the invading streptococcal strain is penicillin resistant. Erythromycin is recommended for penicillin resistant strains or penicillin allergic patients. The sulfonamides are beneficial in treating suppurative infections, but are ineffective against rheumatic fever. Many streptococci demonstrate resistance to the tetracyclines. Gentamycin, cephalosporin and vancomycin are also effective antibiotics. Massive chemotherapy is frequently required for the treatment of many streptococcal infections or diseases.

Streptococcus Pneumoniae

Streptococcus pneumoniae is the most common causative agent of bacterial pneumonia.

MORPHOLOGY/STAINING/PHYSIOLOGY

Streptococcus pneumoniae cells appear as small, slightly elongated, lanced shaped, Gram positive cocci. Because the *Streptococcus pneumoniae* cells frequently appear in pairs, and because the cells are somewhat lance shaped, these bacteria were once referred to as *Diplococcus pneumoniae* and *Micrococcus lancealatus*. Although *S. pneumonia* strains are Gram positive, older cultures may appear Gram negative.

The pneumococci are encapsulated, but their capsule is not as thick as that of *K. pneumoniae*. Milk cultures and blood preparations enhance capsule formation, and, therefore make the capsule more conspicuous with certain capsular stains. On certain media, the capsules give the colonies a mucoid appearance. *Streptococcus pneumoniae* are non-motile, and non-spore forming. Zones of alpha hemolysis are observed on sheep blood agar plates. When grown anaerobically, some *S. pneumoniae* strains produce zones of beta hemolysis.

The *Streptococcus pneumoniae* are nutritionally fastidious, and synthetic media supplemented with vitamins such as biotin, ascorbic acid and nicotinic acid are essential to support their growth.

S. pneumoniae are facultative anaerobes that have a temperature and pH optimum of 37°C and 7.8 respectively.

These pneumococci ferment many sugars and their ability to ferment inulin, as well as their bile solubility (Table 5) are diagnostic criteria to differentiate these bacteria from the alpha hemolytic "green" streptococci.

TABLE 5

SELECTED BIOCHEMICAL TESTS USED TO IDENTIFY THE STREPTOCOCCI

SPECIES	HEMOLYTIC REACTION	LANCEFIELD GROUP	GROWTH at pH 9.6	GROWTH in 6.5-7.5% NaCl	GROWTH at 10°C	GROWTH at 45°C	ARGININE HYDROLYSIS
S. pyogenes	Beta	A	-	-	-	-	+
S. salivarius	Alpha	K	-	-	-	+	-
S. mitis	Alpha	None	-	-	-	+	V
S. lactis	Weakly Alpha or Gamma	N	-	-	-	-	+
S. faecalis	Gamma Few strains are Alpha; some Beta reported	D	+	+	+	+	+
S. faecium	Alpha; some strains Gamma	D	+	+	+	+	+
S. agalactiae	Usually Beta Few Alpha Rarely Gamma	B	-	-	-	-	+
S. bovis	Gamma	D	-	-	-	+	-
S. pneumoniae	Alpha	None	-	-	-	-	+

TABLE 5 (continued)

SPECIES	SODIUM HIPPURATE HYDROLYSIS	GROWTH IN BILE ESCULIN	INULIN FERMENTATION	GROWTH IN 0.1% METHYLENE BLUE MILK
S. pyogenes	-	-	-	-
S. salivarius	-	-	+	-
S. mitis	-	-	-	-
S. lactis	-	+	-	-
S. faecalis	+	+	-	+
S. faecium	V	+	-	+
S. agalactiae	+	-	-	-
S. bovis	-	+	+/-	-
S. pneumoniae	-	+	+	-

+ = positive
- = negative
V = variable

Pure bile salt (sodium deoxycholate), rabbit bile or ox bile may be used for the bile solubility test. Sodium deoxycholate is preferred by many because it can be autoclaved without being denatured.

S. pneumoniae are considered structurally more fragile than most bacteria. This is due to the fact that these pneumococci produce N-acetyl-muramyl-*L* alanine amidase which breaks down their cell wall peptidoglycan and consequently these pneumococci undergo autolysis.

IDENTIFICATION OF STREPTOCOCCUS PNEUMONIAE

Streptococcus pneumoniae may be isolated from transtracheal aspirates, sputum, cerebrospinal fluid, pleural fluid or blood.

Smears should show Gram positive, lance shaped cocci found either in pairs or very short chains. Zones of alpha hemolysis should surround colonies grown on sheep blood agar or other appropriate blood agar preparations. Clinical differentiation of *S. pneumoniae* from the other alpha hemolytic streptococci are listed in Table 6.

TABLE 6

Streptococci	Colony Morphology	Capsule	Sodium Deoxycholate	Optochin	Inulin Fermentation
S. pneumoniae	Small, flat, shiny or mucoid	+	Soluble	Sensitive	+
Alpha Streptococci	Small, raised, smooth, opaque or translucent	–	Insoluble	Resistant	–

In the past, the Quellung (capsular swelling) Reaction was used to identify the pneumococcal capsular type. This is not used much today because the pneumonia of which *S. pneumoniae* is the etiologic agent can be treated effectively with antibiotics without knowing the pneumococcal capsular type.

TREATMENT

Penicillin is the antibiotic of choice unless the *Streptococcus pneumoniae* is not penicillin sensitive and the patient is penicillin allergic. Should this be the case, then methicillin and gentamycin are effective substitutes.

The Neisseria

FAMILY: NEISSERIACEAE
GENUS I: NEISSERIA

Members of the genus Neisseria are Gram negative, non-motile, non-spore forming cocci measuring approximately 0.5-1.0 μm in diameter. Most of the time, the gonococci microscopically appear in pairs, but occasionally they appear singly or as tetrads. Some of the neisseria species are hemolytic and some species are non-hemolytic, but all are fastidious and have complex growth requirements. These bacteria are aerobic or facultatively anaerobic. Characteristically, the neisseria utilize few carbohy-drates and produce catalase and cytochrome oxidase.

Neisseria Gonorrhoeae

Neisseria gonorrhoeae, generally referred to as *Neisseria gonococcus*, is the causative agent of gonorrhea.

MORPHOLOGY/STAINING/PHYSIOLOGY

In smear preparations made from purulent venereal discharges, the gonocococci appear as coffee-bean shaped diplococci with flattened adjacent sides. Each member of the pair has a diamter that measures approximately 0.5 to 1.0 μm. In pus smears, the gonococci frequently are observed within the leukocytes. This is not typical of many Gram negative cocci.

Pure cultures of *N. gonorrhoeae* do not take on the bean-shaped structure, but rather appear as spheres clumped together in any combination. For best results, plates and tubes should contain condensed water and incubation should be in an in-creased CO_2 atmosphere (5-10% CO_2). The neisseria are readily stained, however thick smear preparations and smears made directly from pus have been reported to resist de-colorization. Known Gram positive and Gram negative cultures should be stained si-multaneously with the suspected *N. gonococci* in order to monitor this procedure and ensure consistent and accurate Gram stain results.

PATHOGENICITY

Gonorrhea is a venereal disease transmitted by sexual intercourse. The *Neisseria gonorrhoeae* invade the mucous membranes of the genitourinary tract and cause gonorrhea. Consequently, gonococcal urethritis results in males. Purulent mucoid exudates usually accompany this disease. If untreated, the disease can spread to the prostate, epidi-dymis and rectum.

This disease occurs among homosexuals, and, in many cases, the pharynx, rectum and urethra are the sites of infection. For complete diagnosis, rectal and pharyngeal cultures should be examined and tested along with urethral cultures.

In females, the uterus, ovaries, fallopian tubes and rectum may be infected. Should a recently infected woman give birth, she could transmit the disease to the newborn. Gonorrheal ophthalmia is the most common infection in the newborn. Eye treatment with silver nitrate solution or penicillin ointment prevents eye damage to the newborn.

In old untreated cases, in both males and females, the disease can be spread to other parts of the body and ultimately invade the heart valves, meninges and joints.

Gonorrhea has often been referred to as being a "family" disease because of its indirect spread to children in a family. The infection may be spread to children and young girls via contaminated towels, bedding or other fomites resulting in vulvova-ginitis or conjunctivitis. Vulvovaginities outbreaks are a serious problem among young girls in close contact situations such as summer camps. Except for conjuncti-vitis and vulvovaginitis, gonorrhea is spread by sexual intercourse.

SPECIMEN TYPES AND COLLECTION

Proper specimen collection is vital for proper laboratory diagnosis. This is true for any clinical diagnosis, but extremely so in the case of gonorrhea. Since *N. gonorrhoeae* is excessively sensitive to drying or antiseptics, improperly cleaned glassware, the use of antiseptics in patient preparation, the use of swabs containing inhibitory substances, oversterilized and dry media or improperly prepared transport media could affect proper laboratory diagnosis. The problem is further complicated by the fact that there may be few gonococci at the site of infection and numerous other types of bacteria in the same body area.

URETHRAL SPECIMENS

These should be collected no sooner than one hour after urinating. In males, urethral exudate may be collected. If no exudate is obtainable, then a dry swab or a swab moistened with sterile water is inserted into the urethra.

In females, the urethral area is wiped (do not use soap or disinfectants) with a sterile swab and collect the exudate from the urethra.

Gram stained smears should be made of the collected specimens. No diagnosis of gonorrhea should be made until the isolated colonies, are grown on Thayer-Martin medium or chocolate agar. These same isolates should be: oxidase positive, Gram negative diplococci further confirmed by corbohydrate tests.

ENDOCERVICAL SPECIMENS

Endocervical specimens should be collected using a speculum for direct vision. A swab is used to collect the exudate from the endocervix. If purulent exudate is obtained, and if the Gram stained smears show Gram negative, kidney-shaped diplococci which test oxidase positive, then there may be a strong presumption of a diagnosis of gonorrhea. However, carbohydrate tests and/or commercial tests should be performed for confirmation.

ANORECTAL SPECIMENS

A swab should be used to collect anorectal specimens. The swab should be inserted about one inch into the anal canal. Feces contamination should be avoided. If the swab gets contaminated with feces, repeat the process with another swab. Do not insert the swab too deeply within the anal canal. Specimens may be collected just inside the anal ring. Some physicians perform anoscopy to collect purulent specimens. Clinically diagnose as indicated for uretheral and endocervical specimens.

PHARYNGEAL SPECIMENS

A bacteriological swab may be used to collect specimens from the pharynx. For best results, collect the specimens from the tonsil region and posterior pharyngeal region. Clinically diagnose as indicated in the urethral specimens section.

CONJUNCTIVAL SPECIMENS

A swab may be used to collect conjunctival exudate. Again, identify as previously stated along with growth on proper laboratory media and broths.

OTHER SPECIMENS

Blood, synovial fluid and prostate fluid may also contain *N. gonorrhoeae*. These specimens should be processed in the same manner as the previously mentioned specimens.

CULTURE INOCULATION/TRANSPORT

If immediate processing is not possible, the swabs may be placed in Stuart's transport medium or Transgrow medium. The cultures should be inoculated and incubated as soon as possible. The cultures should not be exposed to extremes in temperature in transport, since *N. gonorrhoeae* is extremely susceptible to temperature changes.

The plates should be incubated at 35°C and kept in a moist and CO_2 enriched environment. A candle jar or CO_2 incubator may be used. Moisture is essential since few *N. gonorrhoeae* grow well in the absence of moisture. Excessive moisture, however, should be avoided to limit the growth of swarmers.

ISOLATION PROCEDURES

Bacteriological cotton swabs may be used to collect pus, exudate and nasopharyngeal specimens. These specimens should be cultures on Thayer-Martin medium. The addition of antibiotics, such as vancomycin and colistin, make the Thayer-Martin medium selective for both *N. gonococci* and *N. meningococci*. Specimens collected from blood, joint fluid or spinal fluid should be plated on Thayer-Martin medium, chocolate blood agar, and Mueller-Hinton agar. Brain-heart infusion broth is used when necessary. The cultures should be incubated in an increased CO_2 environment for 24 hours at 35°C.

IDENTIFICATION PROCEDURES

AGAR PLATE MORPHOLOGY

Colonies are smooth, glistening and translucent on Thayer-Martin medium and chocolate agar plates. Generally, no pigmentation is observed, however, certain serological groups (A and C) appear bluish-gray.

OXIDASE TEST

The oxidase test is based on the presence of a cytochrome oxidase system in bacteria. The cytochrome system is usually produced by all Neisseria, Pseudomonas, and Aeromonas species. These bacteria contain the enzyme, indophenol oxidase, which is capable of oxidizing a redox dye and consequently produce a colony color change.

A loopful of freshly prepared 1.0% tetrametyl-p-phenylenediamine dihydrochloride (or 1.0% N, N-dimethyl-p-phenylenediamine monohydrochloride) is added to suspected isolated colonies. If the colonies produce cytochrome oxidase, the colonies will quickly turn pink and eventually black. Known cytochrome oxidase positive and cytochrome oxidase negative cultures should be tested simultaneously with the suspected colonies in order to determine the freshness and quality of the oxidase test reagent. Many laboratories prepare this reagent every 3-4 days to ensure consistent and accurate results. If the oxidase reagent is not freshly prepared, it should be refrigerated immediately after use. Only platinum loops should be used for the oxidase test, since iron containing loops have been reported to give false positive tests. This is another reason why known positive and negative oxidase cultures should be used as controls.

OXIDASE POSITIVE BACTERIA OTHER THAN NEISSERIA

Since all Pseudomonas, Aeromonas and Neisseria species are oxidase positive, some other criterion must be used to differentiate these from each other. Gram staining characteristics, serological tests, API and TSI results readily distinguish *N. gonococci* from other oxidase positive bacteria.

CARBOHYDRATE TESTS

These tests are performed in 3 or 4 tubes containing 2 to 3 ml of sterile cystine trypticase agar (CTA) supplemented with 1.0% reagent grade glucose, lactose, maltose, sucrose and other selected carbohydrates. A heavy inoculum of each carbohydrate is pipetted onto the surface of the CTA tubes. Some workers suggest that the carbohydrates be stabbed into the upper third of the CTA agar medium. Others feel this is unnecessary. These tubes should be incubated at 35-37°C for 16-20 hours and examined immediately upon removal from the incubator. Inconsistent results may be recorded, if the tubes are not read in the time designated. Conflicting results sometime occur because certain *N. gonorrhoeae* strains may give negative glucose reactions. Should this occur, repeat the CTA inoculation process, but add 10-12% ascitic fluid to stimulate carbohydrate fermentation.

To avoid repeating this process, many clinicians recommend the nongrowth carbohydrate degradation test or the use of rapid commercial carbohydrate fermentation procedures.

Carbohydrate and other Neisseria test information are listed in Table 8.

Carbohydrate fermentation results aid to clinically identify *N. gonorrhoeae*, since this organism utilizes glucose with acid production, but fails to produce acid from lactose, maltose or sucrose.

FLUORESCENT ANTIBODY STAINING

Fluorescent antibody (FA) staining of *N. gonorrhoeae* with current commercial reagents fails to provide consistent and reliable findings because the fluorescein conjugated globulins also cross react with other genera and species as well as with *Neisseria gonorrhoeae*. Their lack of specificity for *N. gonorrhoeae* makes this procedure less reliable than the carbohydrate fermentation test results.

TREATMENT OF GONORRHEA

Antibiotic resistance by *N. gonococci* affects chemotherapy. Generally, *N. gonococci* are sensitive (to some degree) to penicillin, erythromycin, ampicillin, sulfadiazine, chloramphenicol, streptomycin and the tetracyclines.

IMMUNITY

Infection with *N. gonococci* provides little or no immunity to a second or third infection.

Neisseria Meningitidis

N. miningitidis, frequently referred to as *Neisseria meningococcus*, is a causative agent of meningitis, a disease which is characterized by the inflammation of the meninges. *N. meningococcus* is a common inhabitant of the nasopharynx of healthy carriers. Invasion of the bloodstream can result in bacterial meningitis.

MORPHOLOGY/STAINING/PHYSIOLOGY

Morphologically, *N. meningitidis* is similar to *N. gonorrhoeae*. *N. meningitidis* is a Gram negative, diplococcus which is fastidious upon primary isolation. Blood agar or chocolate agar are the media of choice. Primary or fresh isolates of most strains are usually encapsulated. No hemolysis is observed on blood agar. Biochemically most *N. meningitidis* strains produce acid from glucose and maltose. However, on occasion, some strains fail to produce acid on either glucose or maltose or both carbohydrates. The meningococcus is aerobic and facultatively anaerobic. Increased atmospheric CO_2 is not essential during incubation, but it does enhance growth in some strains. *N. meningitidis* is extremely susceptible to dehydration, therefore a moist environment is essential for growth. Condensation in tubes and plates can provide the moisture needed for culture growth and survival. Temperature fluctuation should be avoided, since this bacterium cannot deviate much from 35°C.

Serologically, *N. meningitidis* is divided into 4 groups designated as A, B, C, and D. Groups B and C are recovered from healthy carriers and those infected with *N. meningitidis*.

ISOLATION/DIAGNOSIS

N. meningitidis may be recovered and isolated from the nasopharynx, spinal fluid, or blood. The Gram stain demonstrates Gram negative, kidney shaped diplococci, many of which are within polymorphonuclear leukocytes. The isolated meningococci are oxidase positive, and may be identified by carbohydrate fermentation tests and agglutination with polyvalent antiserum. The Quellung or capsular swelling reaction may also be used to identify the encapsulated strains.

TREATMENT

For many years, the sulfonamides were the drugs of choice in the treatment of bacterial meningitis of *N. meningitidis* origin. Increased resistance to the sulfonamides, through the years, now make penicillin, ampicillin and streptomycin the most effective drugs.

IMMUNITY

Group B and C meningococci have been a major public health concern. Immunization with a vaccine against serogroup C meningococci has been extremely effective. Serogroup C vaccine is now used in the U. S. No effective vaccine has been found against Group B meningococci and this serogroup is still a public health concern.

Other Neisseria

Although *N. gonorrhoeae* and *N. meningitidis* are the medically significant Neisseria, several other Neisseria species are recognized. The less known species also are oxidase positive and morphologically similar to the meningococcus and gonococcus and therefore, may be diagnostically confused with the more pathogenic and well known species. Table 7 lists other Neisseria species and their sources.

Although three of the four less known Neisseria have been isolated from clinical specimens, their actual involvement as pathogens remains to be classified and elaborated.

TABLE 7

OTHER NEISSERIA	SOURCES
Neisseria sicca	Nasopharynx
Neisseria subflava	Nasopharynx and in exceptional cases in CSF of meningitis patients
Neisseria flavescens	Blood in septecemic cases; CSF meningitis cases
Neisseria mucosa	Rhinopharynx--not implicated as a pathogen

Species Related to Neisseria

FAMILY: NEISSERIANCEAE
GENUS: BRANHAMELLA

Branhamella Catarrhalis

Branhamella catarrhalis has been recovered from mucous membranes of meningitis patients and venereal exudates. This Gram negative, aerobic bacterium is encapsulated, does not produce acid from carbohydrates, is oxidase, DN ase and catalase positive and reduces nitrates to nitrites. Branhamella catarrhalis is sensitive to penicillin, streptomycin and the tetracyclines.

FAMILY: NEISSERIACEAE
GENUS: ACINETOBACTER

The Acinetobacter genus is made up of small, plump Gram negative coccobacilli that appear in pairs or short chains. These strict aerobes are not nutritionally fastidious and have an optimum pH of 7.0, and an optimum temperature ranging between 30-32°C. The Acinetobacter species are oxidase negative and catalase positive. *Acinetobacter calcoaceticus* is the only species designated in Bergey's Manual of Determinative Bacteriology (8th Edition). This organism has been recovered from soil and water samples as well as clinical specimens obtained from healthy carriers and the sick. The pathogenicity of *Acinetobacter calcoaceticus* is questionable, but it is believed to be an opportunistic pathogen.

The Enteric Bacilli

FAMILY: ENTEROBACTERIACEAE

Throughout the years numerous taxonomic schemes have been used to classify the enterobacteriaceae. Clinicians frequently employ the Edwards and Ewing classification while academicians often use Bergey's Manual of Determinative Bacteriology. For comparative and reference purposes these two taxonomic schemes will be listed in Table 7.

TABLE 8

MORPHOLOGICAL AND PHYSIOLOGICAL DIFFERENTIATION OF CERTAIN NEISSERIACEAE ACID PRODUCTION FORM

	Pigment	Capsule	Glucose	Maltose	Sucrose	Increased CO_2	$NO_3 \rightarrow NO_2$	Growth at 22°C
Neisseria gonorrhoeae	* -	-	+	-	-	Vital	-	-
Neisseria meningitidis	-	+/-	+	+	-	Enhances Growth	-	-
Neisseria sicca	** +/-	+/-	+	+	+	Not Essential	-	+/-
Neisseria subflava	+	+	+	+	+/-	Not Essential	-	+/-
Neisseria flavescens	+	-	-	-	-	Not Essential	-	+
Neisseria mucosa	-	+	+	+	+	Not Essential	+	+
Branhamella catarrhalis	-	+	-	-	-	Not Essential	+	+
Acinetobacter calcoaceticus	-	+/-	+/-	+/-	-	Not Essential	-	N/D

*N gonorrhea is classically listed as non-pigmented, but serogroups A and C have formed bluish-gray colonies
  on Thayer-Martin medium.
**+/- = some strains positive, some strains negative.
+ = positive
- = negative
N/D = Not Determined

TABLE 9

CLASSIFICATION OF THE FAMILY ENTEROBACTERIACEAE

BERGEY'S MANUAL OF DETERMINATIVE BACTERIOLOGY, 1974, 8th Edition	EDWARDS AND EWING

Genus I   Escherichia
           E. coli
	Tribe I Escherichieae
	Genus I Escherichia
	          E. coli

Genus II   Edwardsiella
           E. tarda
	Genus II Shigella
	          S. dysenteriae
	          S. flexneri
	          S. boydii
	          S. sonnei

Genus III Citrobacter
            C. freundii
            C. intermedius
	Tribe II Edwardsielleae
	Genus I Edwarsiella
	          E. tarda

Genus IV   Salmonella
 	
           Subgenus I
 	
           S. cholerae-suis
           S. hirschfeldii
           S. typhi
           S. paratyphi-A
           S. schottmuelleri
           S. typhimurium
           S. enteritidis
           S. gallinarum
 	
           Subgenus III
 	
           S. salamae
 	
           Subgenus III
 	
           S. arizonae
	Tribe III Salmonelleae
	Genus I Salmonella
	          S. cholerae-suis
	          S. typhi
	          S. enteritidis
	
	Genus II Arizona
	          A. hinshawii
	
	Genus III Citrobacter
	          C. freundii
	          C. diversus

Genus Shigella
 	
           Sh. dysenteriae
           Sh. flexneri
           Sh. boydii
           Sh. sonnei
	Tribe IV Klebsielleae
	
	Genus I Klebsiella
	          K. pneumoniae
	          K. ozaenae
	          K. rhinoscleromatis

Genus VI Klebsiella
 	
           K. pneumoniae
           K. ozaenae
           K. rhinoscleromatis
	Genus II Enterobacter
	
	          E. cloacae
	          E. aerogenes
	          E. hafnia
	          E. agglomerans

GENUS VII   Enterobacter

        E. cloacae
        E. aerogenes

Genus VIII Hafnia

        H. alvei

Genus IX   Serratia

        S. marcescens

Genux X   Proteus

        P. vulgaris
        P. mirabilis
        P. morganii
        P. rettgeri
        P. inconstans

Genus XI   Yersinia

        Y. pestis
        Y. pseudotuberculosis
        Y. enterocolitica

Genus XIII Erwinia*

A.   Amylovora Group
B.   Herbicola Group
C.   Carotovora Group

*Members of this genus are plant patho-
gens; however, the Herbicola group has
one bacterium, E. herbicola, which has
been considered a human pathogen.

Genus III Serratia

        S. marcescens
        S. liquifaciens
        S. rubidaea

Tribe V   Proteeae

Genus I   Proteus

        P. vulgaris
        P. mirabilis
        P. morganii
        P. rettgeri

Genus II   Providencia

        P. stuartii
        P. alcalifaciens

Tribe VI   Yersineae

Genus I   Yersinia

        Y. enterocolitica
        Y. pseudotuberculosis
        Y. pestis

Tribe VII Erwineae*

Genus I   Erwinia

Genus II   Pectobacterium

*Members of Tribe VII are plant pathogens.

MORPHOLOGY/STAINING/PHYSIOLOGY

The enteric bacilli include the intestinal commensals such as the colon bacilli
and Proteus; the enteric pathogens such as Salmonella and Shigella: the respiratory
pathogen, Klebsiella, and the plague bacterium, Yersinia.

The enterics are morphologically similar. All are Gram negative, motile bacilli
which measure about 1.0-3.5 µm in length and 0.5 to 0.8 µm in width. Microscopically,
these bacteria appear singly, in pairs, in small clusters, and occasionally, in short
chains.

The enterobacteriaceae are aerobic and facultatively anaerobic, catalase positive
and oxidase negative. Furthermore, the members of this family do reduce nitrates to
nitrites. All of the enterics ferment glucose with acid or with acid and gas production.

Despite the large number of species included in the family Enterobacteriaceae, bench workers should be aware of the colony traits of the enterics on blood agar.

On blood agar preparations, the enteric bacilli form large, smooth, circular colonies which may or may not be hemolytic.

PIGMENTATION ON DIFFERENTIAL AND SELECTIVE MEDIA

Differential and selective media are employed to distinguish the lactose fermenting enteric bacilli from the non-lactose fermenting enterics. Colored colonies on solid media indicate lactose fermenters and colorless colonies indicate non-lactose fermenters.

Since some of the enteric bacilli are motile and others are non-motile, motility tests also provide diagnostic information. Those strains that are flagellated demonstrate peritrichous flagellation. The enterobacteriaceae may be either encapsulated or non-encapsulated, aerobic or facultatively anaerobic.

Conventionally, the suspected isolates are plated out on a selection of the following. The choice of differential and selective media may vary from laboratory to laboratory. Other media not listed here may also be used.

TABLE 10

MEDIA	GENERA	COLONY APPEARANCE
Mac Conkey Agar	Escherichia Enterobacter Klebsiella	Brick Red Colonies (Lactose Fermented)
	Salmonella Shigella	Uncolored, Transparent Colonies (Lactose Not Fermented)

Eosin Methylene Blue	Escherichia
	Enterobacter
	Klebsiella
		Pinkish Colonies With Dark Or
		    Blackish Centers – OR –
		Colonies Show a Green Metallic
		    Sheen
		(Lactose Fermented in Both Bases)

	Salmonella Shigella Proteus	Colorless, Transparent Colonies (Lactose Not Fermented)

TABLE 10 (continued)

MEDIA	GENERA	COLONY APPEARANCE
Xylose Lysine Desoxycholate Agar (XLD)	Salmonellae	Red Colonies With or Without Black Centers Depending on Species
	Shigella Providence	Red Colonies
	Some Pseudomonas Proteus rettger:	False Positive Red Colonies
	Escherichia Citrobacter Klebsiella Enterobacter Proteus	Yellow Colonies
Salmonella and Shigella Agar (SS)	Salmonellae Shigellae Proteus	Colorless Colonies
	Escherichia Enterobacter Klebsiella	Generally Inhibited But Colonies That Do Grow Are Red in Color
Desoxycholate Citrate Agar	Salmonella typhi	Translucent Colonies With a Bluish Cast
	Other Salmonellae	Opaque Colonies--May Have Brown Centers
	Shigellae	Opaque Colonies With Round, Smooth Edges
	Escherichia Enterobacter Klebsiella	Generally Inhibited Colonies That Do Form Appear Red
Bismuth Sulfite Agar (BS)	Salmonella typhi Coliform Bacteria	Black Colonies Inhibited

The six media mentioned are only a few among a long list of isolation, selective and differential media available to study the cultural traits of the enteric bacilli. Enrichment broths, such as tetrathionate, GN or selenite should be used before plating on solid media, particularly if there are few bacteria in the specimen. Most laboratories use a non-selective medium such as MacConkey agar in conjunction with two or three selective and/or differential media available.

Triple Sugar Iron Agar (TSI) Kligler Iron Agar (KIA) or Lysine Iron Agar (LIA) slants, in conjunction with other biochemical tests and serological tests, are used to confirm the identification of the enteric bacilli using convential laboratory test procedures.

PIGMENTATION

Pigmentation on selective or differential media may serve for diagnostic purposes. Colorless colonies are indicative of non-lactose fermenters and may be pathogenic. Colored colonies indicate lactose fermentation.

Colorless or colored colonies on selective and differential media provide basic identification.

PRELIMINARY CLINICAL IDENTIFICATION

Suspected isolates on selective or differential media should be inoculated into the following:

1. Simmons citrate medium
2. SIM motility medium
3. Tryptone broth (for indole test)
4. Triple Sugar Iron Agar (TSI) and/or Kligler Iron Agar (KIA) and Lysine Iron Agar (LIA) slants
5. Urea broth (or use urea discs)
6. Methyl red Vogess Proskauer (MRVP medium)

The results of the above tests will provide preliminary information necessary to identify the enteric bacilli. Confirmation of the enterics is dependent, usually, upon serological and biochemical test results.

BIOCHEMICAL DISTINCTION

The coliform bacteria (e. g. Escherichia) rapidly ferment lactose with acid and gas production. Characteristically, rapid fermenters produce changes in media within 24-48 hours (or sooner) if incubated at 35-37°C. The so-called pathogenic enterics (e.g., Salmonellae and Shigellae) usually fail to ferment lactose. Consequently, lactose fermentation may be beneficial for primary differentiation. However, primary differentiation results are not absolute, since some coliform bacteria and certain Shigellae are delayed or late lactose fermenters. It should be noted that mannitol fermentation is the basis for differentiating the Shigellae species. Other biochemical tests are used to differentiate the enteric bacilli. As previously stated, TSI, KIA, and LIA slants may be used to differentiate the enterobacteriaceae on the basis of carbohydrate fermentation, gas, acid and hydrogen sulfide production. The carbohydrate content of each is listed on Table 11.

TABLE 11

MEDIA	CARBOHYDRATE CONTENT	CARBOHYDRATE INDICATOR DYE	OPTIMUM INCUBATION TIME	TEMPERATURE
Triple Sugar Iron Agar (TSI)	Glucose Lactose Sucrose	Phenol red	18-24 hours	35-37°C
Kligler Iron Agar (KIA)	Glucose Lactose	Phenol red	18-24 hours	35-37°C
Lysine Iron Agar (LIA)	Glucose	Brom cresol purple	18-24 hours	35-37°C

TRIPLE SUGAR IRON AGAR

TSI contains three carbohydrates in the following concentration: 1.0% lactose, 0.1% glucose and 1.0% sucrose. The enteric bacilli will ferment one, two or all three of these carbohydrates. Carbohydrate fermentation occurs with or without acid and gas production.

To obtain characteristic results on TSI, a sufficient inoculum should be obtained from the center of an isolated clone, grown on either isolation, selective or differential media, and the TSI slant should be streaked, and the butt stabbed. A straight inoculating needle is recommended for the stab.

The control TSI slant (uninoculated) is red in appearance due to the alkalinity of the prepared medium (pH 7.3). Inoculated slants should be examined after 18-24 hours of incubation at 35-37°C.

To determine delayed or late lactose fermentation, many clinicians recommend that, when possible, the suspected tubes be re-incubated and re-examined every 24 hours for 7 days.

When a sugar is fermented and acid is produced, the TSI slant changes from red to yellow due to the lowered pH. The type of sugar(s) fermented determines the location of the color change. The fermentation pattern is representative of a specific genus or species.

Table 12 illustrates possible fermentation patterns exhibited by certain Enterobacteriaceae and one Pseudomonodaceae, Pseudomonas.

Carbohydrate reactions on TSI are listed on Table 13.

Many laboratories, using the conventional procedures for identifying the enteric bacilli use Triple Sugar Iron Agar (TSI) and/or Lysine Iron Agar (LIA) and Kligler Iron Agar (KIA) stabs simultaneously and, in conjunction with, other bacteriological, differential and selective preparations as well as serological tests.

TABLE 12

REACTION PATTERNS ON TSI AGAR SLANTS

| POSSIBLE BACTERIAL GENERA | BUTT/SLANT REACTIONS | | PRODUCTION | | MOTILITY |
	BUTT	SLANT	H_2S	GAS	
Salmonella typhi	Y	R	+	−	+
Salmonella enteritidis	Y	R	+	−	+
Salmonella paratyphi	Y	R	−	+	+
Salmonella typhimurium	Y	R	+	+	+
Shigella dysenteriae	Y	R	−	−	−
Shigella sonnei	Y	R	−	−	−
Enterobacter cloaca	Y	Y	−	+	+
Enterobacter aerogenes	Y	Y	−	+	−
Escherichia coli	Y	Y	−	+	+/−
Klebsiella pneumoniae	Y	R	−	+/−	−
Proteus vulgaris	Y	Y	+	+	+
Proteus mirabilis	Y	Y/R	+	+	+
Proteus morganii	Y	R	−	+/−	+
Proteus rettgeri	Y	R	−	+/−	+/−
Pseudomonas aeruginosa	R	R	−	−	+

Y = acid production
R = no change in butt or slant
+ = no positive reaction
− = negative reaction
+/− = variable, positive or negative

TABLE 13

INTERPRETATION OF REACTIONS ON TSI

OBSERVATION	REACTION
Yellow Butt/Red Clant (Acid) (Alkaline)	Glucose Fermentation
Yellow Butt/Yellow Slant (Acid) (Acid)	Sucrose Fermentation -or- Lactose Fermentation -or- Sucrose <u>and</u> Lactose Fermentation
Red Butt/Red Slant (Alkaline) (Alkaline)	No Carbohydrate Fermentation

Black Butt--sometimes
    entire agar blackens
	Hydrogen Sulfide Production
	Extent of blackening depends on
	    amount of H_2S produced

Bubbles or splits in agar	Gas Production

Stab results provide presumptive identification of the enterics, but biochemical and serological results together provide confirmation of the Enterobacteriaceae and related bacteria.

Conventionally, these stab, biochemical and serological results confirmed the identification of the Enterobacteriaceae and related bacteria. However, in the last 10-12 years several commercial multitest kits have been marketed. Each multitest system is unique and provides rapid *Enterobacteriaceae* procedures. These commercially developed multitest systems have been compared with the conventional multiple test methods employed to identify the Gram negative isolates obtained from clinical specimens suspected to be *Enterobacteriaceae*.

Although there are several rapid and practical multitest kits on the market, only one of the systems will be discussed at length. To date, several investigators have reported that the API SYSTEM (Analytab Products, Division of Ayerst Laboratories, Inc.) is highly reliable, accurate and simple to perform. Consultation with numerous medical microbiologists in several laboratories confirm these findings. Bench workers have repeatedly attested to the accuracy, reliability, and simplicity of the API System in identifying the *Enterobacteriaceae* and other Gram negative bacteria obtained from clinical specimens.

BACKGROUND INFORMATION

In 1970, API introduced API 20E, which is a preset battery of 23 biochemical tests. Later in 1973, API introduced a numerical identification approach, the PROFILE RECOGNITION SYSTEM (PRS). The PRS was based on the study of 25,000 results obtained worldwide on the API 20E System.

By 1975, API compiled 27,829 results in its API Profile Register. The National Institute of Health (NIH) in 1975 compared its computer data with the 27,829 results in API and confirmed 99.36% of API's 27,829 results.*

Subsequently, API developed a computer identification system of its own and has made this data readily available for clinical laboratories using the API 20E system and other API systems.

In 1976, API further expanded its data base by adding nonfermentative Gram-negative bacteria and fermentative Gram-negative bacteria not belonging to the *Enterobacteriaceae* family.

The API System is included in this section to indicate to the prospective Medical Technologist and practicing clinician, not familiar with multitest systems that:

1. Multiple test procedures may be reduced to a single test system.

2. A battery of diverse tests may be performed to identify the *Enterobacteriaceae*.

3. The multiple test system does not sacrifice accuracy and precision for rapidity.

4. The classification of the *Enterobacteriaceae* varies and that results should be recorded accordingly and consistently (see the Edward and Ewing, Bergey's Manual of Determinative Bacteriology, and API classifications in text) depending upon the test procedures employed, and the classification used.

5. Clinicians must follow the manufacturer's instructions METICULOUSLY to obtain accurate results.

Enterobacteriaceae (API 20E)

The API 20E System is a standardized, miniaturized version of conventional procedures for the identification of *Enterobacteriaceae* and other Gram-negative bacteria. It is a ready-to-use, microtube system designed for the performance of 23 standard biochemical tests from a single colony of bacteria on plating medium. Used in conjunction with the APT Profile Recognition System, it is intended to enable laboratory personnel to identify members of the family *Enterobacteriaceae* and other Gram-negative bacteria accurately and easily.

Studies made, with cultures isolated from clinical specimens, have established API 20E as the most complete commercially available system for identification and speciation of *Enterobacteriaceae*. Clear-cut reactions, ease of reading and interpretation, permit valid comparison of results obtained each day in a particular laboratory, as well as valid comparison of results obtained in different laboratories worldwide.

CHEMICAL AND PHYSICAL PRINCIPLES

The API 20E System consists of microtubes containing dehydrated media. These media are reconstituted by adding a bacterial suspension, incubated so that the organisms react with the contents of the tubes and read when the various indicator systems are affected by the metabolites or added reagents, generally after 18-24 hours incubation at 35-37°C. The principles involved for each of the reactions are given on the next page.

---

*Statistic obtained from the API 20E Analytical Profile Index, 1977.

SPECIMEN COLLECTION AND PROCESSING

Regardless of their source, specimens should be transported to the laboratory immediately after collection and processed as soon as possible following their receipt. Although methods for processing specimens may vary somewhat from laboratory to laboratory, proper selection of adequate plating media and conditions of incubation are very important. Most workers employ blood agar plates along with MacConkey's or Eosin Methylene Blue agar or a similar combination for specimens of extraintestinal origin, and use a variety of differential and selective media for stool specimens.

PREPARATION OF BACTERIAL SUSPENSION

1. Add 5 ml of 0.85% saline, pH 5.5 - 7.0 to a sterile test tube.

2. Gently touch the center of a well isolated colony (2-3 mm or larger in diameter) with the tip of a wooden applicator stick. Insert the applicator stick into the tube of saline and, with the tip of the stick at the base of the tube, rotate the stick in a vortex-like action. Recap the tube.
    ALTERNATE PROCEDURE: With a flamed inoculation loop, carefully touch the center of a well-isolated colony (2-3 mm or larger in diameter) and thoroughly mix the inoculum with the tubed saline.

INOCULATION OF THE STRIPS

---cupule
---tube

The API 20E strip contains 20 microtubes each of which consists of a tube and a cupule section.
(See illustration).

1. Remove the cap from the tube containing the bacterial suspension and insert a 5 ml Pasteur pipette.

2. Tilt the API 20E incubation tray and fill the tube section of the microtubes by placing the pipette tip against the side of the cupule.

3. Fill both the TUBE and CUPULE section of the CIT, VPI, and GEL tubes.

4. After inoculation, completely fill the cupule section of the ADH, LDC, ODC and URE tubes with mineral oil.

5. Using the excess bacterial suspension, inoculate an agar slant or plate as a purity check and for oxidase testing, serology, and/or additional biochemical testing. Incubate the slant or plate for 18-24 hours at 35-37°C.

INCUBATION OF THE STRIPS

1. After inoculation, place the plastic lid on the tray and incubate the strip for 18-24 hours at 35-37°C in a non-CO_2 incubator.

2. Weekend incubation: the biochemical reactions of the API 20E should be read after 18-24 hours incubation. If the strips cannot be read after 24 hours incubation at 35-37°C, the strips should be removed from the incubator and stored at 2-8°C (refrigerator) until the reactions can be read.

IDENTIFICATION OF ORGANISMS

Identification of the organisms can be made either with the aid of the differential charts, contained in the kit or by using the Profile Recognition System.

When differential charts are used to determine the identity of cultures, the aggregate reactions given by the strains should be considered as a whole. Even when this is done, however, the conclusions reached may differ from laboratory to laboratory. API suggests use of the specific procedures.

For rapid identification at species and biotype levels, the API Profile Recognition System (PRS) Computer Service is available. A unique data base, compiled from strains of the collections of several institutions as well as type and neotype cultures, allows very precise statistical calculation and thus the identification of less co-monly occuring microorganisms. The PRS Computer Service can now broaden the concept of standardization of the interpretation of the results obtained with API products worldwide. (See table on following pages).

LIMITATIONS

The API 20E System allows the easy performance of 23 present biochemical tests. Interpretation of the results requires a competent microbiologist who should use his/her judgment, knowledge and other confirmatory tests when required before deciding on the identity of a bacterium. For other Gram-negative bacteria, additional biochemical tests may occasionally be required. Some of the following additional characteristics should also be considered including: source of specimen, history of the patient, colonial and microscopic morphology, serology and antimicrobial susceptibility patterns.

API differential charts have been derived from type and neotype cultures and strains from various collections. The percentages obtained on API may differ from percentages appearing in published material based on macromethods. For example, erease test found on API is a Ferguson formulation which is less sensitive than Christensen's formulation which is widely used in existing macrotechniques. Reactions recorded as delayed positive with macromethods generally are shown as negative on the API chart for *Enterobacteriaceae* since this chart is based on results obtained after 18-24 hours of incubation.

On rare occasions, the glucose reactions for organisms such as *Klebsiella* or *Protus* may revert, in which instances a bluish-green color is seen. This reaction may be recorded as a false negative reaction. Such occurrences are reflected in the percentages reported on the differential chart.

The API data presented in pages 33 to 36 of this text has been obtained from the API Profile Recognition System and the July 1980 API 20E Instruction booklet. The API data contained in this text was printed with permission of Analytab Products, Division of Ayerst Laboratories, Plainview, NY.

NOTE: ALL OF THE FOLLOWING API TABLES ARE REPRINTED WITH PERMISSION OF ANALYTAB PRODUCTS, DIVISION OF AYERST LABORATORIES, PLAINVIEW, NEW YORK.

API TABLE 1

SUMMARY OF CHEMICAL AND PHYSICAL PRINCIPLES OF THE TESTS ON THE API 20E

| TUBE | CHEMICAL/PHYSICAL PRINCIPLES | COMPONENTS | | REF. |
		REACTIVE INGREDIENTS	QUANTITY	
ONPG	Hydrolysis of ONPG by beta-galactosidase releases yellow orthonitrophenol from the colorless ONPG; ITPG (isopropylthio-galactopyranoside) is used as inducer.	ONPG ITPG	0.2 mg 8.0 μg	12 13 14
ADH	Arginine dihydrolase transforms arginine into ornithine, ammonia and carbon dioxide. This causes a pH rise in the acid-buffered system and a change in the indicator from yellow to red.	Arginine	2.0 mg	15
LDC	Lysine decarboxylase transforms lysine into a basic primary amine, cadaverine. This amine causes a pH rise in the acid-buffered system and a change in the indicator from yellow to red.	Lysine	2.0 mg	15
ODC	Ornithine decarboxylase transforms ornithine into a basic primary amine, putrescine. This amine causes a pH rise in the acid-buffered system and a change in the indicator from yellow to red.	Ornithine	2.0 mg	15
CIT	Citrate is the sole carbon source. Citrate utilization results in a pH rise and a change in the indicator from green to blue.	Sodium Citrate	0.8 mg	21
H2S	Hydrogen sulfide is produced from thiosulfate. The hydrogen sulfide reacts with iron salts to produce a black precipitate.	Sodium Thiosulfate	80.0 μg	6
URE	Urease releases ammonia from urea; ammonia causes the pH to rise and changes the indicator from yellow to red.	Urea	0.8 mg	7
TDA	Tryptophane deaminase forms indolepyruvic acid from trypto-phane. Indolepyruvic acid produces a brownish-red color in the presence of ferric chloride.	Tryptophane	0.2 mg	22
IND	Metabolism of tryptophane results in the formation of indole. Kovacs' reagent forms a colored complex (pink to red) with indole.	Tryptophane	0.4 mg	10
VP	Acetoin, an intermediary glucose metabolite, is produced from sodium pyruvate and indicated by the formation of a colored complex. Conventional VP tests may take up to 4 days, but by using sodium pyruvate, API has shortened the required test time. Creatin intensifies the color when tests are positive.	Sodium Pyruvate Creatine	2.0 mg 0.9 mg	3
GEL	Liquefaction of gelatin by proteolytic enzymes releases a black pigment which diffuses throughout the tube.	Kohn Charcoal Gelatin	0.6 mg	9
GLU MAN INO SOR RHA SAC MEL AMY ARA	Utilization of the carbohydrate results in acid formation and a consequent pH drop. The indicator changes from blue to yellow.	Glucose Mannitol Inositol Sorbitol Rhamnose Sucrose Melibiose Amygdalin (l +) Arabinose	2.0 mg 2.0 mg 2.0 mg 2.0 mg 2.0 mg 2.0 mg 2.0 mg 2.0 mg. 2.0 mg	5 6 12
Oxidase	The enzyme cytochrome oxidase oxidizes cytochrome c. Oxidase reagent (N, N, N', N', tetramethyl-p-phenylenediamine) is oxidized by cytochrome c resulting in a purple compound.			11
GLU Nitrate Reduction	Nitrites form a red complex with sulfanilic acid and N, N-dimethyl-alpha-naphthylamine. In case of negative reaction, addition of zinc confirms the presence of unreduced nitrates by reducing them to nitrites (pink-orange color). If there is no color change after the addition of zinc, this is indicative of the complete reduction of nitrates through nitrites to nitrogen gas or to an anaerogenic amine.	Potassium Nitrate	80.0 μg	6
MAN INO SOR Catalase	Catalase releases oxygen gas from hydrogen peroxide.			24

API TABLE 2

SUMMARY OF RESULTS — 18-24 HOUR PROCEDURE

TUBE	INTERPRETATION OF REACTIONS			
	POSITIVE		**NEGATIVE**	**COMMENTS**
ONPG	Yellow		Colorless	(1) Any shade of yellow is a positive reaction. (2) VP tube, before the addition of reagents, can be used as a negative control.
ADH	Incubation 18-24 h	Red or Orange	Yellow	Orange reactions occurring at 36-48 hours should be interpreted as negative.
	36-48 h	Red	Yellow or Orange	
LDC	18-24 h	Red or Orange	Yellow	Any shade of orange within 18-24 hours is a positive reaction. At 36-48 hours, orange decarboxylase reactions should be interpreted as negative.
	36-48 h	Red	Yellow or Orange	
ODC	18-24 h	Red or Orange	Yellow	Orange reactions occurring at 36-48 hours should be interpreted as negative.
	36-48 h	Red	Yellow or Orange	
CIT	Turquoise or Dark Blue		Light Green or Yellow	(1) Both the tube and cupule should be filled. (2) Reaction is read in the aerobic (cupule) area.
H$_2$S	Black Deposit		No Black Deposit	(1) H$_2$S production may range from a heavy black deposit to a very thin black line around the tube bottom. Carefully examine the bottom of the tube before considering the reaction negative. (2) A "browning" of the medium is a negative reaction unless a black deposit is present. "Browning" occurs with TDA positive organisms.
URE	18-24 h	Red or Orange	Yellow	A method of lower sensitivity has been chosen. *Klebsiella, Proteus* and *Yersinia* routinely give positive reactions.
	36-48 h	Red	Yellow or Orange	
TDA	Add 1 drop 10% Ferric chloride			(1) Immediate reaction. (2) Indole positive organisms may produce a golden orange color due to indole production. This is a negative reaction.
	Brown-Red		Yellow	
IND	Add 1 drop Kovacs' Reagent			(1) The reaction should be read within 2 minutes after the addition of the Kovacs reagent and the results recorded. (2) After several minutes, the HCl present in Kovacs' reagent may react with the plastic of the cupule resulting in a change from a negative (yellow) color to a brownish-red. This is a negative reaction.
	Red Ring		Yellow	
VP	Add 1 drop of 40% Potassium hydroxide, then 1 drop of 6% alpha-naphthol.			(1) Wait 10 minutes before considering the reaction negative. (2) A pale pink color (after 10 min.) should be interpreted as negative. A pale pink color which appears immediately after the addition of reagents but which turns dark pink or red after 10 min. should be interpreted as positive.
	Red		Colorless	
Motility				Motility may also be observed by hanging drop or wet mount preparation.
GEL	Diffusion of the pigment		No Diffusion	(1) The solid gelatin particles may spread throughout the tube after inoculation. Unless diffusion occurs, the reaction is negative. (2) Any degree of diffusion is a positive reaction.
GLU	Yellow or Gray		Blue or Blue-Green	**Fermentation** (*Enterobacteriaceae, Aeromonas, Vibrio*) (1) Fermentation of the carbohydrates begins in the most anaerobic portion (bottom) of the tube. Therefore, these reactions should be read from the bottom of the tube to the top. (2) A yellow color at the bottom of the tube only indicates a weak or delayed positive reaction.
MAN INO SOR RHA SAC MEL AMY ARA	Yellow		Blue or Blue-Green	**Oxidation** (Other Gram-negatives) (1) Oxidative utilization of the carbohydrates begins in the most aerobic portion (top) of the tube. Therefore, these reactions should be read from the top to the bottom of the tube. (2) A yellow color in the upper portion of the tube and a blue in the bottom of the tube indicates oxidative utilization of the sugar. This reaction should be considered positive **only** for non-*Enterobacteriaceae* gram-negative rods. This is a negative reaction for fermentative organisms such as *Enterobacteriaceae*.
Oxidase	Place one drop of 1% tetramethyl-p- phenylenediamine dihydrochloride on filter paper			(1) Oxidase reagents should be prepared fresh weekly.
	Dark Purple		Colorless or Light Purple	
GLU Nitrate Reduction	After reading GLU reaction, add 2 drops 0.8% sulfanilic acid and 2 drops 0.5% N, N dimethyl- alpha-naphthylamine			(1) Before addition of reagents, observe GLU tube (positive or negative) for bubbles. Bubbles are indicative of reduction of nitrate to the nitrogenous (N$_2$) state. (2) A positive reaction may take 2-3 minutes for the red color to appear. (3) Confirm a negative test by adding zinc dust. A pink-orange color after 10 minutes confirms a negative reaction. A yellow color indicates reduction of nitrates to nitrogenous (N$_2$) state.
	NO$_2$ N$_2$ gas	Red Bubbles: Yellow after reagents and zinc	Yellow Orange after reagents and zinc	
MAN INO SOR Catalase	After reading carbohydrate reaction, add 1 drop 1.5% H$_2$O$_2$			(1) Bubbles may take 1-2 minutes to appear. (2) Best results will be obtained if the test is run in tubes which have no gas from fermentation.
	Bubbles		No bubbles	

(Column between GLU/MAN carbohydrate rows and COMMENTS, reading vertically: COMMENTS FOR ALL CARBOHYDRATES)

API TABLE 3

SUMMARY OF RESULTS — SAME DAY PROCEDURE

TUBE	POSITIVE	NEGATIVE	COMMENTS
ONPG	Yellow	Colorless	(1) Any shade of yellow is a positive reaction. (2) VP tube, before the addition of reagents, can be used as a negative control.
ADH	Red or Orange	Yellow	Any shade of orange or red is a positive reaction.
LDC	Red or Orange	Yellow	Any shade of orange is a positive reaction.
ODC	Red or Orange	Yellow	Any shade of orange or red is a positive reaction.
CIT	Turquoise or Dark Blue	Light Green or Yellow	(1) Both the tube and cupule should be filled. (2) Reaction is read in the aerobic (cupule) area. (3) Any shade of blue should be interpreted as positive.
H_2S	Black deposit	No Black Deposit	(1) H_2S production may range from a heavy black deposit to a very thin black line around the tube bottom. Carefully examine the bottom of the tube before considering the reaction negative. (2) A "browning" of the medium is a negative reaction unless a black deposit is present. "Browning" occurs with TDA positive organisms.
URE	Red or Orange	Yellow	(1) A method of lower sensitivity has been chosen. *Proteus* and *Yersinia* routinely give positive reactions. (2) Any shade of orange or red should be interpreted as positive.
TDA	Add 1 drop 10% Ferric chloride Golden Brown/ Red Brown	Yellow	Immediate reaction
IND	Add 1 drop Kovacs' Reagent Pink-Red Ring	Yellow	(1) The reaction should be read within 2 minutes after the addition of the Kovacs' reagent and the results recorded. (2) After several minutes, the HCl present in Kovacs' reagent may react with the plastic of the cupule resulting in a change from a negative (yellow) color to a brownish-red. This is a negative reaction.
VP	Add 1 drop of 40% Potassium hydroxide, then 1 drop of 6% alpha-naphthol Pink-Red	Colorless	(1) Wait 10 minutes before considering the reaction negative. (2) A pale pink color (after 10 min.) should be interpreted as negative. A pale pink color which appears immediately after the addition of reagents but which turns dark pink or red after 10 min. should be interpreted as positive.
Motility			Motility may also be observed by hanging drop or wet mount preparation.
GEL	Diffusion of the pigment	No Diffusion	(1) The solid gelatin particles may spread throughout the tube after inoculation. Unless diffusion occurs, the reaction is negative. (2) Any degree of diffusion is a positive reaction.
GLU	Yellow or Gray (at the bottom of tube or throughout tube)	Blue, Blue-Green or Green	**COMMENTS FOR ALL CARBOHYDRATES** Fermentation (*Enterobacteriaceae, Aeromonas, Vibrio*) (1) Fermentation of the carbohydrates begins in the most anaerobic portion (bottom) of the tube. Therefore, these reactions should be read from the bottom of the tube to the top. (2) A yellow color at the bottom of the tube only indicates a weak or delayed positive reaction.
MAN INO SOR RHA SAC MEL AMY ARA	Yellow/Yellow-Green (at bottom of tube or throughout tube)	Blue, Blue-Green or Green	Oxidation (Other Gram-negatives) (1) Oxidative utilization of the carbohydrates begins in the most aerobic portion (top) of the tube. Therefore, these reactions should be read from the top to the bottom of the tube. (2) A yellow color in the upper portion of the tube and a blue in the bottom of the tube indicates oxidative utilization of the sugar. This reaction should be considered positive only for non-*Enterobacteriaceae* Gram-negative rods. This is a negative reaction for fermentative organisms such as *Enterobacteriaceae*. NOTE: With the 20E 5 hr., only fermentations should be interpreted as positive.
GLU Nitrate Reduction	After reading GLU reaction, add 2 drops 0.8% sulfanilic acid and 2 drops 0.5% N, N dimethyl-alpha-naphthylamine NO$_2$ — Red / Yellow N$_2$ gas — Bubbles; Yellow after reagents and zinc / Orange after reagents and zinc		(1) Before addition of reagents, observe GLU tube (positive or negative) for bubbles. Bubbles are indicative of reduction of nitrate to the nitrogenous (N$_2$) state. (2) A positive reaction may take 2-3 minutes for the red color to appear (3) Confirm a negative test by adding zinc dust. A pink-orange color after 10 minutes confirms a negative reaction. A yellow color indicates reduction of nitrates to nitrogenous (N$_2$) state.

API TABLE 4

DIFFERENTIATION OF *ENTEROBACTERIACEAE*

Uapi® figures indicate the percentage of positive

		ONPG	ADH	LDC	ODC	CIT	H₂S	URE	TDA	IND	VP
Escherichieae	Escherichia coli	98.7	2.9	82.8	75.7	0	1.0	0	0	97.2	0
	Shigella dysenteriae	14.7	0	0	0	0	0	0	0	32.0	0
	Sh. flexneri	0.9	0	0	0.9	0	0	0	0	36.2	0
	Sh. boydii	.7.6	0	0	3.4	0	0	0	0	32.2	0
	Sh. sonnei	87.6	0	0	92.9	0	0	0	0	0	0
Salmonelleae	Edwardsiella tarda	0	0	99.9	99.9	0	94.4	0	0	99.0	0
	Citrobacter freundii	99.0	33.8	0	39.3	61.5	60.7	0	0	7.4	0
	C. diversus	97.5	63.6	0	98.8	91.0	0	0	0	98.8	0
	C. amalonaticus	95.0	40.0	0	98.0	77.0	0	0	0	100	0
	Salmonella spp.	1.9	69.2	96.2	95.7	75.4	85.7	0	0	3.0	0
	Sal. typhi	0	5.8	99.0	0	0	8.3	0	0	0	0
	Sal. cholerae suis	0	18.4	98.0	98.0	4.1	65.3	0	0	0	0
	Sal. paratyphi A	0	0	0	100	0	0.6	0	0	0	0
	Arizona – S. arizonae	98.7	48.0	96.1	97.4	50.6	98.1	0	0	0	0
Klebsielleae	Klebsiella pneumoniae	99.0	0.2	74.8	0.9	75.0	0	63.6	0	0	92.4
	Kl. oxytoca	99.0	0	86.7	0	86.7	0	60.0	0	100	92.4
	Kl. ozaenae	90.0	23.3	32.2	1.1	40.0	0	6.7	0	0	0
	Kl. rhinoscleromatis	0	0	0	0	0	0	0	0	0	0
	Enterobacter aerogenes	99.5	0	98.8	99.0	88.7	0	0.3	0	0	93.6
	Ent. cloacae	99.0	93.5	0.1	97.3	90.5	0	0.4	0	0	96.6
	Ent. agglomerans	97.9	1.0	0	0	54.2	0	5.0	5.5	32.8	34.4
	Ent. gergoviae	94.0	0	28.8	100	82.0	0	100	0	0	95.2
	Ent. sakazakii	100	99.0	0	85.7	85.7	0	0	0	5.0	78.7
	Serratia liquefaciens	98.1	0.6	87.4	99.0	88.7	0	5.0	0	0.7	52.8
	Ser. marcescens	94.2	0	98.5	95.6	79.9	0	29.0	0	0	60.9
	Ser. rubidaea	99.0	0	68.5	0	81.5	0	3.3	0	0	63.5
	Ser. odorifera 1	95.0	0	99.0	100	95.0	0	0	0	100	50.0
	Ser. odorifera 2	95.0	0	99.0	0	90.9	0	0	0	100	54.5
	Ser. fonticola	99.0	0	83.3	99.0	16.7	0	0	0	0	0
	Ser. plymuthica	99.0	0	0	0	50.0	0	0	2.0	0	77.5
	Hafnia alvei	71.1	1.8	100	100	10.6	0	1.0	0	0	15.4
Proteeae	Proteus vulgaris	0.5	0	0	0	41.2	83.1	98.9	99.6	88.9	0
	Prot. mirabilis	0.2	0.6	2.0	98.4	57.8	83.3	99.0	98.7	1.9	2.4
	Providencia alcalifaciens	0	0	0	0	97.5	0	0	99.0	99.0	0
	Prov. stuartii	0	0	0.8	0	85.1	0	0	91.7	97.1	0
	Prov. stuartii Ure +	1.0	0	0	0	68.6	0	100	75.7	88.6	0
	Prov. rettgeri	1.0	0	0	0	70.7	0	99.0	99.0	97.4	0
	Morganella morganii	0.5	0	0.5	99.0	2.2	0	99.0	91.8	97.2	0
Yersiniae	Yersinia enterocolitica	81.1	0	0	90.1	0	0	93.7	0	69.4	0
	Y. intermedia	95.1	0	0	100	0	0	97.6	0	97.6	2.4
	y. fredericksenii	95.6	0	0	100	0	0	100	0	99.0	0
	Y. pseudotuberculosis	77.1	0	0	0	13.3	0	96.2	0	0	0
	Y. pestis	68.6	0	0	0	0	0	0	0	0	8.6
	Y. ruckeri (25C)	73.5	0	93.9	95.9	0	0	0	0	0	0
	API Group 1	91.7	0	56.7	90.0	91.7	0	0	0	99.0	0
	API Group 2	100	22.2	45.0	0	0	0	0	0	0	0

BY BIOCHEMICAL TESTS PROVIDED ON API 20E®

reactions after 18-24 hours of incubation at 35-37°C.

API 20E													Supplementary Tests**			
GEL	GLU	MAN	INO	SOR	RHA	SAC	MEL	AMY	ARA	OXI	NO₂	N₂ GAS	MOT	MAC	OF-O	OF-F
0	99.9	99.0	0.5	94.4	87.9	41.8	67.1	9.2	90.8	0	99.7	0	62.1	100	100	100
0	94.1	2.0	0	18.6	21.6	0	0	0	21.6	0	99.7	0	0	100	100	100
0	99.0	91.8	0	24.0	2.6	0	24.9	0	61.6	0	99.8	0	0	100	100	100
0	99.1	94.1	0	55.9	0.8	0.8	14.4	0	76.3	0	100	0	0	100	100	100
0	99.9	99.0	0	2.2	80.0	0	0	0	93.8	0	100	0	0	100	100	100
0	100	0	0	0	0	0	0	0	1.1	0	100	0	98.2	100	100	100
0	100	99.8	17.5	98.8	91.1	68.2	72.6	42.2	99.5	0	98.6	0	95.7	100	100	100
0	100	100	4.5	92.6	95.1	24.7	1.2	96.3	95.1	0	100	0	92.9	100	100	100
0	100	100	0	100	100	19.4	23.0	95.0	97.0	0	99.0	0	99.0	100	100	100
0	99.9	98.7	33.7	93.2	93.1	2.3	78.2	0	94.6	0	100	0	94.6	100	100	100
0	99.9	99.0	0	100	0	0	94.4	0	0	0	100	0	100	100	100	100
0	99.9	99.0	0	89.8	95.9	0	20.4	0	0	0	100	0	100	100	100	100
0	99.9	99.0	0	99.0	99.0	0	96.9	0	99.0	0	100	0	94.6	100	100	100
0	100	99.0	0	99.0	96.1	0	64.9	0	99.0	0	100	0	100	100	100	100
0.2	99.0	100	96.5	99.0	97.9	100	100	100	100	0	100	0	0	100	100	100
1.0	99.0	99.0	96.7	99.0	96.7	99.0	96.7	99.0	96.7	0	100	0	0	100	100	100
0	97.8	92.2	61.1	44.4	66.7	21.1	83.3	90.0	67.8	0	92.0	0	0	100	100	100
0	96.2	100	83.0	64.2	39.6	39.6	18.9	92.5	1.9	0	100	0	0	100	100	100
0.4	100	100	92.8	97.0	100	98.1	100	100	99.0	0	100	0	97.3	100	100	100
0.6	99.0	99.0	13.4	96.4	85.3	99.0	96.3	99.0	99.0	0	100	0	94.5	100	100	100
1.7	99.2	98.7	22.3	30.2	79.4	73.1	58.0	75.2	93.7	0	85.9	0	89.4	100	100	100
0	100	98.2	19.3	0	100	98.2	100	100	100	0	100	0	100	100	100	100
0	100	100	72.0	0	99.0	99.0	99.0	99.0	99.0	0	100	0	94.0	100	100	100
60.4	100	100	71.7	98.7	22.4	100	77.5	100	93.8	0	100	0	93.3	100	100	100
85.5	100	100	71.0	91.3	0	98.5	68.1*	97.1	15.9*	0	95.8	0	98.6	100	100	100
62.9	96.7	98.9	42.4	4.3	2.3	84.8	86.6	94.6	85.8	0	100	0	88.0	100	100	100
99.0	100	100	100	100	100	100	100	100	100	0	99.0	0	99.0	100	100	100
99.0	100	100	100	100	100	0	100	100	100	0	99.0	0	87.5	100	100	100
0	100	100	83.3	100	66.7	0	100	100	90.0	0	99.0	0	99.0	100	100	100
95.0	100	90.0	100	50.0	5.0	100	100	90.0	100	0	99.0	0	95.0	100	100	100
0	100	95.2	0	1.0	71.5	0	2.9	11.5	95.2	0	100	0	93.0	100	100	100
52.8	97.3	0.5	1.3	0	2.7	89.6	0	65.2	0.5	0	100	0	94.7	100	100	100
76.6	96.3	0.4	0	0.4	0	0.7	0.1	1.0	0.2	0	93.8	0	95.9	100	100	100
0	99.0	2.5	2.5	0	0	2.5	0	0	2.9	0	100	0	96.5	100	100	100
0.4	99.0	0.8	99.0	0	0	3.7	0	0.8	3.3	0	100	0	87.0	100	100	100
0	100	14.0	85.7	0	0	62.9	0	0	0	0	100	0	87.0	100	100	100
0.4	99.0	84.1	78.8	0	41.2	34.4	0	33.4	1.5	0	98.8	0	94.4	100	100	100
0	97.0	0.2	0	0	0	0.3	0	0	1.2	0	88.5	0	87.7	100	100	100
0	99.0	99.1	25.2	98.2	5.4	90.1	0.9	92.8	76.6	0	98.7	0	0	100	100	100
0	100	100	63.4	95.1	100	100	100	100	46.3	0	98.7	0	0	100	100	100
0	100	100	11.1	95.6	100	100	0	97.8	57.8	0	98.7	0	0	100	100	100
0	98.1	97.1	0	0	77.1	0	9.5	0	29.6	0	95.0	0	0	100	100	100
0	99	97.1	0	71.4	0	0	0	11.4	0	0	47.9	0	0	100	100	100
0	83.7	95.9	0	0	0	0	0	0	0	0	50	0	0	100	100	100
0	100	91.7	0	5.0	85.0	66.7	87.0	100	90.0	0	95.0	0	97.0	100	100	100
0	100	100	0	0	83.3	5.6	94.4	94.4	100	0	100	0	100	100	100	100

**These tests may be required for differentiation of *Enterobacteriaceae* from other Gram-negative bacteria.

*Positive by oxidative metabolism.

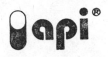

DIFFERENTIATION OF <u>ENTEROBACTERIACEAE</u> AND GRAM-NEGATIVE BACTERIA BY BIOCHEMICAL
figures indicate the percentage of positive reactions after

	ORGANISM	ONPG	ADH	LDC	ODC	CIT	H₂S	URE	TDA	IND	VP
Escherichieae	E. coli	98.2	1.0	90.2	67.3	0	1.0	0	0	85.0	0
	Shigella dysenteriae	27.8	0	0	0	0	0	0	0	33.0	0
	Sh. flexneri	5.3	0	0	0	0	0	0	0	15.0	0
	Sh. boydii	5.0	0	0	0	0	0	0	0	20.0	0
	Sh. sonnei	96.7	0	0	80.0	0	0	0	0	0	0
	Edwardsiella tarda	0	0	99.0	99.0	0	55.0	0	0	100	0
Salmonelleae	Salmonella sp.	1.9	1.0	89.2	95.4	15.4	76.9	0	0	3.1	0
	Sal. typhi	0	0	90.0	0	0	0.1	0	0	0	0
	Sal. paratyphi A	0	0	0	100	0	0.2	0	0	0	0
	Arizona-S. arizonae	94.7	1.0	95.0	98.5	15.0	85.0	0	0	0	0
	Citrobacter freundii	97.0	10.0	0	60.0	10.0	81.0	0	0	6.0	0
	C. diversus-Levinea	97.0	10.0	0	90.0	10.0	0	0	0	91.0	0
	C. amalonaticus	97.0	10.0	0	95.0	10.0	0	0	0	99.0	0
Klebsielleae	Klebsiella pneumoniae	99.0	0	80.0	0	13.9	0	10.0	0	0	72.0
	K. oxytoca	98.0	0	83.0	0	13.0	0	10.0	0	100	60.0
	K. ozaenae	85.0	0	38.0	0	1.0	0	0	0	0	0
	K. rhinoscleromatis	0	0	0	0	0	0	0	0	0	0
	Enterobacter aerogenes	99.0	0	98.0	98.0	8.9	0	0	0	0	56.0
	Ent. cloacae	97.0	51.9	0	65.0	9.0	0	0	0	0	80.0
	Ent. agglomerans	90.0	0	0	0	5.4	0	0	0	50.0	20.0
	Ent. gergoviae	99.0	0	61.0	99.0	8.2	0	75.0	0	0	75.0
	Ent. sakazakii	97.0	51.6	0	59.0	8.6	0	0	0	4.0	85.0
	Serratia liquefaciens	85.0	0	85.0	95.0	8.9	0	1.0	0	0	50.0
	Ser. marcescens	83.0	0	88.0	94.0	8.0	0	1.0	0	0	58.0
	Ser. rubidaea	96.0	0	60.5	0.1	8.2	0	0	0	0	70.0
	Ser. odorifera 1	99.0	0	95.0	100	9.5	0	0	0	90.0	63.0
	Ser. odorifera 2	99.0	0	92.0	0	9.1	0	0	0	90.0	80.0
	Hafnia alvei	60.0	0	99.0	99.0	1.0	0	0	0	0	25.0
Proteeae	Proteus vulgaris	0.5	0	0	0	4.1	75.3	91.0	95.0	75.3	0
	Prot. mirabilis	1.0	0	0	90.0	5.8	66.0	97.0	90.0	1.0	0
	Providencia alcalifaciens	0	0	0	0	9.8	0	0	95.0	94.0	0
	Prov. stuartii	1.0	0	0	0	8.5	0	0	95.0	86.0	0
	Prov. stuartii URE +	1.0	0	0	0	6.9	0	99.0	99.0	95.0	0
	Prov. rettgeri	1.0	0	0	0	7.1	0	80.0	95.0	90.0	0
	Morganella morganii	1.0	0	0	87.0	0.2	0	78.0	92.0	92.0	0
Yersiniae	Yersinia enterocolitica	81.0	0	0	36.0	0	0	59.0	0	54.0	0.4
	Y. pseudotuberculosis	80.0	0	0	0	0	0	88.0	0	0	0
	Y. pestis	93.0	0	0	0	0	0	0	0	0	1.0
	API Group 1	99.0	0	58.8	99.C	9.2	0	0	0	99.0	0
	API Group 2	99.0	2.0	7.3	0	0	0	0	0	0	0
Other Gram-negatives	Pseudomonas maltophilia	62.0	0	5.0	0	7.6	0	0	0	0	0
	Ps. cepacia	61.0	0	5.0	5.0	7.5	0	0	0	0	1.0
	Ps. paucimobilis	40.0	0	0	0	1.0	0	0	0	0	0
	A. calco. var. anitratus	0	0	0	0	2.8	0	0	0	0	1.0
	A. calco. var. lwoffii	0	0	0	0	0	0	0	0	0	0.1
	CDC Group VE-1	90.0	1.0	0	0	7.7	0	0	0	0	1.0
	CDC Group VE-2	0	0	0	0	7.9	0	0	0	0	1.0

API TABLE 5 (continued)

SOME NON-ENTEROBACTERIACEAE
TESTS PROVIDED ON API 20E®
5 hours of incubation at 35-37°C

GEL	GLU	MAN	INO	SOR	RHA	SAC	MEL	AMY	ARA	OXI
0	100	98.4	0.1	95.5	84.5	41.1	88.4	0.1	95.0	0
0	100	0.1	0	0	22.2	0	61.1	0	16.7	0
0	100	94.7	0	78.9	0	0	21.1	0	36.8	0
0	100	60.0	0	53.3	1.0	0	33.3	0	66.7	0
0	100	99.0	0	39.9	80.0	0	50.0	0	96.7	0
0	100	0	0	0	0	0	50.0	0	1.1	0
0	100	98.7	4.6	95.2	95.4	4.6	96.9	0	94.5	0
0	100	99.0	0	99.0	1.8	0	100	0	27.0	0
0	100	99.0	0	99.0	99.0	0	40.0	0	80.0	0
0	100	99.0	0	87.0	96.1	0	89.5	0	95.0	0
0	100	98.0	1.0	96.0	87.0	59.0	77.0	30.0	98.0	0
0	100	97.0	14.5	88.0	99.0	51.0	47.0	34.0	99.0	0
0	100	97.0	0.1	93.0	99.0	29.4	53.0	80.0	93.8	0
0	100	98.0	30.0	95.0	91.0	99.0	99.0	98.0	99.0	0
1.0	100	99.0	29.0	92.0	98.0	99.0	99.0	98.0	99.0	0
0	100	69.0	1.0	76.0	69.0	15.0	92.0	99.0	84.0	0
0	100	99.0	1.0	86.0	53.0	33.0	66.0	99.0	95.0	0
0	100	99.0	28.0	90.0	90.0	85.0	97.0	96.0	98.0	0
0	100	99.0	1.0	92.0	90.0	98.0	92.0	65.0	95.0	0
0	100	99.0	1.0	80.0	60.0	60.0	70.0	70.0	95.0	0
0	100	99.0	1.0	8.3	99.0	99.0	99.0	99.0	99.0	0
0	100	99.0	4.0	8.5	90.0	95.0	90.0	76.0	95.0	0
60.0	100	99.0	1.0	99.0	30.0	85.0	80.7	80.0	92.9	0
72.0	100	96.0	1.0	97.0	2.0	98.0	37.0	72.0	18.0	0
75.6	100	99.0	10.0	75.0	13.4	99.0	82.6	96.0	85.8	0
62.0	100	99.0	10.0	99.0	85.0	100	99.0	90.0	99.0	0
78.0	100	99.0	10.0	99.0	95.0	0	99.0	85.4	99.0	0
0	99.0	99.0	0	35.0	75.0	0	50.0	30.0	95.0	0
75.3	100	0	0.1	0	0	83.0	1.0	20.0	4.0	0
93.0	100	0	0	0	1.0	9.6	10.0	1.0	27.0	0
0	100	0	0	0	0	0	0	0	25.0	0
0	100	0	8.0	0	0.8	3.7	34.0	0	30.0	0
0	100	15.0	5.0	0	0.5	65.0	20.0	0	20.0	0
0	100	85.0	1.0	30.0	40.0	5.0	0	40.0	10.0	0
0	98.0	0	0	0	0	0	0	0	1.0	0
0	100	99.0	1.0	95.0	9.0	78.0	40.4	31.0	76.6	0
0	100	94.0	0	76.0	58.0	0	5.0	0	52.0	0
0	93.0	87.0	0	56.0	0	0	0.6	25.0	87.0	0
0	100	99.0	0	75.4	82.4	82.4	94.1	97.0	94.1	0
0	100	99.0	0	2.3	30.8	5.6	90.0	38.5	92.3	0
50.0	0.5	0	0	0	0	0	0	0	22.0	4.8
46.0	33.0	1.0	0	1.0	0	7.0	0	1.0	1.0	90.7
0	0.5	0	0	0	0	0.5	0	0	0.5	50.0
0.1	85.0	0	0	0	0	0.1	77.0	0	60.0	0
0	0	0	0	0	0	0	0	0	0	0
1.3	33.0	0	1.0	0	1.0	0.1	1.0	1.0	16.0	0
0.1	4.5	0	1.0	0	0	0	1.0	0	5.0	0

The Vibrios

FAMILY: VIBRIONACEAE
GENERA: VIBRIO AEROMONAS

GENERAL CHARACTERISTICS

The members of the family Vibrionaceae are Gram negative facultative anaerobic rods. The non-encapsulated rods are either straight or curved and measure approximately 2.0 - 3.0 µm in length and 0.5 µm in width. Most Vibrionaceae are motile by polar flagellation, but non-motile species do exist.

These bacteria are not nutritionally fastidious and will grow on most general purpose media, however NaCl is required for growth. Some species or biotypes will not grow unless NaCl is in the growth medium. Most grow best in a 3.0% to 4.0% NaCl concentration.

The optimum temperature and pH ranges are 18-37°C and 6.0-9.2 respectively. As a group the Vibrionaceae are oxidase positive, urease negative and convert NO_3 to NO_2.

The two most clinically significant Vibrios are *V. cholerae* and biotypes, and *V. parahaemolyticus.*

MORPHOLOGY/STAINING/PHYSIOLOGY

V. cholerae is a curved rod which measures approximately 1.5 to 3. µm x 0.5 µm. The rods may microscopically appear singly or in pairs as "S" shaped cells.

V. cholerae is Gram negative, bears a single short polar flagellum, and is non-spreforming.

V. cholerae requires an alkaline and aerobic environment for growth. Best growth results are observed when this bacterium is cultivated in a medium having an alkaline pH (7.8-8.2).

Despite their alkaline requirement, *V. cholerae* are not fastidious and grow well in peptone broth.

Biotypes of Vibrio Cholerae

Until several years ago, *V. cholerae* was believed to be the agent primarily responsible for cholera. Today, it is clearly recognized that biotypes exist.

The *V. cholerae* biotype cholerae and *V. cholerae* biotype El Tor are also pathogenic. Table 14 differentiates *V. cholerae* from the biotypes.

INFECTION

Ingestion of *V. cholerae* is essential for infection. The incubation period varies from person to person. Symptoms have been reported from 24 hours to 3-5 days after ingestion.

CLINICAL DIAGNOSIS

The rice water stools contain numerous *V. cholerae* organisms and these are quite apparent in Gram stained smears. Specimens may be collected either with rectal swabs

TABLE 14

TEST	V. CHOLERAE	V. CHOLERAE BIOTYPE CHOLERAE	V. CHOLERAE BIOTYPE EL TOR
Soluble tube Hemolysin (Greig test)	+	–	Variable
Antibiotic	Novobiocin Sensitive	Polymyxin B Sensitive	Polymyxin B Resistant
Phage IV Sensitivity	+	+	–
Hemolysis on Blood Agar	+	–	–

+ = Positive
– = Negative

or a rectal catheter and placed into either a buffered salt solution or alkaline peptone water. The specimens may be subcultured in either enrichment broths or directly plated on selected alkaline media (pH 8.2–8.6) such as thiosulfate–citrate–bile salt sucrose agar (TCBS) or alkaline nutrient agar (ANA) (pH 8.2–8.4) containing 0.5 to sodium taurocholate. After 24 hours of incubation at 35–37°C, the colonies grown on TCBS are yellow with opaque centers and transparent edges. Selected isolated colonies from either TCBS or ANA may be inoculated on Kligler iron agar and also used for a slide agglutination test with O group I antisera. A positive slide agglutination with O group I antiserum and red slant, yellow butt, no gas reaction on KIA confirm the presence of an O group I vibrio bacterium.

Fluorescent antibody (FA) techniques are also used to a limited extent to identify the vibrios.

VIRULENCE

A protein enterotoxin is apparently responsible for the virulence of *V. cholerae*.

TREATMENT

Intravenous administration of isotonic bicarbonate solution is essential to replenish body fluids and prevent electrolyte imbalances. Saline should be administered intravenously until diarrhea ceases. The tetracyclines seem to be the drug of choice.

IMMUNITY

Contraction and recovery from cholera provides a limited immunity to a second infection. Immunity seems to last from six months to one year. Numerous reinfections have been reported.

EPIDEMIOLOGY

Poor sanitation standards play a key role in the dissemination of *V. cholerae*, since ingestion of these organisms is essential for infection.

Improved wastewater disposal and potable water supplies would greatly reduce the incidence of this disease in endemic areas since in these areas cholera is primarily waterborne.

Vibrio Parahaemolyticus

V.parahaemolyticus has been recovered from contaminated fish, shell fish, and marine sediments and is responsible for gastroenteritis, as a result of having ingested contaminated fish and shell fish. *V. parahaemolyticus* is halophilic and requires 6-8% NaCl for growth, but is inhibited in a 10% NaCl medium. The inhibitory action of the 10% NaCl solution differentiates *V. parahaemolyticus* from another marine vibrio, *V. agarlyticus* which does grow in the higher salt concentration.

FAMILY: VIBRIONACEAE
GENUS: AEROMONAS

The Aeromonas have characteristics which may cause workers to confuse them with some Pseudomonas, Enterobacteriaceae, and Vibrios. Care should be taken to avoid confusion.

MORPHOLOGY/STAINING

Aeromonas species are Gram negative rods bearing rounded ends. The Aeromonas are facultative anaerobes which are motile due to polar flagellation.

As a group, the aeromonas hydrolyze casein, liquify gelatin and produce phosphatase, oxidase and catalase.

V. hydrophila causes red leg in frogs and appears to be an opportunistic pathogen for fresh water fish.

The Pseudomonas

FAMILY: PSEUDOMONODACEAE
GENUS: PSEUDOMONAS

The members of the genus Pseudomonas are common inhabitants of soil, water, and decomposing organic matter. These organisms are straight or curved Gram negative rods which measure 1.5 µm in length by .5 to 1.0 µm in width. One property demonstrated by various Pseudomonas is their ability to utilize various organic compounds as sole or prime carbon sources. Some Pseudomonas species form diffusible fluorescent pigments.

Pseudomonas Aeruginosa

MORPHOLOGY/STAINING/PHYSIOLOGY

Pseudomonas aeruginosa is a motile, non-encapsulated and non-sporeforming, Gram negative rod which measures approximately 1.5 to 3.0 µm in length and 0.4 to 0.5 µm in width. *Pseudomonas aeruginosa* is not nutritionally fastidious, requires an aerobic environment, but may grow anaerobically if nitrate (NO_3) is in the growth medium. Acid is produced from glucose, gelatin is liquified, and indole is not produced. *Pseudomonas aeruginosa* produces two pigments: pyocyanin and a yellowish-green pigment. Pyocyanin, a deep blue pigment, is unique to this bacterium. Chloroform can be used to extract pyocyanin from aqueous solutions. The yellowish-green pigment is water soluble and cannot be extracted with chloroform.

PATHOGENICITY

For years, *Pseudonomas aeruginosa* was considered relatively medically insignificant. This is no longer the case. *Pseudonomas aeruginosa* has been implicated in suppurative lesions, mastoiditis, eye infections, urinary tract infections, pneumonia, endocarditis, and bacteremia. *Pseudonomas aeruginosa* gained recognition in the last few years primarily because of its involvement in post surgical and burn infections.

VIRULENCE

An exotoxin which inhibits protein synthesis seems to be the most toxic component elecited by *Pseudonomas aeruginosa*. The exotoxin is a single polypeptide chain which is heat-labile and protein in nature. It is also important to note that mucoid strains of this bacterium form slime in vivo. Since this slime inhibits phagocytosis, it is considered as a virulence factor.

TREATMENT

Pseudonomas related infections are not readily treated because of the microorganism's resistance to antibiotics. Some strains demonstrate multiple antibiotic resistance. Polymyxin, although resistant by some strains, still remains the antibiotic of choice.

LABORATORY DIAGNOSIS

Biochemical tests, serological tests, phage typing and pyocyanin identification or pyocyanin typing have been useful in clinically diagnosing *Ps. aeruginosa*.

Pseudonomas Mallei

Pseudonomas mallei causes glanders disease in horses, mules, goats, sheep and swine. This disease may be transmitted to domestic animals. The alimentary tract seems to be the portal of entry for this microorganism. Depending on the animal infected, the disease may be chronic or acute and fatal. Horses seem to be more seriously affected by glanders and fatality rates are relatively high due to glanders disease.

PATHOGENICITY

It is believed that animal trainers, workers or veterinarians have contracted glanders via cuts and abrasions on the skin. Glanders is of serious concern to those coming in contact with infected animals primarily because most infections have been fatal to humans. Death has been reported within a few days or up to 4 weeks following infection.

The Brucellae

GENUS: BRUCELLA

MORPHOLOGY/STAINING/PHYSIOLOGY

Members of the genus Brucella are Gram negative coccobacilli which measure approximately 0.7 to 1.5 μm by 0.5 to 0.6 μm. Microscopically these short rods appear singly or in short chains. These bacteria are non-motile, non-encapsulated and non-spore forming.

Nutritionally, the members of the genus Brucella require vitamins such as biotin, thiamin and niacin or amino acids as growth factors.

The Brucellae species are strict aerobes which are catalase positive, generally oxidase positive, indole negative. Some strain grow best in a 5-10% CO_2 environment.

PATHOGENICITY

Dogs, goats, swine and cattle are primarily susceptible to Brucella. Fetal death and/or abortions occur in pregnant female animals infected with Brucella. Infected male animals are reported to have testicular atrophy and epididymitis. *B. suis* is usually responsible for the infection in swine and dogs; B. abortus has been isolated from infected swine and cattle; *B. melitensis* also has been recovered from cattle; and B. canis (considered by many to be a *B. suis* biotype) has been recovered from infected dogs.

Brucella suis, Brucella abortus and *Brucella melitensis* are pathogenic to humans. In humans these brucellae are usually cause generalized infections and the microorganisms may be recovered from the blood. Localized infections have been the apparent cause of pulmonary infections, pulmonary lesions, endocarditis and meningitis.

LABORATORY DIAGNOSIS

B. abortus requires a minimum of 5% CO_2 for growth where the other brucellae species do not have a CO_2 growth requirement. Small blue-gray colonies can be observed on trypticase soy agar plates. Glucose, lactose and sucrose fermentation tests will help differentiate the brucellae from other Gram negative rods, since the brucellae only weakly ferment glucose and no other carbohydrate. Most of the other Gram negative rods either will be late lactose fermenters or sucrose fermenters. Again, motility tests may be employed to differentiate the brucellae from some of the other Gram negative rods, since none of the brucellae are motile and some other Gram negative rods are motile.

Fluorescent antibody (FA) staining techniques, phage typing, agglutination reactions with specific antisera, H_2S production, urea hydrolysis, oxidase production, growth in thionine and basic fuchsin aid in the diagnosis of brucellosis.

TREATMENT

The tetracyclines are effective for treatment of brucellosis.

Bordetella

GENERAL CHARACTERISTICS/SPECIES

Members of the genus Bordetella are small coccobacilli which measure approximately 0.4 to 1.0 μm by 0.2 to 0.3 μm and which microscopically appear singly, in pairs or in very short chains. The Bordetella are strict aerobes which resemble Haemophilus, but which do not require the X or V factors for growth. Nutritionally, however, many of the Bordetella do require cysteine, methionine and nicotinic acid. Three Bordetella species are recognized: *Bordetella pertussis, Bordetella parapertussis* and *Bordetella bronchiseptica*.

Bordetella Pertussis

MORPHOLOGY/STAINING/PHYSIOLOGY

Bordetella pertussis, frequently referred to as the Bordet-Gengou bacillus, is a coccobacillus which measures about 0.4 to 9.0 μm by 0.2 to 0.3 μm and which may be microscopically observed singly or in pairs. Smears made from broth cultures may demonstrate a short chain arrangement. *B. pertussis* is non-spore forming, non motile, but is covered by a sheath that is capsule-like. The capsule-like sheath fails to swell in antiserum. Large, opaque, smooth pearl colonies are apparent on Bordet-Gengou agar plates incubated 35-37° for 72 hours. The colonies turn brownish in color when the plates are left in the incubator beyond 72 hours. Penicillin is added to the Bordet-Gengou agar plates to inhibit a mixed flora. *Bordetella pertussis* is a fastidious microorganism which will not grow in peptone broth unless blood is added. It is believed that the blood inactivates the fatty acids contained in the peptone broth. The fatty acids usually inhibit the growth of *B. pertussis*. This bacterium is not biochemically active: citrate and urea are not utilized, nitrate is not reduced to nitrite, indole is not utilized and carbohydrates are not fermented.

SPECIMEN COLLECTION

SWAB TECHNIQUE

Nasopharyngeal swabs are recommended for collecting B. pertussis from patients with whooping cough. The swab containing the collected specimen should be streaked over penicillin containing Bordet-Gengou agar.

COUGH PLATE

The patient coughs directly into Bordet-Gengou agar plates. Spray droplets adhere to the moist agar.

The cough plate is the traditional specimen collection method and is frequently used if there is a difficulty in getting the swab through the nostril.

Specimens should be collected during the first stage of the disease. Negative plate results may be obtained from specimens during the later stages of the disease. Generally, the nasopharyngeal swab cultures give a greater number of positive diagnostic results than the cough plates.

PATHOGENICITY

Bordetella pertussis is the causative agent of whooping cough, a disease which is worldwide in distribution and which afflicts both children and adults.

LABORATORY DIAGNOSIS

Cultures, collected with either the nasopharyngeal swab or the cough plate, are streaked on Bordet-Gengou agar and incubated at 35-37°C for about 72 hours. Large, opaque colonies serve to differentiate *Bordetella pertussis* from *Haemophilus influenzae*. Furthermore, the X and V factors are unnecessary for the growth of *B. pertussis*. The *B. pertussis* bacilli, contained within exudates, may be clinically identified by using fluorescent antibody (FA) staining techniques or by employing agglutination tests.

EPIDEMIOLOGY

Whooping cough is a highly communicable disease which can be transmitted from infected persons via fomites contaminated with oral or nasal secretions or by direct contact with the ill. The disease is more serious in young children and the mortality rate due to whooping cough is greatest in children under five years of age. In the young children, mucous blocks the bronchi resulting in anoxia.

TREATMENT

The tetracyclines, ampicillin and chloramphenicol are recommended for treatment of whooping cough.

IMMUNITY

Recovery from whooping cough provides permanent protection. Second attacks are not common, but should a second attack occur, it is generally milder in children and greater in severity in adults.

Bordetella Parapertussis

A bacillus closely resembling *B. pertussis* has been isolated from exudates of whooping cough patients. This recovered bacillus is *Bordetella parapertussis*. *B. parapertussis* is not as nutritionally fastidious as *B. pertussis* and can grow in general purpose laboratory media. *B. parapertussis* is somewhat more biochemically active in that it utilizes urea and citrate. *B. parapertussis* grows well on Bordet-Gengou agar and its growth on agar plates causes a change in the color of the agar preparation. A brownish color appears in the agar beneath or around the colonies. Tyrosinase is reported to be responsible for the color change.

Bordetella Bronchiseptica

This bacterium has been isolated from respiratory infections resembling whooping cough. However, this microorganism differs from *B. pertussis* in that it is motile with peritrichous flagellation, is catalase and urease positive, utilizes citrate as a sole carbon source and reduces nitrates to nitrites. This bacterium resembles *B. pertussis* in that it grows on Bordet-Gengou agar and does not ferment carbohydrates. Also, *B. bronchiseptica* can cross agglutinate with *B. pertussis* and *B. parapertussis* since the Bordetella share a common O antigen. *B. bronchiseptica* has been recovered from the respiratory tract of swine, rabbits and guinea pigs and has been the causative agent of bronchopneumonia in these animals.

Francisella

MORPHOLOGY/STAINING/PHYSIOLOGY

The Francisella bacteria are small pleomorphic Gram negative, non-motile rods. The optimum growth temperature is 35-37°C and a strict aerobic environment is essential for growth. Carbohydrate fermentation is evidenced by acid production gas and is not fermented. As a group, the Francisella are soluble in sodium lauryl sulfate, are catalase negative and hydrogen sulfide positive.

Bergey's Manual of Determinative Bacteriology (8th Edition) lists two species: *Francisella tularensis* and *Francisella novicida*. These two species are differentiated on the basis of pathogenicity as well as serological and biochemical tests.

Francisella Tularensis

MORPHOLOGY/STAINING/PHYSIOLOGY

F. tularensis (formerly Pasteurella tularensis) is a Gram negative, non-motile pleomorphic rod which measures approximately 0.2 to 0.6 μm by 0.2 μm. General purpose laboratory media must contain enrichment for this bacterium to grow. Growth of *F. tularensis* occurs in blood-glucose-cystine agar, glucose-blood agar, glucose serum agar and blood agar preparations. Thiamine heart agar is also a satisfactory growth medium. Blood-glucose-cystine agar is the medium of choice of many bacteriologists. The blood agar preparations demonstrate a greenish discoloration near the colonies. Growth is slow for primary isolates on all media and may require 3-7 days of incubation for sufficient growth. Subcultures on the same medium grow well in 48-72 hours.

LABORATORY IDENTIFICATION

Isolated colonies, grown on blood-glucose-cystine agar, may be tested for: carbohydrate fermentation, agglutination with specific antisera, fluorescent antibody (FA) staining reactions or phage typing.

PATHOGENICITY

F. tularensis is the causative agent of tularemia, a disease common to rodents. Blood sucking arthropods (ticks) may indirectly transmit the disease to humans. Laboratory workers or veterinarians may directly contract the disease by handling infected animals. Most workers have been infected while working with either infected rabbits or guinea pigs.

Tularemia has occurred in all sections of the United States.

TREATMENT

Streptomycin is the antibiotic of choice in the treatment of tularemia. The tetracyclines are also effective, but to a lesser extent than streptomycin. *F. tularensis* demonstrates antibiotic resistance, therefore sensitivity testing is highly recommended.

Francisella Novicida

This microorganism produces tularemia-like lesions in white mice and guinea pigs and is not pathogenic to humans. *F. novicida* grows well on primary isolation and may be differentiated from *F. tularensis* on the basis of pathogenicity and serological and biochemical tests.

Pasteurella

Pasteurella Multocida

Pasteurella multocida, formerly called *Pasteurella septica*, is a Gram negative coccobacillary pleomorphic rod. Pasteurella multocida may be encapsulated or non-encapsulated. Hemolysis is not apparent on blood agar, but a brownish discoloration of the blood agar preparation is apparent when heavily inoculated and profuse growth is apparent. A characteristic odor can also be detected from agar plates with heavy growth. Some biochemical characteristics of *Pasteurella multocida* are listed in Table 15.

TABLE 15

CHARACTERISTICS OF PASTEURELLA MULTOCIDA

TEST	RESULTS
Indole	+
H_2S	+
Ammonia	+
Urease	–
Oxidase	+/–*
KCN	+**
Ornithine Decarboxylase	+
Hemolysis on Blood Agar	–

*Most strains are oxidase positive but a few strains were reported negative.
**Most strains grow in KCN.

Pathogenicity

Different strains affect animals in a variety of ways. Strains of *Pasteurella multocida* are highly pathogeric for rabbits, fowl, mice, cattle, sheep, pigs, cats and dogs. Humans become infected as the result of cat or dog scratches or bites. The smooth strains are pathogenic to humans and are usually recovered from wound infections.

TREATMENT

Although *Pasteurella multocida* is a Gram negative bacillus, it is highly suscepti-ble to penicillin in vitro. Erythromycin is also effective in treating infections.

Haemophilus

The genus Haemophilus is comprised of small pleomorphic Gram negative, non-spore-forming, non-motile rods. The Haemophilus bacteria are frequently considered to be hemophilic, i.e., blood loving bacteria. The hemophilic attribute is due to the fact that these bacteria require blood constituents (X and V factors) for life and growth processes. The X factor is associated with hemoglobin while the V factor is associ-ated with whole blood.

The members of this genus are aerobic or facultatively anaerobic. Some strains produce hemolysis on blood agar preparations.

Haemophilus Influenzae

MORPHOLOGY/STAINING/PHYSIOLOGY/PATHOGENICITY

H. influenzae are small Gram negative Bocilli or filaments which may be encapsulated. Six serotypes have been identified by the capsule polysaccharide. *H. influenzae* is believed to be the causative agent of pandemic influenza. Clinically, this bacterium has been recovered from specimens of patients suffering with conjunctivitis, septicemia, osteomyelitis, otitis, and subacute bacterial endocarditis.

Haemophilus haemolyticus is generally a commensal found in the upper respiratory tract of humans. On occasion this bacterium has caused mild to severe sore throats.

Haemophilus parainfluenzae has been recovered from the upper respiratory tract of humans, cats, cattle and sheep. This microorganism is non-pathogenic in the respiratory tract.

Haemophilus parahaemolyticus is a common inhabitant of the upper respiratory tract and frequently has been diagnosed as the etiologic agent of acute pharyngitis, pleuropneumonia and endocarditis in humans.

Haemophilus Paraphrophilus

This bacterium has been recovered from the urogenital tract, vagina, urine, infected appendix, and from purulent lesions of the brain. *H. paraphrophilus* has been implicated in osteomyelitis and subacute endocarditis and respiratory tract infections.

Haemophilus Aphrophilus

Haemophilus aphrophilus has been isolated from blood, spinal fluid, and sputum specimens and is a causative agent of encocarditis, septicemia and meningitis.

Haemophilus Ducreyi

Haemophilus ducreyi is difficult to isolate because of its strict nutritional requirements. Nevertheless, this bacterium has grown on clotted sheep and human blood agar and chocolate blood agar preparations. Some bacteriologists report good growth results on blood agar plates while others report equivalent or better results on chocolate blood agar plates. *H. ducreyi* causes the venereal disease known as soft chancre or chancroid. Smears of lesion specimens which demonstrate small, Gram negative ovoid rods (approximately 1.5 µm by 0.5 µm) occurring in pairs or chains, may serve for presumptive diagnosis of the disease. *H. ducreyi* can be cultivated on freshly clotted rabbit or human blood when incubated at 35-37°C for 7 to 9 days. An increased CO_2 atmosphere is recommended for better results. Smears from the clotted blood medium will show small Gram negative rods in a chain arrangement. Subcultures may be made on chocolate blood agar. Many workers recommend chocolate blood agar slants for maintaining stock cultures.

TREATMENT

Chlortetracycline and streptomycin have been effective in the treatment of the chancroid disease caused by *H. ducreyi*.

Haemophilus Vaginalis

This bacillus is Gram variable and unlike other Haemophilus species it requires neither the X (hemin) or V (niacin adenine nucleotide) factor. Some workers have grown *H. vaginalis* on semisynthetic media containing vitamins (folic acid, biotin,

TABLE 16

SEVERAL CHARACTERISTICS OF HAEMOPHILUS SPECIES

HAEMOPHILUS SPECIES	FACTORS X	FACTORS V	INCREASED CO₂	NO₃→NO₂	HEMOLYSIS	CATALASE	INDOLE	FERMENTATION OF GLUCOSE	SUCROSE	MALTOSE
H. influenzae	+	+	-	+	-	+	+/-	Acid	Acid	Acid +/-
H. parainfluenzae	-	+	-	+	-	+	+/-	Acid	Acid	Acid +/-
H. haemolyticus	+	+	-	+	-	+	+/-	+/-	+/-	+/-
H. parahaemolyticus	-	+	-	+	+	+	-	Acid	-	Acid
H. paraphrophilus	-	+	+	+	-	+	-	Acid	Acid	Acid
H. paraphrohaemoly- ticus	-	+	+	+	+	+	+/-	Acid	Acid +/-	Acid
H. aphrophilus*	+	-	+	+	-	D	-	Acid	Acid	Acid
H. ducreyl	+	-	+	N/D	+/or D	N/D	N/D	N/C	N/D	N/D
H. vaginalis	-	-	+	-	+/-	-	-	Acid	Acid +/-	Acid

*Most H. aphrophilus strains require the X factor for growth, however, some workers have reported the contrary.
N/D = Not determined or not data available.
+/- = Variable results.
D   = Delayed positive result.

thiamine and riboflavin), salts and nucleic acid bases. This species is still said to be haemophilic (blood loving) and grows fairly well on chocolate blood agar with an increased CO_2 environment. *H. vaginalis* may be recovered from genital tract specimens of infected people. This bacterium has been diagnosed as a causative agent of vaginitis, urethritis and postpartum bacteremia. *H. vaginalis* strains have demonstrated antibiotic resistance, but most strains are sensitive to penicillin, erythromycin, neomycin and tetracycline. Some common traits of the Haemophilus species are listed on Table 16.

The Clostridia

FAMILY: BACILLACEAE
GENUS: CLOSTRIDIUM

The members of the genus Clostridium are Gram positive, spore-forming bacilli that, as a group, are nearly all strictly anaerolic. The spore may be placed in a different location within the cells. This characteristic may be used to identify the different Clostridia species.

The taxonomy of the Clostridia is confusing. More than 300 species have been classified as Clostridia over the years. For identification purposes, the Clostridia are divided into four groups. Group classification is dependent upon the location of the spore in the cell and gelatin liquifaction.

The pathogenic Clostridia produce potent exotoxins.

Clostridium Perfringens

MORPHOLOGY/STAINING

C. perfringens is a short, plump, spore forming Gram positive bacillus which occurs singly or in pairs. *C. perfringens* is nonmotile and has a capsule.

Clostridium perfringens is associated with gas gangrene. Other species isolated from cases of gangrene include *C. sporogenes,* and *C. novyi.* *C. perfringens* is a normal inhabitant of the intestinal tract of humans and animals and becomes pathogenic only in cases of intestinal perforation. Any wound contaminated with soil also may be infected with these spore-bearing anaerobes.

Clostridium tetanus is a slender rod which measures 2 to 5 μm in length and 0.3 to 0.8 μm in width. Peritrichous flagellation is present in younger cultures. Spores located at the end of the rod give the appearance of a "drunstick."

Tetanus is the causative agent of tetanus. *C. tetanus* is a very virulent organism producing a fibrinolysin, a hemolysin, and other toxins.

The fibrinolysin is capable of destroying fibrin formed by the body's coagulation mechanism. The hemolysin causes lysis of erythrocytes.

Toxins produced by *C. tetanus* are specific for the nervous system and humans are extremely susceptible to this neurotoxin.

Clostridium botulinum is a Gram-positive bacillus that possesses four to eight flagella.

TABLE 17

BIOCHEMICAL CHARACTERISTICS OF THE CLOSTRIDIA

TESTS	C. PERFRINGENS	C. SPOROGENES	C. SEPTICUM	C. NOVYI A TYPE	C. HISTOLYTICUM	C. TETANUS	C. BOTULINUM ABCDE TYPES	C. BIFFERMENTANS
Indole Production	-	-	-	-	-	V	-	+
Lipase	-	+	-	+	-	-	+	+
Lecithinase	+	-	-	+	-	-	-	+
H₂S	-	+	-	-	d	+	+	d
Digestion of Casein	-	+	-	-	+	-	+	+
FERMENTATION — Glucose	+	+	+	+	-	-	+	+
Lactose	+	-	+	-	-	-	-	-
Maltose	+	V	+	d	-	-	V	+
Mannose	+	-	+	-	-	-	-	V
Raffinose	d	-	-	d	-	ND	-	-
Sucrose	+	d	-	d	!	ND	d	-
Fructose	+	+	+	d	-	ND	+	d
Urease	d	-	-	-	-	ND	-	-
Hemolysis on blood agar	d	+	+	+	+	+	+	V

+ = positive
- = negative
V = variable
d = results differ
ND = not determined

C. botulinum is the cause of "food poisoning" due to a potent exotoxin. There are six known exotoxins designated A, B, C, D, E, F. The toxins act on the myoneural functions and produce death by respiratory paralysis.

Clostridium perfringens grows in meat media but under strictly anaerobic conditions. A Brewer anaerobic jar can be used to maintain anaerobic conditions.

C. perfringens does not form spores easily.

C. tetanus is an obligate anaerobe which loses its ability to produce a toxin when grown microaerophilically.

Clostridium botulinum is a strict anaerobe and is easily cultivated under anaerobic conditions on the usual meat-infusion media. Several types of *C. botulinum* have been isolated. They have been designated as types A, B, C, D, E. Corresponding toxins, designated A through E, are produced by these organisms when grown at optimum temperatures, which in most cases range between 25°C and 37°C.

The organism grows only at a neutral pH or moderate alkalinity.

Outbreaks of botulism are rare in the United States because of the rigid standards for canning and food preservation.

BACTERIOLOGICAL CHARACTERISTICS

Many of the pathogenic species, such as *C. septicum*, *C. sporogenes*, *C. tetanus* and *C. perfringens* show zones of hemolysis on blood agar. A characteristic double-zone of hemolysis is produced by *C. perfringens* when grown on blood agar plates which were incubated in an anaerobic environment.

Microscopy and colony morphology of some Clostridia are distinct and different. Nevertheless, confirmation of the Clostridia species should be based upon biochemical test results and animal virulence tests.

IDENTIFICATION

If spores of a suspected Clostridium species are observed in a mixed thioglycollate broth culture, the spore's resistance to heat may facilitate its isolation and identification. Inoculated broth cultures are placed for 20-30 minutes in a water bath set at 80°C. This temperature setting and exposure time will kill vegetative cells but not spore forming bacteria. The heated broth culture is incubated for 24-48 hours to allow the spore forming Clostridium to grow.

To identify *C. perfringens,* exudate from wounds is collected with sterile swabs and used for smears or cultures. The smears should be examined for larger Gram positive spore forming bacilli. Cultural morphology should be determined.

The *C. botulinum* toxin may be recovered from leftover food or from the serum of infected persons. Blood agar is a good isolation medium. Isolates may be transferred to thioglycollate broth. Toxin elicited from *C. botulinum* is recovered and injected peritoneally into mice, thus causing death.

As stated, biochemical test results aid in the differentiation of the Clostridia species.

Selected biochemical results are found in Table 17.

Bacillus

FAMILY: BACILLACEAE

GENUS: BACILLUS

Members of the genus Bacillus are Gram positive bacilli that are strictly aerobic or facultatively anaerobic. These bacilli measure about 1.0 to 7.0 µm in length by 0.2 to 2.0 µm in width and possess heat resistant endospores. Although most species strongly stain Gram positive, older cultures may tend to appear Gram negative. These bacteria are not nutritionally fastidious and several species produce antibiotics. Most of the species are non-pathogenic but a few species are medically significant.

BACILLUS ANTHRACIS

MORPHOLOGY/STAINING/PHYSIOLOGY

B. anthracis is a Gram positive encapsulated spore forming bacillus. In blood or tissue smears, the bacilli appear singly or in pairs. The spore is not larger than the vegetative cell, therefore *B. anthracis* cells maintain the rod configuration and are not distorted in the same manner as are some of the spore forming Clostridia.

Incubation of cultures at 32-35°C seems to enhance spore formation. *B. anthracis* is aerobic and facultatively anaerobic. Simple laboratory media will support the growth of this bacterium and the addition of enrichments to broths or agar preparations usually do not enhance growth.

Biochemically, this organism ferments glucose, trehalose, sucrose and maltose, fails to produce indole or reduce nitrate, and slowly liquifies gelatin.

PATHOGENICITY

Humans are not the prime target of *B. anthracis*. Anthrax is a disease that primarily affects animals, especially sheep and cattle. Occasionally horses, goats and swine are infected with *B. anthracis* but sheep and cattle are the prime target. *B. anthracis* generally enters the animals via skin abraisons or ingestion of the spores. Humans either inhale the spores or contract the infectious agent through skin cuts, scratches or abrasions. The spores germinate at the site of entry. Eventually, the organisms spread to deeper tissues, the lymphatics and bloodstream. Infections are named according to the affected site: cutaneous anthrax, pulmonary anthrax and intestinal anthrax. Anthrax is an occupational hazard for those who work with animals or animal products. Textile workers have been unsuspecting victims of anthrax.

BACTERIOLOGICAL IDENTIFICATION

Tissue smears demonstrate Gram positive bacilli either singly or in pairs and infrequently in short chains. Isolates on sheep blood agar are non-hemolytic. The isolate is prepared for mouse or guinea pig inoculation to establish animal virulence. If the isolate is *B. anthracis*, the animal dies within five days. A gelatinous edema is observed at the site of injection. Also, once the anthrax bacilli are in the circulatory system, they attack various organs, but the spleen seems to be the prime target. Spleen smears show an abundance of large, Gram positive bacilli.

Further subculturing or biochemical tests are not essential, since none of the other Gram positive, aerobic spore forming bacilli resembling *B. anthracis* can cause such a virulent reaction in the mouse or guinea pig.

TREATMENT

B. anthracis is susceptible to the sulfonamides, penicillin and the tetracyclines. These antibiotics have been effective in the treatment of anthrax.

Bacillus Cereus

B. cereus is morphologically similar to *B. anthracis*, however *B. cereus* is hemolytic on sheep blood agar and *B. anthracis* is non-hemolytic. Further characteristics used to differentiate these two aerobic, spore forming bacilli are found in Table 18.

B. cerus is medically and clinically significant in that it produces an enterotoxin which causes a type of food poisoning in humans.

TABLE 18

CHARACTERISTICS WHICH DIFFERENTIATE B. ANTHRACIS FROM B. CEREUS

BACILLACEAE	HEMOLYSIS ON BLOOD AGAR	CAPSULE	MOUSE OR GUINEA PIG VIRULENCE TEST	CAUSES
B. anthracis	−	+	+	Anthrax
B. cereus	+	−	−	Food poisoning

Listeria

FAMILY: LACTOBACILLAEAE
GENUS: LISTERIA

Members of the genus Listeria are small Gram positive, non-sporeforming, non-encapsulated cocco-bacilli. Smears made from 18-24 hour cultures incubated at 35-37°C show the diphtheroid "picket-fence" arrangement with a few V or Y forms dispersed throughout the smear. Although the members of this genus stain well with the Gram stain, older cultures frequently decolorize.

Peritrichous flagellation is observed in cultures incubated at 25°C, but the number of flagella is reduced or absent in most cultures incubated 35-37°C.

Characteristically, members of the genus Listeria fail to hydrolyze either urea or gelatin, do hydrolyze esculin and do not produce indole.

These bacteria are aerobic to microaerophilic and grow best in a CO_2 (10%) enriched environment.

Listeria Monocytogenes

MORPHOLOGY/STAINING/PHYSIOLOGY

Listeria monocytogenes is a cocco-bacillus which measures approximately 1.0 to 2.0 μm by 0.5 μm. This bacterium is Gram-positive, non-encapsulated, non-sporeforming and appears singly, in pairs, short chains or in a V arrangement.

When incubated at 20 to 25°C, *L. monocytogenes* bears four peritrichously arranged flagella, but the number of flagella may decrease to one, when this same microorganism is incubated at 35-37°C.

L. monocytogenes is beta hemolytic on the proper blood agar preparations and if the incubation temperature is lowered to 4°C, this bacterium may survive for 6 to 7 weeks in a 15-20% NaCl medium.

ISOLATION/IDENTIFICATION

L. monocytogenes may be recovered and isolated from pupulent lesions, blood, cerebrospinal fluid (CSF) and feces. This organism causes septicemia, endocarditis, encephalitis, meningitis, abortions, lesions and abscesses. Deaths have been reported due to L. monocytogenes infections.

Small zones of beta hemolysis are produced on sheep and rabbit blood agar. However, the degree of hemolysis varies from strain to strain, and no hemolysis may be apparent from isolates obtained from feces.

Reflected light sources demonstrate milky, smooth, butyrous colonies on sheep liver extract agar. Black, circular and smooth colonies appear on potassium tellurite agar. On general purpose media, rough (R) and smooth (S) colony types may be observed.

L. monocytogenes is a Gram positive diphtheroid-like bacterium which usually yields the following results:

BIOCHEMICAL CHARACTERISTICS

Bacterium	INDOLE	H$_2$S	NO$_3$→NO$_2$	UREASE	CATALASE	GLUCOSE	MALTOSE	LEVULOSE
L. monocytogenes	−	−	−	−	+	+	+	+

MONOCYTOSIS

Infection with *L. monocytogenes* is characterized by a marked increase in the number of monocytes resulting in a condition referred to as monocytosis. When *L. monocytogenes* cells are introduced into rabbits, their monocyte count increases and constitutes 30% of the total white blood cell count.

DETERMINATION OF PATHOGENICITY

L. monocytogenes causes conjunctivities in rabbits and guinea pigs. Insertion of 2-3 drops of a *L. monocytogenes* culture into the conjunctiva of rabbits or guinea pigs, causes conjunctivitis within a week. The condition disappears, but the condition does confirm the pathogenicity of *L. monocytogenes*. Several of the drugs of choice to treat listeriosis are: erythromycin, tetracycline, ampicillen, and chloramphenicol.

Listeriosis is dangerous and identification is essential for proper treatment. Until recently *L. monocytogenes* was considered relatively medically insignificant. Consequently few laboratories are prepared to deal with this microorganism. Many laboratories send positive *L. monocytogenes* cultures to another laboratory for a second confirmation.

Erysipelothrix

Erysipelothrix rhusiopathiae is the only species in this genus and is the causative agent of erysipeloid. Erysipeloid is a disease which is primarily occupational affecting those who handle contaminated poultry, fish, shellfish and meat products, especially pork. *Erysipelothrix rhusiopathiae* has an affinity for the skin, joints and endocardium. Erysipeloid should NOT be confused with streptococcal erysipelas.

MORPHOLOGY/STAINING/PHYSIOLOGY

Morphologically, *Erysipelothrix rhusiopathiae* exhibits rough and smooth colony types. Smears of cells from rough colonies show filamentous forms while smears of cells from smooth colonies show short, narrow, straight, or slightly curved bacilli. The smooth colonies are small, round, water-clear and glisten on solid media while the rough colonies are larger, granular and curled in appearance.

Erysipelothrix rhusiopathiae is alpha hemolytic on blood agar. In gelatin stabs, the stab portion is bead-like in appearance. Lateral, brush-like, filaments grow from the stab. This organism grows poorly on simple media. The addition of glucose or serum to simple media will enhance growth.

Refelcted light causes the colonies to appear transparent with a bluish sheen. Since this bacterium can tolerate up to 0.5% potassium tellurite, potassium tellurite may be incorporated into an agar preparation. After 24 hours of incubation, on tellurite agar, *Erysipelothrix rhusiopathiae* colonies are pinpoint and grayish. Further incubation will cause these same colonies to increase in size and turn black.

Lactose, glucose and levulose are fermented with acid production. *Erysipelothrix rhusiopathiae* is a facultative anaerobe with microaerophilic tendencies.

TREATMENT

Erysipelothrix rhusiopathiae is the causative agent of swine erysipelas and mouse septicemia. It is an occupational hazard for those working with infected animals. Streptomycin, penicillin and erythromycin are among the drugs that are effective in the greatment of erysipeloid.

RELATIONSHIP WITH LISTERIA

Listeria monocytogenes and *Erysipelothrix rhusiopathiae*, according to many are considered to be closely related although *Erysipelothrix rhusiopathiae* is serologically different from *Listeria monocytogenes*. Differentiation criteria may be found in Table 19.

TABLE 19

CHARACTERISTICS DIFFERENTIATING ERYSIPELOTHRIX RHUSIOPATHIAE
FROM MONOCYTOGENES

CHARACTERISTICS	ERYSIPELOTHRIX RHUSIOPATHIAE	LISTERIA MONOCYTOGENES
Hemolysis on Blood Agar	Alpha	Beta
Cell Wall Components	Lysine, Serine, Glycine, Alanine, and Glutamic Acid	Diaminopimelic Acid, Aspartic Acid, Glutamic Acid, Alanine and Leucine
Esculin Hydrolysis	–	+
Catalase Production	–	+
H_2S	+	–
Acid from Glucose	+	+
Acid from Lactose	+	+/–
Acid from Sucrose	–	+/–
Motility	Non-motile	Motile

Corynebacterium

FAMILY: CORYNEBACTERIACEAE
GENUS: CORYNEBACTERIUM

Members of the genus Corynebacterium are Gram positive, slender rods which occasionally appear "club-shaped" and irregular in arrangement. In stained smears,
these bacteria take on a palisade or picket fence arrangement. Deeply stained granules appear within these bacteria. The metachromatic granules stain intensely with
analine dyes. The Corynebacteria are aerobic and facultatively anaerobic but seem
to grow best in the presence of oxygen. Some pathogenic species of this genus produce exotoxins and as a group they are catalase positive.

Corynebacterium Diphtheriae

MORPHOLOGY/STAINING/PHYSIOLOGY

Three distinct *C. diphtheriae* cultural types are recognized on the basis of their
severity: *C. gravis*, *C. intermedius* and *C. mitis*. Discussion in this section will be
restricted to typical *C. diphtheriae* strains.

Corynebacterium diphtheriae are Gram positive straight or curved rods which are
swollen at one or both ends and consequently appear as a "club" or "dumbbell." The
rods measure approximately 1.0 to 1.7 μm by 0.3 to 0.7 μm, and usually contain deep

staining metachromatic granules. Although this bacterium strongly stains Gram positive, it may tend to decolorize. This is particularly true of older cultures which
may appear Gram negative. The diphtheria bacilli tend to be pleomorphic and this
pleomorphic trait seems to be even more pronounced and frequent when *C. diphtheriae*
is grown on Loeffler's serum medium, a medium which supports the growth of the
diphtheria bacilli.

Although smears of the corynebacteria show a characteristic morphological appearance due to irregular staining of the metachromatic granules with methylene blue, and
the unique picket-fence, V or L shaped arrangement, *C. diphtheriae* cannot be identified on these traits alone. Typical strains demonstrate a fairly broad temperature
range. These bacteria can grow at temperatures ranging from 15-40°C, but they grow
best between 35-37°C. An alkaline medium, with a pH of approximately 7.6-8.0, and
an aerobic environment enhance growth. These bacteria, are aerobic, and facultatively anaerobic but grow best in the presence of oxygen.

Most of the diphtheria bacilli produce acid from glucose and maltose but not
sucrose; do not produce urease, gelatinase and indole; but do produce a lethal
exotoxin.

Diphtheria bacilli stock cultures may remain viable for a fairly extensive time
period. Cultures grown on blood serum have remained viable for four to six months
and ten to twelve months on glucose blood serum. For isolation and differentiation
purposes, potassium tellurite may be added to blood or chocolate blood agar. The
tellurite inhibits other bacterial flora and the diphtheria bacilli colonies appear
grayish-black.

TOXIN RECOVERY

Most *C. diphtheriae* strains produce an exotoxin. Nutritional and environmental
factors greatly influence the production of this potent exotoxin. For optimum toxin
production, cultures of *C. diphtheriae* should contain the required amino acids, other
nutrients, and iron. Iron is believed to be a key component for exotoxin formation.
The medium should have an alkaline pH (7.6-8.0) since an acidic pH inhibits toxin
production. The cultures should be incubated at 35-37°C for a minimum of 8-10 days.

PATHOGENICITY

C. diphtheriae is the causative agent of diphtheria. Diphtheria has always been
considered a childhood disease. The incidence of diphtheria has been on the decrease
for many years, but the number of adult cases, ironically have been on the increase.
This is due undoubtedly to the decrease immunity towards the diphtheria bacillus in
adulthood due to a deminished or limited exposure to the disease in our society.
Regardless of the frequency, dipththeria is contagious and dangerous without early
and proper treatment. The dipththeria bacilli invade the mucous membranes of the
upper respiratory tract and produce a potent exotoxin. The exotoxin is absorbed by
the mucous membranes, and induces an inflammatory reaction that destroys the
epithelium of the mucous membranes. The *C. diphtheriae,* in the course of the disease,
forms a pseudomembrane. The toxin may play a role in the formation of the pseudomembrane, but the spread of the toxin after absorption is by far the more serious
action of the toxin. Since the diphtherial toxin invades the body, diphtheria, like
tetanus, is considered a toxemia. The effects of the toxin on the heart, kidneys
and nerves are the most dangerous aspects of diphtheria. The affect on the body,
particularly the heart and kidneys, depends upon the length of time the disease is
untreated.

BACTERIOLOGICAL IDENTIFICATION

Specimens may be obtained by swabbing the nose, throat or other suspected lesions before antibiotics are administered. Smears are made of the collected specimens and simultaneously Gram stained and stained with alkaline methylene blue. In addition, the specimens are either cultured in an enrichment medium and/or directly plated on Loeffler's serum agar and chocolate tellurite agar. Many laboratories also inoculate into blood agar to isolate and study the diphtheria bacterial colony morphology and to establish whether hemolytic streptococci also may be present in the lesion. Grayish-black colonies on tellurite agar should be Gram stained and subjected to biochemical tests. At times, tellurite reducing stapthylococci have produced "blackish" colonies which could be mistaken for the diphtheria bacilli. This can be detected with a Gram stain.

VIRULENCE DETERMINATION

The guinea pig and rabbit are frequently used to establish the virulence of suspected colonies. Guinea pig A receives 250 units of diphtheria antitoxin 24 hours prior to receiving a subcutaneous injection of *C. diphtheriae*. Guinea pig B does not receive any antitoxin, but is subcutaneously injected with a suspension of the suspected *C. diphtheriae* cells.

If the suspected cells are *C. diphtheriae*, the uninoculated guinea pig would die in approximately 3-5 days following the injection. The autopsy will demonstrate that the adrenal gland enlarged and hemorrhaged . Guinea pig B inoculated with antitoxin will show no clinical symptoms and will survive.

Intracutaneous injections of a saline suspension of suspected colonies injected into the shaved skin area of an uninoculated guinea pig will cause lesions and necrosis in 2-3 days after the injection. This is considered a positive toxicity test.

IMMUNITY

Diphtheria differs from other respiratory diseases in that frequent or long term exposure to *C. diphtheriae* forms a solid immunity to this disease and its clinical symptoms.

Other Corynebacteria (Diphtheroids)

The diphtheroid bacilli are morphologically similar to *C. diphtheriae* and frequently are mistaken for the diphtheria bacilli. Bergey's Manual of Determinative Bacteriology (8th Edition) lists nine diphtheroid species. Of these nine species listed, only 3 are found in humans:

1. *Corynebacterium xerosis*
2. *Corynebacterium pseudodiphtheriticum*
3. *Corynebacterium pseudotuberculosis*

C. xerosis is believed to be a common inhabitant of the skin and mucous membranes of humans. It is considered non-pathogenic despite the fact that it has been recovered from numerous conjunctivitis conditions. It is believed that *C. xerosis* is a non-pathogenic inhabitant of the conjunctival sac.

C. pseudodiphtheriticum is commonly found in the nasopharyngeal mucosa of humans. Upon preliminary microscopic examination, this non-pathogen may be suspected of being

TABLE 20

REACTIONS USED TO DIFFERENTIATE CERTAIN CORYNEBACTERIACEAE

C. DIPHTHERIAE AND DIPHTHEROIDS	ACID PRODUCTION FROM			HEMOLYSIS ON BLOOD AGAR
	GLUCOSE	MALTOSE	SUCROSE	
C. diphtheriae	+	+	-	*+/-
C. pseudodiphtheriticum	-	-	-	-
C. pseudotuberculosis	+	+	+/-	+
C. xerosis	+	+	+	-
C. pyogenes	+	+	-	+
C. striatum	+	+	-	**+

*C. diphtheriae hemolysis on blood agar varies depending upon the C. diphtheriae type in question, e.g., C. gravis (-), C. intermedius (-), and C. mitis (+).
**Slight hemolysis observed near deep colonies.

C. diphtheriae. However, since *C. pseudodiphtheriticum* is morphologically shorter and broader than *C. diphtheriae*, fails to produce a soluble toxin and does not ferment glucose or produce acid from any carbohydrate, it may be distinguished from *C. diphtheriae* on these criteria.

C. pseudotuberculosis produces an exotoxin different from the *C. diphtheriae* exotoxin. This bacillus has been isolated from abscesses and purulent lesions in horses, sheep, goats, and other warm blooded animals. Some reports suggest that this organism occasionally causes similar infections in humans.

Bergey's Manual of Determinative Bacteriology (8th Edition) in addenda list two diphtheroids worthy of discussion: *C. pyogenes* and *C. striatum*.

C. pyrogenes is a Gram positive, beta hemolytic, rod which measures approximately 0.3 to 2.0 μm by 0.2 μm. These short rods form streptococcal-like chains and on occasion have been mistaken for beta hemolytic streptococci until further testins is performed.

Mutants of *C. pyogenes* form larger colonies on agar preparations and are referred to as *C. haemolyticum* by many workers. Biochemical studies have been performed to show the similarities and dissimilarities between *C. pyogenes* and its mutant *C. haemolyticum.*

Corynebacterium striatum has been isolated from the nasopharynx of humans. This organism is slightly hemolytic on blood agar and may be morphologically confused with *C. diphtheriae* until biochemical tests are performed. See Table 20 for biochemical reactions of certain Corynebacteriaceae.

The Spirochetes

ORDER: SPIROCHAETALES

FAMILY: SPIROCHAETACEAE
GENUS: TREPONEMA

Members of the genus Treponema are motile Gram-negative, helical, spiral bacilli which measure about 5.0 to 18.0 μm in length and 0.1 to 0.5 μm in width. The treponemas are strict anaerobes. In vitro studies indicate that they are catalase, oxidase, urease and Voges-Proskauer negative.

Fibrils are at the end of the spiral bacilli. Although the terminal fibrils have no role in motility, they aid to microscopically identify the treponema bacilli primarily in dark field microscopy. Motility is due to the twisting action of the spiral treponema.

TREPONEMA PALLIDUM

T. pallidum is not particularly resistant and laboratory studies are further complicated by the fact that virulent *T. pallidum* bacteria have never been cultivated in artificial laboratory media, tissue cultures or chick embryos. Cells are unable to replicate when inoculated on artificial media.

Once removed from the infected individual, or infected laboratory animal, the *T. pallidum* survival time is limited. This organism is strongly dependent upon environmental conditions for survival. The treponemas are highly sensitive to soaps, disinfectants, bile salts and drying.

PATHOGENICITY

T. *pallidum* is the causative agent of syphilis. Syphilis is transmitted by sexual intercourse with an infected person. The treponemas leave the site of infection and invade deeper body tissues.

PRIMARY STAGE

The primary lesion, a small ulceration, appears on the mucosa of the genital tissues, 2 to 8 weeks after contracting the infectious agent. The ulcer enlarges and hardens. This encrusted ulcer is referred to as a CHANCRE. When the encrusted chancre is raised or removed, fluid containing T. *pallidum* organisms can be recovered for darkfield microscopy and further testing. The chancre heals and is no longer apparent. The infected falsely feel that they are well and that the infection was localized. This is false since the treponemas invade tissues and later cause a generalized infection, referred to as the secondary stage of the disease.

If untreated, the secondary and tertiary stages may occur. Eventually, skin lesions, containing the treponemas, are apparent throughout the body and liver, spleen, lymph nodes, brain, walls of arteries, skin and mucosal surfaces are invaded. The syphilis organisms are also in the blood, but difficult to demonstrate clinically.

In the untreated, internal lesions, called gummatas, are formed in numerous organs and on the skin. The liver may become infected resulting in syphilitic cirrhosis. The treponemas may weaken the walls of the aorta and cause an aneurysm. Brain and spinal cord damage may also result. These latter symptoms may occur years after the initial infection.

LABORATORY DIAGNOSIS

Darkfield microscopy is used for preliminary diagnosis of the primary stage of syphilis. Serous fluid, containing T. *pallidum* is obtained from beneath the primary chancre and examined, unstained. Typical slender spirals measuring 5.0 to 15.0 μm long and about 0.2 μm wide are observed by darkfield microscopy. Since T. *pallidum* cannot be grown on synthetic laboratory media, syphilis must be confirmed by serological means. This is particularly true during the later stages of syphilis. Confirmation is dependent upon antigen-antibody reactions. Blood (serum) plasma and cerebrospinal fluid are tested for antigen-antibody reactions. The kind of antigen used denotes the test performed. That is, tests performed with normal tissue or other specimens are specified as NONTREPONEMAL TESTS or reagin tests, while tests using treponemas or treponemal extracts as antigens to determine antibody reactions, are listed as TREPONEMAL TESTS.

Commonly used nontreponemal tests include the rapid plasma reagin (RPR) test and the Venereal Disease Research Laboratory (VDRL) test. Although these two nontreponemal antigen tests are neither extremely sensitive nor specific for syphilis, they are simple to do, fairly inexpensive, quite consistent and reliable and can diagnose for syphilis during all stages of infection.

Many laboratories cannot perform all tests to confirm syphilis. These laboratories may send serum or cerebrospinal fluid specimens to state or reference laboratories for confirmation. In addition to the tests mentioned, many reference laboratories employ fluorescent antibody (FA) techniques to detect and confirm the presence of treponemas.

TREATMENT

Penicillin is still the drug of choice in treating syphilis. Penicillin seems
more effective when treating primary syphilis. Proper antibiotic treatment is essential to maintain a high serum antibiotic level. Should the infected person be
allergic to penicillin, then the tetracyclines are recommended. In many cases, side
effects have been observed during antibiotic treatment. It is believed that drug
destruction of *T. pallidum* cells, causes the release of an endotoxin which produces
a toxicity-like reaction in the patient. This reaction is apparent when treating
patients during the primary and secondary stages of infection.

Treponema Pertenue

T. pertenue is the causative agent of yaws, a disease which is common in tropical
countries. Yaws is an infectious disease which causes skin lesions. The disease is
spread by contact with an infected person. The spirochete may be recovered from skin
lesions and the lymph nodes. Darkfield microscopy may be used to demonstrate
T. pertenue.

The primary yaws lesion generally appears on the lower leg or foot. Usually, the
genital area is not the primary site of infection. Secondary and tertiary yaws
lesions appear. The frequency of tertiary lesions is limited.

CLINICAL DIAGNOSIS

Morphologically, *T. pertenue* resembles *T. pallidum*. Patients with yaws are
serologically positive for syphilis.

However, *T. pertenue* is non-venereal in transmission and the yaws primary lesion
appears as a papule and not a chancre. *T. pertenue* very rarely forms tertiary lesions and stains more readily with Giemsa stain than does *T. pallidum*. Virulent
T. pertenue strains fail to grow in vitro.

TREATMENT

Penicillin and tetracyclines are effective in the treatment of yaws. Penicillin,
however, is the drug of choice.

Treponema Carateum

T. carateum is the causative agent of pinta or carate, a skin disease occurring
primarily in Mexico. *T. carateum* may be recovered from skin lesions and lymph nodes.
Smears of the lesion specimen and lymph node aspirates may be stained with Giemsa.
Fresh specimens may also be examined with darkfield microscopy.

The disease has three stages of development with varied cutaneous damage.
Hyperpigmentation may be observed during the earlier stages of infection and ultimately depigmentation and numerous cutaneous changes occur during the tertiary stage.

TREATMENT

Pinta or carate may be treated with penicillin.

CULTURES

To date, *T. carateum* microorganisms are unable to grow in vitro.

TRANSMISSION

Contact with an infected person seems to be the prime mode of transmission. Studies show lesion fluid contains *T. carateum* organisms. These bacteria may infect another person upon contact and entrance via skin abrasions or cuts.

Treponema Vincentii (Borelia)

T. vincentii, formerly *Borrelia vincentii*, is found in the oral cavity. It is not clear whether this bacterium is pathogenic or whether combined with other oral treponemas such as *T. orale*, and *T. denticola*, it may be implicated in Vincent's disease (trench mouth).

Under anaerobic conditions, *T. vincentii* grows in meat peptone extract preparations. Ascitic fluid or serum enhance growth and either is essential for growth.

Biochemically, *T. vincentii* is H_2S and indole positive (weak reaction), hydrolyzes gelatin and fails to hydrolyze esculin.

Leptospira

ORDER: SPIROCHAETALES

GENUS: LEPTOSPIRA

Bergey's Manual of Determinative Bacteriology (8th Edition) lists one species of Leptospira and that is *Leptospira interrogans*.

The cells of Leptospira are long and helical measuring approximately 6.0 to 20.0 μm in length and 0.1 μm in diameter. This genus is strictly aerobic and motile. *L. interrogans* is readily observable with darkfield microscopy.

The optimum growth temperature for Leptospira ranges from between 28-38°C. This genus grows well in vitro, but growth is enhanced in liquid or semi-solid media.

Many believe that Leptospira can live as a parasite in human kidney tubules for many years and then ultimately induce infection to become pathogenic. The kidneys are Leptospira's prime target. Nephritis and eventually kidney lesions occur due to Leptospira.

CLINICAL DIAGNOSIS

Clinical diagnosis of leptospirosis is based upon the isolation of the Leptospira and upon the immune response to the infection.

Isolates may be obtained from urine, blood or cerebrospinal fluid. The spirochete is readily seen with darkfield illumination. Many laboratories are not prepared to confirm leptospirosis. After establishing the morphological traits of Leptospira it is recommended that isolates be sent to state or specialized laboratories.

TREATMENT

Antibiotic treatment of leptospirosis has been far from satisfactory. Treatment
with erythromycin, streptomycin, and penicillin have, to date, yielded the best
results.

Mycobacterium

FAMILY: MYCOBACTERIACEAE
GENUS: MYCOBACTERIUM

Members of the genus Mycobacterium are bacilli which measure approximately 1.0 to
9.5 μm in length and 0.2 to 0.6 μm in width. Although the Mycobacteria are considered
to be Gram positive, they resist staining with this technique. The Mycobacteria, as
a group, are devoid of spores and capsules, and are non-motile.

Some Mycobacteria strains have simple nutritional requirements while other strains
are fairly fastidious. All strains are aerobic. The Mycobacteria are acid-fast.
The term acid-fast is designated to the Mycobacteria on the basis of their staining
characteristics. The Mycobacteria resist staining due to their high lipid content.
Consequently special staining procedures are required to allow dyes to penetrate these
bacilli. However, once stained, the Mycobacteria resist decolorization with acid
alcohol and hence the foundation for designating these as acid-fast bacilli.

Mycobacterium Tuberculosis

MORPHOLOGY/STAINING/PHYSIOLOGY

In tissues and exudate specimens, the *Mycobacterium tuberculosis* bacilli are
straight or slightly curved and measure about 2.0 to 4.0 μm in length and 0.3 to
1.5 μm in width. Longer filaments or smaller or club-shaped cell types are apparent
in culture smears. The tubercle bacilli occur either singly, in small clusters, or
in masses.

The tubercle bacillus is aerobic and fails to grow in the absence of oxygen.
Primary isolates, plated on Lowestein-Jensen (LJ) agar and incubated at 35-37°C,
show growth in 14 to 21 days. Plates of Middlebrook 7H10 medium, inoculated and
incubated at 35-37°C show growth in 12 to 16 days. An enrichment containing oleic
acid, bovine albumin dextrose and beef catalase may be added to the 7H10 medium to
facilitate growth. This enrichment medium may be obtained commercially and is
referred to as Middlebrook 7H10 agar with OADA enrichment.

The Middlebrook 7H10 medium facilitates early detection of the tubercle bacilli
because the medium is clear. The medium allows easy differentiation of mixed colony
types and contaminants are slower to alter or destroy this medium. This medium also
readily shows the "cording" of the tubercle bacilli. However, it is essential to note
that the Middlebrook 7H10 medium must be FRESH. An increased CO_2 environment (5.0 -
10.0%) stimulates the growth of tubercle bacilli cultures. Also, since *M. tuberculosis* is a relatively slow grower, malachite green is added to Lowenstein-Jensen and
Middlebrook 7H10 preparations to inhibit the growth of non-mycobacteria. Biochemically, *M. tuberculosis* rapidly reduces nitrate, is niacin positive, and is weakly
catalase positive. The catalase activity is lost if the cultures are heated at 68°C.

PATHOGENICITY

Mycobacterium tuberculosis is a causative agent of tuberculosis. The tubercle
bacillus enters the body via the respiratory tract, the alimentary tract, the genitourinary tract, and the conjunctiva of the eye. Infected persons (when sneezing,
coughing or expectorating) can form infectious aerosols. The infectious aerosol
droplets contaminate dust and can be inhaled by susceptible persons. Fomites, such
as towels, tissues, utensils, glasses or clothing may also contaminate susceptibe
individuals. Once in the host, the tubercle bacilli produce primary and secondary
lesions within the tissue. The circulatory and lymphatic systems disseminate the
bacilli throughout the system and practically no organ is spared invasion. Although
the lungs seem to be the prime target for the tubercle bacilli, the spleen, liver,
kidneys, bones, lymph nodes, meninges and gastrointestinal tract infections are not
uncommon. The systemic spread of the tubercle bacilli is more common in children
than in adults.

The tissue lesions formed by *M. tuberculosis* are called tubercles. The tubercles
contain the infectious bacilli. If these tubercles break, the bacilli may spread to
form more infections. If the tubercles encase or seal, the bacilli are sealed off
by calcification or by fibrosis.

IMMUNITY/RESISTANCE

Recovery from tuberculosis provides some resistance to a second attack. This
resistance seems to be due to the body's increased ability to localize and destroy
the tubercle bacilli. Despite the fact that the individual's system produces antibodies against the tubercle bacilli, the antibody titer is low and the antibodies
apparently fail to increase resistance to a subsequent infection. The increased
protection provided is cell-mediated. The macrophages acquire a great ability to
ingest the tubercle bacilli. The macrophages develop this ability during the course
of the initial infection. The following will serve to clarify:

If a guinea pig receives an injection of virulent *M. tuberculosis* cells, the
guinea pig will develop a local lesion within two weeks, and the infection will spread
from the lymph nodes throughout the guinea pig's system.

If a second injection of virulent tubercle bacilli were administered two days
after the initial injection, the same results would occur. However, if the second
injection were given 2 to 3 weeks after the first injection, the second injection
would cause a marked local inflammation reaction within one or two days. Generally,
the area lymph nodes do not contain the tubercle bacilli. Therefore, the guinea pig
is resistant to the second infecting dose of *M. tuberculosis*. The host's acquired
resistance is known as KOCH'S PHENOMENON.

Koch also noted that subsequent to the initial infection, the hypersensitivity
reaction could be obtained by injections containing dead bacilli or "old tuberculin".
"Old tuberculin" consists of a filtrate of a glycerol broth culture in which the
tubercle bacilli, were cultured. No local response is elicited after the subcutaneous
injection of either the dead bacilli or the "old tuberculin" into a guinea pig with
no previous history of tuberculosis. The hypersensitivity response induced by the
tuberculosis infection is helpful in diagnosing tuberculosis for it is the principle
upon which the tuberculin skin test is based.

CLINICAL IDENTIFICATION

Sputum, urine, gastric washing, tissue specimens as well as joint, pleural, cerebrospinal or pericardial fluid, and feces specimens may be brought to the laboratory

for diagnosis of tuberculosis. Proper specimen collection and processing are essential to identify *M. tuberculosis*.

STAINS/SMEARS

As previously stated, the Mycobacteria stain poorly with the Gram stain, since lipids and waxes prevent the Gram stain from penetrating the bacilli. The Ziehl-Neelsen carbolfuchsin stain or the Kenyoun carbolfuchsin staining procedure overcome the staining difficulties. The Truant fluorochrome staining technique is also used by many laboratories. In this procedure, fluorescent dyes (auramine and rhodamine) are used to stain smears. Fluorescent microscopy is used to examine these smears. The acid fast bacteria (Mycobacteria and Nocardia) appear as bright yellow bacilli. Since no antigen-antibody reaction is involved in the Truant procedure, this cannot be considered as a typical FA technique. Many workers confirm positive-fluorochrome smears with the Ziehl-Neelsen or Kinyoun staining procedures. Positive Ziehl-Neelsen, Kinyoun or fluorochrome results do not confirm the presence of the tubercle bacilli, but rather indicate the presence of ACID FAST BACILLI. A positive acid fast stain constitutes only PRESUMPTIVE identification of *M. tuberculosis*.

Cultural studies and animal virulence tests are used to establish the pathogenicity of the recovered organisms.

ACID-FAST BACILLI PIGMENTATION

Runyon classified the medically relevent strains of Mycobacteria into four groups:

GROUP I PHOTOCHROMOGENS

The members of this group produce a lemon-yellow pigment in the presence of light. The photochromogens are involved in human pulmonary infection. *Mycobacterium kansasii*, the yellow bacillus, is the most frequently isolated from pulmonary infections. When incubated in the dark, *M kansasii* colonies are a cream colored but become lemon-yellow when put in a lighted environment. These bacilli grow best at 35-37°C. Growth is apparent after 14 to 21 days of incubation at the previously indicated temperature.

GROUP II SCOTOCHROMOGENS

Mycobacterium scrofulaceum is representative and characteristic of the scoto-chromogens in that it is a yellow or orange to deep red pigment whether cultivated in the dark or in the presence of light. Generally, *M. scrofulaceum* is considered to be non-pathogenic however occasionally, it has been implicated in rare pulmonary disease and lymphadenitis in children.

GROUP III NONPHOTOCHROMOGENS

The nonphotochromogens are non-pigmented and do not become pigmented upon exposure to light. The most important members of the nonphotochromogens are *M. avium* and *M. intracellulare*, which cause a chronic pulmonary disease, and *M. xenopi*, causative agent of pulmonary disease.

GROUP IV RAPID GROWERS

The rapid growers, when incubated at 25°C or 35°C, demonstrate growth in 3 to 5 days. The members of this group include *M. fortuitum* and *M. chelonei*. Both of these bacteria cause pulmonary disease. *M. fortuitum* is more frequently recovered from pulmonary infections than is *M. chelonei*. *M. ulcerans* is also included with the rapid growers. This organism causes skin ulcers in humans.

BIOCHEMICAL TESTS

Several biochemical tests are used to differentiate the Mycobacteria. These include the niacin test, the nitrate reduction test, the catalase activity test, the test for Tween 80 hydrolysis, and the sodium chloride tolerance test.

NIACIN TEST: Niacin production is detected by a color reaction with cyanogen bromide and aniline. The test may be performed as follows: (1) Pipette 1.0 ml of sterile saline to a 3-week or older culture slant. No niacin-containing additive, such as penicilin, should be in the medium; (2) the saline should remain in the slant for 30 minutes; (3) transfer a portion of the saline to a small screw-capped test tube; (4) add an equal portion of aniline and cyanogen bromide solution to the saline extract; (5) a yellow color will appear instantly if niacin is present. This test should be performed in a well-ventilated area.

NITRATE REDUCTIONS: This test is useful in differentiating slower growing organisms (*M. tuberculosis* and *M. kansasii*) from Group II Mycobacteria.

CATALASE ACTIVITY TEST: All acid-fast bacilli produce catalase. Reduced catalase production may be apparent. This decrease is correlated with a lessening of virulence of the organism against the guinea pig. It is possible to subgroup the acid-fast bacilli on the basis of their catalase activity at different temperatures and pH. At a temperature of 68°C and a pH of 7.0, the catalase of HUMAN and BOVINE tubercle bacilli is selectively inactivated. Under the same conditions, all other acid-fast species are catalase positive. Catalase activity may be determined as follows: (1) prepare a 1.1 mixture of 10 percent Tween 80 and 30% NaOH. Both should be at room temperature; (2) add 0.5 ml of the mixture to the Lowenstein-Jensen slant. Bubbling indicates a positive catalase test; (3) to test catalase activity at 68°C, add several loops of mycobacteria from a slant to 0.5 ml of a phosphate buffer solution (pH 7.0) in a test tube; (4) incubate this mixture in a waterbath at 68°C for 30 minutes; (5) add 0.5 ml of the Tween-peroxide mixture to the buffered growth solution; (6) bubbling is indicative of a positive reaction.

TWEEN 80 TEST: Certain mycobacteria species can hydrolyze Tween 80 to oleic acid. Neutral red is used as a pH indicator and pink to amber colors are obtained. The neutral red indicator is reddish at an acidic pH, becomes amber in the substrate and changes to pink or reddish in a positive reaction. The test procedure is as follows: (1) one loopful of an actively growing L-J culture is placed into a tube containing Tween 80 substrate (M/15 phosphate buffer, pH 7.0, 100 ml containing 0.5 ml Tween 80 and 2.0 ml of 0.1 percent aqueous neutral red) and incubate this at 35°C; (2) set up a control tube using *M. kansasii* (a known positive) along with an uninoculated (negative control) tube. The tubes are allowed to incubate for 5 days prior to testing, and replaced in the incubator, if no reaction is observed; (3) on the 12th day of incubation the tubes are again examined for a color change.

SODIUM CHLORIDE TOLERANCE TEST: The procedure is helpful in distinguishing the rapid-growing Mycobacteria (positive) from the slow growers (negative). The medium is prepared by adding NaCl in a final concentration of 5% to Lowenstein-Jensen slants. A light suspension of organisms is prepared and 1 ml is inoculated into the surface of the NaCl medium and a control slant containing no NaCl. The slants are incubated at 35°C and examined every week for 4 weeks. Growth on both slants is indicative of a positive salt tolerance test.

VIRULENCE TEST

The presence of acid-fast bacilli, upon direct examination, and of typical colonies on agar is strong evidence of tuberculosis. Demonstration of specific lesions in laboratory animals is not necessary, but is useful in confirmation. The guinea pig virulence test is one method of providing this information. Many clinical laboratories are not equipped to perform animal virulence tests. When facilities are lacking, cultures should be shipped to reference laboratories for confirmation. For shipment, cultures should be placed in equal volumes of trisodium phosphate solution.

CULTURE TECHNIQUES

N-ACETYL-L-CYSTINE METHOD SOLUTIONS: (Digestion and decontamination of sputum for *Mycobacterium tuberculosis*).

1. Prepare a volume of digestant by adding equal volumes of 1N (4.0%) NaOH and 0.1 M 2.9%) sodium citrate • $2H_2O$ with 0.25 gm of N-acetyl-L-cysteine powder for every 50 ml of combined solution, that is, 25 ml + 25 ml + 0.25 gms. The solution is self-sterilizing but deteriorates rapidly, and should therefore, be used within 24 hours.

2. In a safety hood, transfer about 10 ml of sputum or bronchial secretion to a sterile 50-ml, screwcapped, centrifuge tube.

3. Add an equivalent amount of the digest to the specimen. Mix well with a mixer. Digestion generally occurs in 5 to 30 seconds. Avoid extreme agitation for this may inactive the digest by oxidizing it.

4. Transfer a portion of sputum to a 15-ml centrifuge tube and centrifuge for 10 minutes at 3000 rpm.

5. Pour off the supernatant and allow tube to stand in an inverted position on a paper towel or filter paper in order to drain the sediment.

6. Taansfer the creamy white sediment to a slide. Air dry and stain by the Ziehl-Neelsen or Kinyoun method.

N-ACETYL-L CYSTEINE SODIUM HYDROXIDE CULTURE METHOD: (The use of NALC as a mucolytic recommended as a mild decontaminant and digestion procedure).

1. Collect the sputum (an early-morning, deep-cough specimen) and transfer approximately 10 ml to a 50-ml, sterile conical, screw capped tube.

2. Add an equal volume of NALC (with sodium hydroxide solution).

3. Mix in a mixer for 10 to 20 seconds to complete digestion. Gently agitate the mixer, because violent mixing can cause the NALC to deteriorate.

4. Stand at room temperature for 15 minutes so that decontaminating can occur.

5. Fill the tube within one-half inch of the top with Sorensen buffer, pH 6.8, or sterile distilled water.

6. Centrifuge at 3000 rpm for 15 minutes. Decant the supernatant fluid into a vessel containing a phenol disinfectant. Wipe the mouth of the tube with a cotton ball soaked with 5 percent phenol. Do not discard the sediment.

7. Make a smear using a sterile, cotton-tipped applicator stick or a wire loop. Spread the sediment on an area about the size of a penny. Stain by the Ziehl-

Neelsen method and determine the approximate number of acid-fast-bacilli per oil-immersionfield.

8. Pipet 1 ml of a 0.2% bovine albumin to the sediment. Shake gently to mix. Refrigerate overnight. If the sediment is small, add the albumin to the sediment before making the smear.

9. Make a 1:10 dilution of this sediment by adding 10 drops of it to 4.5 ml of sterile water.

10. Inoculate the proper media, with 0.1 ml of the sediment for each plate. Plate two tubes using undiluted and diluted sediment preparations for incubation at 35°C to 37°C.

TREATMENT

Streptomycin is among the drugs which are effective in the treatment of tuberculosis.

Mycobacterium Leprae

FAMILY: MYCOBACTERIACEAE
GENUS: MYCOBACTERIUM

MORPHOLOGY/STAINING/PHYSIOLOGY

M. leprae is morphologically similar to *M. tuberculosis*. The leprosy bacilli are strongly acid fast and at times stain evenly and at other times are beaded in appearance. Innumerable attempts have been made to cultivate pathogenic *M. leprae* bacilli on artificial laboratory media. To date investigators have not been able to cultivate viable, pathogenic acid fast leprosy bacilli obtained from human infected tissues. However, some non-cultivable leprosy bacilli, obtained from human infected tissues, did grow and replicate in mice footpads.

PATHOGENICITY

Mycobacterium leprae, also called Hansen's bacillus, is the causative agent of leprosy. *M. leprae* is only a human pathogen. No other animal or soil is known to be infected with the leprosy bacillus. The armadillo seems susceptible and presently is being used for experimental studies. Humans are faily resistant to leprosy. Nevertheless, leprosy cases are still reported in some Asiatic countries and in South America.

The leproma, the characteristic leprosy lesion, occurs on the body and is responsible for the distorted tissue appearance.

There are two types of leprosy: tuberculoid and lepromatous. The leprosy bacilli may be recovered from the lesions of both types of leprosy. The skin and nerves are the prime targets in tubercular leprosy. All body parts are vulnerable in lepromatous leprosy, but the major sites include the skin, nerves, eyes, respiratory tract, kidneys, liver and spleen.

TABLE 21

BIOCHEMICAL PROPERTIES USED TO DIFFERENTIATE CERTAIN MYCOBACTERIA

MYCOBACTERIA	NIACIN PRODUCTION	CATALASE PRODUCED (mm) 740	750	NITRATE REDUCTION	TWEEN 80 HYDROLYSIS +5(DAYS)+10	GROWTH IN 5% NaCl	PIGMENT DARK	PIGMENT LIGHT	GROWTH AT 37°C	45°C	MEDICAL SIGNIFICANCE
M. tuberculosis	L	L	P	L	N	P	P	P	+	−	Tuberculosis
M. kansaii	P	L	L	L	L	P	P	L	+	−	Pulmonary disease, similar to, but milder than tuberculosis
M. sacrofulaceum	P	L	L	O	P	P	L	L	+	−	Rare pulmonary disease; lymphadenitis in children
M. avium	P	L	P	P	P	P	P	O	+	+/− 0	Chronic pulmonary disease
M. intracellulare	P	L	P	P	P	P	P	P	+	−	Chronic pulmonary disease
M. xenopi	P	L	P	P	P	P	O	O	+	+	Pulmonary disease
M. fortuitum	P	L	L	N	O	L	P	P	+	−	Pulmonary disease
M. chelonei	V	L	L	P	P	N	P	P	+	−	Pulmonary disease
M. ulcerans	P	L	L	P	P	ND	P	P	−	−	Skin ulcers

L = 85 to 100% of the strains are positive
M = 75 to 84% of the strains are positive
N = 50 to 74% of the strains are positive
O = 15 to 49% of the strains are positive
P = 0 to 14% of the strains are positive
V = variable results (+/−)
N/D = not determined

TRANSMISSION

The mode of transmission of leprosy is uncertain. Nasal secretions of patients with lepromatous leprosy contain an excessively high number of leprosy bacilli. Aerosals and fomites may be modes of dissemination, but no sound evidence supports this finding.

Acid-fast staining of smears from nasal secretions or skin lesion specimens are useful to establish the presence of these bacilli in suspected leprosy victims.

TREATMENT

The sulfones, such as diaminodiphenyl sulfone (DDS or Dapsone) are the drugs of choice in the treatment of leprosy.

Nocardia

FAMILY: NOCARDIACEAE
GENUS: NOCARDIA

Members of the genus Nocardia belong to the order Actinomycetales and are there-fore characterized by their branching filaments which develop into short or fairly long mycelia. The extent of mycelial development categorizes the members of this genus into three groups. The Nocardia are Gram-positive, non-motile, obligate anaerobes which may or may not be acid fast. Several species are pigmented. Some species have coccoid or bacillary mycelia. The coccoid cells are referred to as either chlamydospores or microcysts.

Most of the Nocardia species are isolated from soils, and a few from marine sedi-ments. Several species are pathogenic to humans. *Nocardia asteroides* and *Nocardia brasiliensis* are the recognized etiological agents of nocardiosis. *Nocardia aste-roides* is an opportunistic pathogen which affects the chronically ill or debilitated. Many consider *Nocardia brasiliensis* more virulent than *Nocardia asteroides* for *N. brasiliensis* is the frequent cause of pulmonary mycetoma which may spread sys-temically. Recently, *Nocardia caviae* has been reported as the etiologic agent of systemic infection. The differentiating characteristics of these three Nocardia species may be found in Table 22.

TABLE 22

*CHARACTERISTICS WHICH HELP TO DIFFERENTIATE CERTAIN NOCARDIA SPECIES

NOCARDIA SPECIES	ACID FAST	COLONY MORPHOLOGY ON NUTRIENT AGAR	AERIAL HYPHAE ON NUTRIENT AGAR	GROWTH IN 7.0% NaCl
Nocardia brasiliensis	+	Granular, orange-buff, piled or heaped in appearance	Scant white aerial hyphae at edge of colonies	-
Nocardia asteroides	+	Granular, yellow-orange, heaped and folded in appearance	Thin hyphae at edge of colonies	+
Nocardia caviae	+	Granular, buff to drab pink, heaped, folded and crusty in appearance	Thin and off-white in older cultures	+

*Many include Nocardia with the mycotic infections, however, because of the acid fast trait of the three Nocardia listed on this table, these have been included here and purposefully following the Mycobacteria.

BIBLIOGRAPHY AND RECOMMENDED READINGS

Buchanan, R. E. and N. E. Gibbons (co-editors), *BERGEY'S MANUAL OF DETERMINATIVE BACTERIOLOGY*. Eighth Edition 1974. The Williams and Wilkins Co., Baltimore.

Finegold, Sydney M., Martin, William J., and Elvyn G. Scott. *BAILEY AND SCOTT'S DIAGNOSTIC MICROBIOLOGY*. Fifth Edition 1978. The C. V. Mosby Company, St. Louis.

Freeman, Bob A. *BURROWS TEXTBOOK OF MICROBIOLOGY*. Twenty-first Edition 1979. W. B. Saunders Company, Philadelphia.

Fuerst, Robert. *MICROBIOLOGY IN HEALTH AND DISEASE*. Fourteenth Edition 1978. W. B. Saunders Company, Philadelphia.

Lenette, E. H., Spaulding, E. H. and J. P. Truant. *MANUAL OF CLINICAL MICROBIOLOGY*. Second Edition 1974. American Society for Microbiology, Washington, D. C.

MacFaddin, Jean F. *BIOCHEMICAL TESTS FOR IDENTIFICATION OF MEDICAL BACTERIA*. 1976. The Williams and Wilkins Company, Baltimore.

Moffet, Hugh L. *CLINICAL MICROBIOLOGY*. 1975. J. B Lippincott Company, Philadelphia.

Myruik, Q. N., Pearsall, N. N., and R. S. Weiser. *FUNDAMENTALS OF MEDICAL BACTERIOLOGY AND MYCOLOGY*. 1976. Lea and Fhbiger, Philadelphia.

Schuhardt, Vernon T. *PATHOGENIC MICROBIOLOGY*. 1978. J. B. Lippincott Company, Philadelphia.

Volk, Wesley A. *ESSENTIALS OF MEDICAL MICROBIOLOGY*. 1978. J. B. Lippincott Company, Philadelphia.

Chapter 2

Fundamental Clinical Mycology

LORRAINE D. DOUCET, CSC, PhD.
Medical Technology Program Director
Professor of Biology
Notre Dame College
Manchester, New Hampshire

OUTLINE

THE SUPERFICIAL MYCOSES
    Tinea Versicolor   Cladosporium werneckii
                                Growth Rate
                                KOH Preparation
                                Recurrence
    Tinea nigra (Cladosporium species)
    Black Piedra   Piedraia hortae
                                Growth Rate
                                Morphology
                                Treatment
    White Piedra   Trichosporon cutaneum
                                Growth Rate
                                Morphology
THE CUTANEOUS MYCOSES
    Media and Nutritional Requirements of the Dermatophytes
    Dermatophyte Characteristics
        Trichophyton
        Microsporum
        Epidermophyton
THE SUBCUTANEOUS MYCOSES
    Chromomycosis
    Sporotrichosis
    Characteristics of Subcutaneous Fungi
THE SYSTEMIC MYCOSES
    General Characteristics
    Histoplasmosis
    Isolation of Histoplasma capsulatum
        Dimorphism
    Blastomycosis
        Isolation of B. dermatitidis
        Diagnosis
        Dimorphism
    Cocidioidomycosis
        General Characteristics
        Isolation of C. immitis
        Lactophenol cotton blue preparation
        Identification
OPPORTUNISTIC FUNGI
    Candida
    Aspergillus
    Rhizopus

INTRODUCTION

Although the pathogenicity of certain fungi was recognized in the early 19th century, many laboratory personnel still find themselves with limited academic preparation or scant clinical experience in isolating and identifying the pathogenic fungi. In the past, the lack of emphasis on Mycology, in both academic and clinical training programs, could have been due to: (1) the structural complexity of the fungi; (2) their relatively limited involvement in serious disease; and (3) the infrequent occurrence of mycoses as compared to bacterial infections.

For many years, it appeard as though Mycology was the "forgotten" component of microbiology.

Today, however, mycoses (diseases of fungal etiology) are on the increase. Prolonged or massive use of broad spectrum antibiotics as well as immunosuppressive therapy have lowered body defenses and have allowed the opportunistic fungi to infect normally resistant hosts. Clinical laboratories are, of late, reporting a sharp increase of opportunistic fungus infections, especially systemic mycoses. Consequently, many practicing microbiologists have had to "hit the books" to find identifying characteristics. This section will deal with some of the more important pathogenic fungi and yeasts. The simplicity of this chapter is intentional and designed to introduce the untrained in Mycology to the basic aspects of the field.

This chapter is not intended to challenge the "large texts" in Mycology, but is an attempt to: (1) emphasize the importance of Diagnostic Mycology upon the prospective medical technologist or the practitioner untrained in Mycology, (2) stress its relevance in modern medicine; and (3) at least briefly stop students and/or clinicians from working with that "fuzzy stuff" with only a "ho-hum" approach.

FUNDAMENTAL LABORATORY MYCOLOGY

BASIC INFORMATION

Fungi consist of molds and yeasts. Molds are generally identified by the "fuzzy" or "hairy" appearance of their colonies. Yeast colonies are soft and appear either creamy, dry or wrinkled. Yeast colonies look more like bacterial colonies.

Molds are filamentous and the filaments grow upward or downward into the agar in which they were inoculated. The filaments that shoot upward give the fungi their characteristic "fuzzy" appearance. A single filament is called a *hypha*. Two or more filaments are called *hyphae*. All the hyphae, growing upward or downward, collectively are called a *mycelium* (or mycelia). The hyphae growing upward make up the *aerial mycelium* while the hyphae growing downward are referred as a *vegetative mycelium*. The hyphae may or may not have cross walls. The cross walled hyphae are said to be *septate* and the non-cross walled are aseptate.

The fungi are *heterotrophic* and utilize organic materials as nutrients. The vegetative mycelia secrete enzymes into their substrate to break down molecules to be assimilated into the hyphae cell walls.

The *aerial mycelia* bear spores which are produced either *asexually* or *sexually*. Sexually reproducing fungi have structures that facilitate fertilization and nuclear fusion resulting in the formation of *oospores*, *ascospores* or *zygospores*.

Fungi that demonstrate sexual reproduction are called *perfect* fungi while the fungi that reproduce asexually are termed *imperfect* fungi.

The mycelia of the imperfect fungi are involved in spore formation.

Most of the clinically important fungi produce asexual spores. Molds are usually identified by: (1) spore characteristics; and (2) modes of reproduction, but dermatophytes often are identified by colony morphology.

The thallus (plant body) itself or the conidiophores (which are part of the thallus) may form asexual spores.

Since spore formation is an important factor for identifying the fungi, sporulation types will be briefly discussed.

Spores produced from the thallus itself are called *Thallospores*. *Arthrospores*, *chlamydospores* and *blastospores* are *thallospores*.

THALLOSPORES: These spores develop from the vegetative mycelium directly.

ARTHROSPORES: These spores are formed due to the fragmentation of the mycelium into thick-walled, cylindrical spores.

CHLAMYDOSPORES: These spores are formed when cells of septated hyphae or pseudohyphae "round up" and become thicker than other cells of the hyphae. Chlamydospores may form within, or the end (terminal) or on a short branch of the hyphae. *Candida albicans* produces chlampydospores and these have diagnostic significance. Some molds also produce chlamydospores, but these are of little diagnostic value.

BLASTOSPORES: Blastospores are buds produced from mother cells. The daughter cell extrudes from the mother cell. Elongated budding cells which have not detached from the mother cell are called pseudohyphae.

Many molds have specialized vegetative hyphae that produce spores. The spores are called *conidia* and the hyphae producing them are termed *conidiophores*. The conidia are asexual spores.

Aseptate hyphae (sporangiophores) produce asexual spores called *sporangiospores*.

FIGURE 1

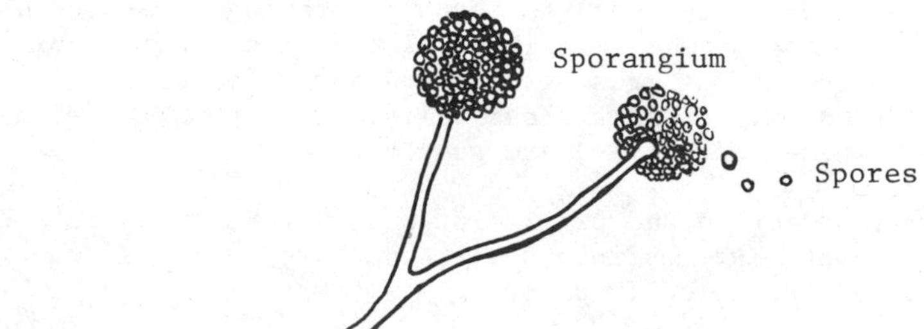

Sporangium

Spores

FIGURE 2

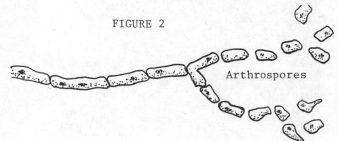

Arthrospores

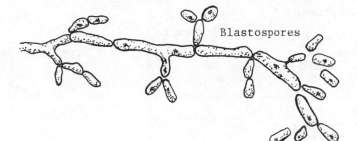

Blastospores

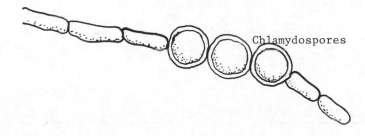

Chlamydospores

EXAMINATION OF MOLD CULTURES

The following is suggested to facilitate the morphological identification of molds. The following should be observed each time a mold is examined:

I. GROSS CHARACTERISTICS

    A. The type of media employed.
    B. The age of the culture--incubation time and temperature.
    C. Colony appearance--flat--wrinkled--grooved.
    D. Pigmentation.
    E. Colony Quality

        1. Cottony
        2. Smooth

    3. Powdery and soft
    4. Granular (gritty)
    5. Colony size

II. MICROSCOPIC CHARACTERISTICS

   A. Hyphae

      1. Diameter
      2. Pigmented or non-pigmented
      3. Septated or non-septated

   B. Conidiophore

      1. Unbranched
      2. Branched

   C. Conidia

      1. Size and structure

   D. Determine whether:

     arthrospores, chlamydospores, or blastopores are present (when applicable)

   E. Determine whether:

     ascospores are present or absent (when applicable)

Knowledge of the gross appearance of some of the medically important fungi (opportunistic fungi, dermatophytes, and fungi responsible for subcutaneous and systemic diseases) help and facilitate the identification of isolates as seen in Table 1.

EXAMINATION OF MOLDS

1. Direct Microscopic Examination

All specimens may be examined directly for fungi. This should be done simultaneously with culture preparations and should not replace culturing the fungi. Direct examination may provide significant information concerning the fungus that will later be identified on agar preparations.

2. Potassium Hydroxide Preparation (10-20%)

Fairly strong alkaline solutions serve to differentiate fungi from organic substances which might confuse the two. In alkali, many of the organic materials are changed to an almost clear background, thereby making the fungi more visible and obvious.

   A. A few drops of 10-20% KOH solution are placed in the center of a clean glass slide.

   B. Some of the specimen (purulent material, scraping or tissue fragment) is placed in the KOH. A teasing needle is to be used to spread the specimen and give a thin preparation.

TABLE 1

MORPHOLOGICAL CHARACTERISTICS OF CERTAIN FUNGI AND YEASTS*

CHARACTERISTICS	POSSIBLE FUNGI OR YEASTS
Olive-black to black colonies; suede aerial mycelium; compact, raised colonies; obvious folding; grow in 2-3 weeks	Phialophora verrucosa; Fonsecae Pedrosoi Cladosporium carrionii
Black to gray-black colonies; smooth colonies-- not fuzzy but may have some areas of suede type aerial mycelium	Cladosporium werneckii; Wangiella (Phialophora) dermatitidis
Suede to wooly, brightly colored mycelium; may have a powdery appearance intermittent with aerial mycelium	Trichothecium sp.; Trichoderma sp.; Penicillium spp.; Fusarium spp.; Aspergillus spp. (except Aspergillus niger)
Suede to wooly aerial mycelium; white surface, however the back may be pigmented	Trichophyton rubrum; Trichophyton terrestre; Histoplasma capsulatum; Blastomyces dermatitidis; Coccidioides immitis; Geotrichum candidum
Yeast-like, creamy colonies, Pigmentation may be present	Candida spp.; Cryptococcus spp.; Sporothrix schenckii (yeast form); Blastomyces dermatitidis (yeast form); Paracoccidioides brasiliensis (yeast form)
Suede colony with rose colored surface; a rose colored water soluble pigment diffuses throughout the medium	Trichophyton gallirae

*Isolates were grown on Sabouraud dextrose agar containing neopeptone (pH 5.5-6.0) for 7-21 days.

C.   Place a coverslip over the mixture and heat gently over a flame. Remove the
     slide from the flame just before the mixture reaches the boiling point. This
     process may have to be repeated for nail specimens. The nail specimen must
     be soft enough to be able to press the materials out of the nail.

D.   The preparation may then be examined under low and high power. If molds are
     present in the specimens, hyphae segments, granules, spherules, spores or
     budding yeasts should be evident in KOH. Do not use cotton swabs in preparing
     slides of suspected mycotic agents, since the cotton filaments could be con-
     fused with hyphae.

3.   The India Ink Preparation

A.   Place a drop of India ink on a glass slide.

B.   Centrifuged spinal fluid sediment is added to the India ink. Usually a loop-
     ful of sediment is sufficient.

C.   Mix the sediment into the India ink and cover with a coverslip. If the India
     ink is too dark for proper observations, it may be diluted.

     Spinal fluid and urine sediments may be examined with the India ink prepara-
     tion. India ink readily demonstrates the cryptococcus capsule and facilitates
     its identification.

4.   The Lactophenol Cotton Blue Preparation

     The lactophenol cotton blue preparation is used to stain for chitin or cellulose.
     The cell walls of fungi are mainly chitin and wet mounts can be used in this
     preparation to examine microscopic features.

5.   The PAS Preparation

     The periodic acid-Schiff (PAS) preparation is used to show fungi in tissue homo-
     genates, body fluids and exudates.

6.   Gram Staining Technique

     The Gram stain (Hucker's modification) may be used to demonstrate yeast cells and
     mycelial components in some specimens. This stain does not show fungi in speci-
     mens. All fungi are Gram positive.

7.   Other Staining Preparations

     Wrights stain, or Giemsa stain, may be employed to demonstrate the yeast forms of
     Histoplasma capsulatum in bone marrow and blood specimens. H. capsulatum may be
     unnoticed in unstained specimens.

PRIMARY ISOLATION MEDIA

Appropriate media must be used to allow the growth of the fungal species that
will be found in clinical specimens. Once inoculated, the plates, screw cap vials,
tubes or bottles should be incubated at either 25°C or 37°C. If 25°C incubators are
not available and the room temperature is 25°C then these plates may be left at ambient temperature. Some media preparations should contain chloramphenicol and/or
cycloheximide which inhibit bacteria and saprophytic fungi respectively. Some agar

preparations should be devoid of cycloheximide and chloramphenicol, since these anti-biotics do prevent the growth of some pathogenic fungi. The two media which best support the growth of fungi are: Sabouraud dextrose agar (SDA) and brain heart infusion agar (BHI). BHI supports the growth of the more fastidious fungi such as Blastomyces dermatitidis.

The commercially available agar preparations for molds are:

1. Plain Sabouraud Dextrose Agar (SDA)

2. Sabouraud Dextrose Agar with cycloheximide and chloramphenicol

3. Plain Brain Heart Infusion Agar

4. Brain Heart Infusion Agar with cycloheximide and chloramphenicol

MACROSCOPIC EXAMINATION

Media preparations should be examined every 2 or 3 days for fungal growth. Rapid growers should be apparent in 4 to 6 days but slow growers may be noticeable in 15 to 21 days. The characteristics listed in the EXAMINATION OF MOLD CULTURES section should be noted and reported. In addition to these, however, care should be taken to observe growth or the absence of growth on the antibiotic containing media. Furthermore, if the slant contains more than one fungus, the various fungal types should be aseptically streaked (on either a plate unless coccidioides is suspected, or a slant) for isolation purposes.

Also, many microbiologists recommend that cultures should not be discarded for 4 to 6 weeks. In this time some fungi were subcultured to obtain isolates. Nevertheless, this prolonged incubation will ensure the growth of slow growers. Care should be taken to avoid contamination.

LABORATORY SAFETY IN HANDLING CULTURES

Microbiologists have to decide whether they will use petri dishes, test tubes, culture bottles or culture dishes, to recover fungi from clinical specimens. Many workers prefer not to use petri dishes for primary isolation for fear the isolate may be the causative agent of systemic mycoses.

The agar surface area is limited in culture bottles and tubes and this is considered a disadvantage by many workers. Many workers resort to culture dishes. These have a fairly large surface area and adequate aeration. Anaerobic conditions should be avoided. Also, the culture dishes can contain 30-40 ml of agar. This amount of agar is needed to avoid drying, since slow growers may be incubated for 3-5 weeks. Furthermore, dehydration, drying and splitting of the media can be delayed or avoided by placing a pan of water on the bottom of the incubator and the plates can be inserted in cellophane bags or taped with a tape which is permeable to oxygen.

There are still other laboratory directors who do not recommend the use of either culture dishes or petri dishes for primary isolation of fungi from clinical specimens. These clinicians feel that there is a great risk of contaminating the laboratory environment and personnel when plates are used.

Many laboratories enforce the wearing of a mask for personnel working in mycology and insist that culture plates be opened in well vented microbiological hoods.

RECOMMENDED INCUBATION TEMPERATURE

In the past, it was recommended that primary isolates be incubated at 37°C to obtain the yeast form of suspected dimorphic fungi and to also isolate duplicate agar preparations at 25°C. Recent findings do not support the continuation of this practice. The more recent trend is to recover fungi from specimens on media incubated at 25°C. Isolates suspected of being dimorphic are then subcultured on appropriate media and incubated at 37°C to induce the yeast form of this suspected dimorphic culture.

DIMORPHIC FUNGI--CONVERSION IN CULTURE MEDIUM

The yeast phase of dimorphic fungi may serve to differentiate the fungi from one another. Mycelial fungi which are suspected dimorphic forms may be tested as follows:

A. Inoculate mycelial growth onto a brain heart infusion agar slant. The BHI slant should be freshly prepared and moist. If there is insufficient moisture, add a few drops of sterile water of BHI broth to the slant. The mycelial growth should remain on the slant. Screw capped tubes should be used to avoid drying.

B. Incubate the slant at 37°C. Check the slants daily and loosen the caps to prevent anaerobic conditions. The caps should be tightened after to prevent drying or contamination.

C. If yeast does not form and only mycelia grow, subculture as before, but on another BHI slant. Sometimes several transfers are needed to recover the yeast form.

YEAST IDENTIFICATION

Yeast may be recovered from clinical specimens and primary isolates may be obtained on isolation media. Isolates may then be:

A. Examined in a sterile diluted water mount to determine cell size or observe budding. If ascospores are present, many laboratories send the culture to a reference laboratory.

B. Examined in an India ink preparation to determine whether the yeast is encapsulated. The capsule appears as a halo around the cells. The halo is clearly and consistently demarcated against a blackish background. The presence or absence of capsules is not always of paramount importance in yeast identification for some capsules fail to be noticed. Also, spinal fluid containing white blood cells frequently confuses the untrained examining India ink preparations. WBC's repel the India ink particles creating an irregular halo around the white cells. Although this halo is not uniformly surrounding the white cells as is the yeast capsule, it may be recorded as a yeast capsule.

C. Checked for purity with Candida BCG agar (DIFCO) and blood agar preparations. The blood agar plates are used when bacterial contaminants are suspected. A small inoculum can be recovered from isolated yeast colonies on the blood agar plates and streaked on Sabouraud dextrose agar plates containing chloramphenicol only.

D. Examined morphologically on morphology agar preparations for yeast (rice extract agar or corn meal agar) without glucose.

The addition of 3.0% Tween 80 to either the rice extract agar or corn meal agar increases the formation of chlamydospores by *Candida albicans*. Pseudohyphae production is also increased. Since these two media complement each other, and since different candida species react differently on each, bi-plates (2 compartment plates) containing 8-10 ml of each media are recommended for chlamydospore, pseudohyphae and blastospore production by candida species. An inoculation loop is used to streak 24-72 hour old cultures into the morphology media. Two streaks are made along the agar across the length of the plate. Do not dig into the agar. Coverslips are arranged over a portion of the streaks, but the streaks overlap the coverslips. The plates should be incubated at 20-25° for 24 hours. If the room temperature is about 20-25°C, then ambient temperature will do, but care should be taken to avoid temperature fluctuation, since chlamydospore production is limited or inhibited around 30°C. Identification or morphological characteristics facilitates the selection of physiological or biochemical tests.

Fermentation tests, carbon assimilation studies, and nitrate assimilation studies are used to identify yeasts when the previously listed identification preparations have failed. Many of these physiological and biochemical tests are not routine clinical procedures, therefore the reader is referred to Clinical Procedure Manuals in Mycology for detailed information. Furthermore, commercially prepared rapid test kits are available to identify fungi and yeasts. These have proven reliable and rapid. Many clinicians recommend these for identification purposes.

GERM TUBE TEST FOR YEASTS

Once the yeast is recovered from a clinical specimen and isolated, a small inoculum of the isolate is suspended in a vial containing 0.5-1.0 ml of either human or sheep serum and incubated at 37°C for 2 to 3 hours. Following incubation, an aliquot sample is pipetted from the serum, placed on a slide, covered with a coverslip and examined microscopically. If the germ tubes are present, they should be visible under low magnification.

FIGURE 3

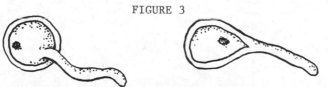

Spore and germ tube; the formation of a hypha.

FUNGI PREPARATION FOR MICROSCOPIC EXAMINATION

There are three recognized procedures to study fungi. Each procedure has advantages and disadvantages.

1. Tease Mount Procedure

2. Tape Procedure

3. Slide Culture Procedure

Tease Mount Procedure

Remove a small section of a colony and transfer it to the center of a slide, containing lactophenol cotton blue. The colony section must be well teased for microscopic examinations. The disadvantage of this procedure is the inability to maintain consistency in examining mold components--especially hyphae or fruiting bodies. The teasing of the mold section makes this difficult. This is however, a rapid and widely used procedure.

TABLE 2

SELECTED PHYSIOLOGICAL PROPERTIES OF SOME YEASTS FOUND IN CLINICAL SPECIMENS

YEAST	CARBOHYDRATES FERMENTED				CARBOHYDRATES ASSIMILATED				UREASE PRODUCTION	NITRATE REDUCTION	GERM TUBES	CAPSULE
	GLUCOSE	MALTOSE	LACTOSE	SUCROSE	GLUCOSE	MALTOSE	LACTOSE	SUCROSE				
Candida albicans	G*	G	-	-	+	+	-	+	-	-	+	-
Candida krusei	G	-	-	-	+	-	-	-	(-) Rarely (+)	-	-	-
Candida stellatoides	G	G	-	-	+	+	-	+	-	-	+	-
Candida parapsilosis	G	-	-	-	+	+	-	+	-	-	-	-
Cryptococcus neoformans	-	-	-	-	+	+	-	+	+	-	-	+
Cryptococcus laurenti	-	-	-	-	+	+	+	+	+	-	-	+
Cryptococcus gastricus	-	-	-	-	+	+	Rarely (+)	-	+	-	-	+
Torulopsis glabrata	Acid Gas				+	-	-	+	-	-	-	-
Torulopsis stellata	Acid Gas			Acid Gas	+	-	-	+	-	-	-	-
Torulopsis candida	Acid & Gas or only gas	-		Acid & Gas or only acid	+	+	+/-	+	-	-	-	-
Saccharomyces cerevisiae	Acid Gas	Acid Gas	-	Acid Gas	+	+	-	+	-	-	-	-

TABLE 2 (continued)

YEAST	CARBOHYDRATES FERMENTED				CARBOHYDRATES ASSIMILATED				PRODUCTION UREASE	NITRATE REDUCTION	GERM TUBES	CAP- SULE
	GLUCOSE	MALTOSE	LACTOSE	SUCROSE	GLUCOSE	MALTOSE	LACTOSE	SUCROSE				
Candida parapsilosis	G	-	-	-	+	+	-	+	-	-	-	-
Trichosporon cutaneum	-	-	-	-	+	+ Rarely (−)	+ Rarely (−)	+	+	-	-	-
Trichosporon pullulans	-	-	-	-	+	+	+	+	+	+	-	-

*Gas production is the only indicator of fermentation.

Tape Procedure

A completely transparent 4 cm tape strip is looped back over itself with sticky side out. The sticky portion of the tape is gently pressed to the surface of a fungal colony so as to permit the aerial mycelium to adhere to the adhesive surface of the tape. The tape is then placed in a drop of lactophenol cotton blue contained on a slide. The aerial mycelium may be examined microscopically. This procedure is difficult to use in narrow lipped-tubes or bottles. Also, moist yeast colonies and fungi, with limited aerial mycelia, are difficult to adhere on to the tape. Many prefer this procedure to the tease method since hyphae and spores remain intact.

Slide Culture Procedure

This is not a rapid procedure but it is considered by many to be the best microscopic examination technique.

Blocks of Sabouraud dextrose agar, measuring approximately 1 x 2 cm, are cut out of an SDA agar preparation approximately 4 mm deep (10–15 ml SDA). The agar is cut with either a sterile scalpel or thin spatula.

A. This extracted agar section is placed into a second sterile petri dish containing a sterile V or U shaped glass rod supporting a sterile slide.

B. Using a heavy gauge inoculating needle, inoculate the four sides of the agar block with the selected fungus.

C. Cover the preparation with a sterile coverslip.

D. Add sterile water to the bottom of the petri dish but be certain the water level does not reach the slide.

E. Cover the dish and incubate at 25°C or ambient temperature.

F. Examine the colony growth microscopically at regular and planned intervals.

G. When the growth stage desired is reached, remove the coverslip from the agar block preparation and place the coverslip into a drop of lactophenol cotton blue on the center of another slide.

H. Carefully remove the block from the original slide and discard the block in an antifungal agent such as phenol.

I. On the original slide, place a drop of lactophenol cotton blue on the site where the block was removed and where mycelial growth remains. Cover the mycelial growth and lactophenol cotton blue with a coverslip. The two microscopic slides (G + I) preparations may be preserved with fingernail polish.

NOTE: Highly pathogenic fungi, e.g., Coccidioides immitis or Histoplasma capsulatum, should not be grown on slide cultures!

SPECIMEN COLLECTION AND PROCESSING

Molds (fungi and yeasts) can be recovered from body tissues and fluids. Recovery and isolation of these molds are dependent upon proper specimen collection and processing.

TABLE 3

FLOW CHART OF PROCEDURES TO HELP IDENTIFY YEASTS

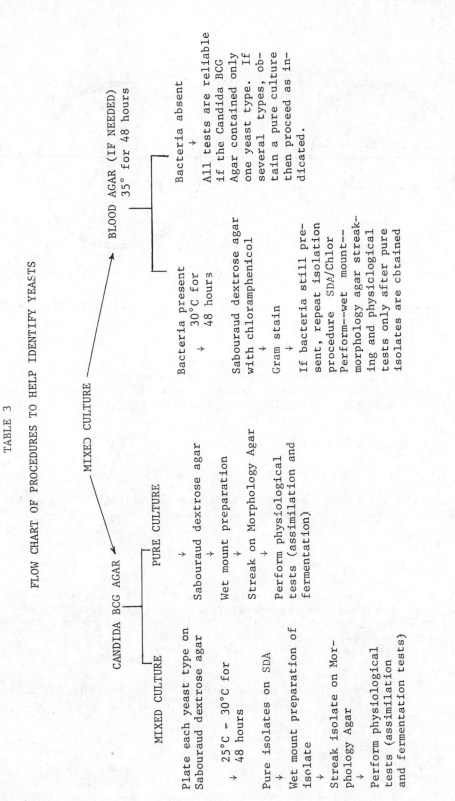

MIXED CULTURE

CANDIDA BCG AGAR

MIXED CULTURE
→ Plate each yeast type on Sabouraud dextrose agar
→ 25°C – 30°C for 48 hours
Pure isolates on SDA
→ Wet mount preparation of isolate
→ Streak isolate on Morphology Agar
→ Perform physiological tests (assimilation and fermentation tests)

PURE CULTURE
→ Sabouraud dextrose agar
→ Wet mount preparation
→ Streak on Morphology Agar
→ Perform physiological tests (assimilation and fermentation)

BLOOD AGAR (IF NEEDED) 35° for 48 hours

Bacteria present
→ 30°C for 48 hours
Sabouraud dextrose agar with chloramphenicol
→ Gram stain
→ If bacteria still present, repeat isolation procedure SDA/Chlor Perform—wet mount—morphology agar streaking and physiological tests only after pure isolates are obtained

Bacteria absent
→ All tests are reliable if the Candida BCG Agar contained only one yeast type. If several types, obtain a pure culture then proceed as indicated.

FIGURE 4

SLIDE CULTURE PROCEDURE

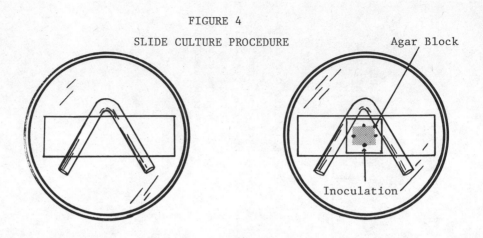

1. Biopsy Specimen

    A. Liver: a small portion of liver tissue should be inserted directly into BHI broth or Sabhi broth and sent to the laboratory. The liver specimen should be dissolved in the broth.

    B. Tissues other than liver: other tissues should be placed in a sterile container and sent to the laboratory. The gross character of the tissue is examined. The presence of purulent lesions or necrosis is reported. Several thin smears are made. The following tests are performed as needed: KOH, PAS stain, F.A., or India ink preparations.

        The biopsy specimens are prepared as follows:

        --cut the tissues into small pieces with sterile scissors

        --pipette 0.5 to 1.0 ml of the hemogenate into Brain heart infusion broth and plates

        --incubate

2. Bone Marrow Specimens

    Approximately 0.3 ml of bone marrow is collected in a heparin containing syringe. Several smears are made from bone fragments. All parts of the remaining specimen are inoculated into Brain heart infusion (BHI) broth and several agar plates of BHI. Some laboratories prefer Sabhi agar to BHI agar.

3. Blood

    Once the blood is properly collected and an appropriate anticoagulant is used, mold recovery procedures begin. The different culture methods used for mold recovery are:

    (1) membrane filter technique (8 ml blood)
    (2) agar slants/broths

(1) The membrane filter technique is rapid and has yielded excellent results for yeast recovery from blood.

(2) BHI slants/BHI broths also give good recovery results. The blood/broth ratio in a broth culture ranges from 1:10 to 1:20. A higher blood volume is not recommended. The blood/broth must be well mixed. Incubate at about 25°C for at least 28-30 days. Certain Candida and Torulopsis strains appear in blood cultures only after 25-30 days.

The type of anticoagulant and the wash solutions used are critical to the results. Many laboratories use sodium, polyanethol sulfonate (.03-.05% SPS) to inhibit clotting. Check a procedure manual before attempting the MF technique.

No matter how experienced the mycologist, isolation and identification is unlikely unless the specimen is properly collected and sent immediately to the laboratory. Also, for blood analysis, several blood smears should be made, stained with PAS and examined. Wright's or Giemsa stains detect the yeast forms of H. Capulatum in blood and CSF.

BRONCHIAL ASPIRATE

The bronchial aspirate should be brought to the laboratory as soon as possible. An aliquot of the aspirate is used for:

1. KOH preparation

2. PAS stain and any other stain preparation deemed necessary.

SKIN

The area to be removed is cleaned with 70% alcohol. The edge of a lesion is scraped with a sterile scalpel or thin edged spatula and placed in a sterile container.

PUS

Pus from a lesion may be aspirated aseptically and immediately sent to the laboratory.

CEREBROSPINAL FLUID (CSF)

The CSF should be aspirated aseptically and the collected specimen should be centrifuged at 2000 rpm for 15 minutes. DO NOT decant the supernate with a sterile pipette; recover a small amount of the sediment contained in the bottom of the centrifuge tube. An aliquot sample of the sediment is used for:

1. Smears (PAS - India ink - Gram stain - Giemsa stain or Wright's stain)

2. Media inoculation (BHI or Sabhi agar, BHI broth).

If the membrane filter technique is used, the sediment is mixed with the supernate.

SPUTUM

Lung material is essential for proper diagnosis. Saliva is undesirable. Early morning specimen are recommended. The specimen should be brought to the laboratory soon after collection and processed quickly. Delay in culturing may cause the bacteria present in the sputum to outgrow the fungi. Also, saprophytic fungi may interfere with the culture process.

Nocardia and Mycobacteria may be present in sputum specimen.

THRUSH LESIONS OF THE MOUTH

A tongue depressor (split lengthwise) can be used to scrape an oral lesion. It is necessary to scrape the infected mucous membrane. In the laboratory, a portion of the lesion is placed on a slide containing a drop of KOH. In the KOH, the lesion material is teased with a sterile needle, covered with a coverslip and examined microscopically for the presence of blastospores and pseudohyphae.

Another sample of the lesion material is collected on an inoculating loop and streaked over chloramphenicol containing SDA agar plates. The plates are incubated either at room temperature or 25°C. Plates should be kept for at least 7-10 days before discarding.

VAGINAL SPECIMEN

1. Swab to collect material from the vagina. The swabs may be inserted into a tube containing SDA broth and immediately brought to the laboratory.

2. Inoculate chloramphenicol containing SDA agar plates.

3. Tease another portion of the specimen in a KOH preparation.

4. Cover slide.

5. Examine

HAIR/SKIN/NAIL SPECIMENS

Hair, scraped skin scales, nail clippings or scrapings are collected and brought to the laboratory. Nail fragments and/or large skin scrapings may have to be cut or minced prior to inoculating into media.

The pathogenic fungi grow less quickly than the non-pathogenic fungi, therefore the incubation time for most pathogens is longer in duration. Some pathogenic fungi require 4-6 weeks of incubation before reaching maturity.

The fungi are heterotrophic and generally are not considered nutritionally fastidious.

Sabouraud dextrose agar (SDA) is probably the most widely used to maintain stock cultures. Most dermatophyte and systemic fungi morphological traits have been made on SDA and consequently this medium is used and is a standard medium in diagnostic laboratories.

CLASSIFICATION ARRANGEMENT

The pathogenic fungi discussed will be grouped according to the body site they infect.

Superficial Mycoses

The superficial fungi invade only the outermost layers of the skin (stratum corneum). The infected host does not react to this type infection.

Cutaneous Mycoses

The cutaneous fungi infect only the superficial layers (stratum corneum) of the skin. The resulting infections are more serious than those categorized as superficial mycoses. The dermatophytes and the dermal Candidas are included with the cutaneous mycoses. The dematophyte infections are the most frequent infections of fungal etiology.

Subcutaneous Mycoses

Subcutaneous fungi invade subcutaneous tissues. Clinical diseases referred to as chromomycosis, mycetoma and sporotrichosis are examples of subcutaneous mycotic infections.

Systemic Mycoses

The systemic fungi are the most dangerous of the pathogenic fungi and can be fatal to the host. The lungs are usually the portal of entry, however, the infective agents can spread to the rest of the body. The dimorphic fungi which are the causative agents of histoplasmosis, coccidioidomycosis, and blastomycosis as well as the opportunistic fungi responsible for aspergillosis, cryptococcosis and mucormycosis are included in this category. Cryptococcosis is a yeast.

The Superficial Mycoses

1. Tinea Versicolor (Pityriasis versicolor)

Tinea versicolor is a fairly frequent superficial fungal infection of the skin. It is worldwide in distribution, but most common in tropical areas. The infection is characterized by yellow to brown scaly spots over the trunk area. Sometimes the face, neck and legs demonstrate scaling. Only the keratin, or outer portion of the skin is affected, therefore inflammation and lesions are absent.

CAUSATIVE AGENT

The etiologic agent of Tinea versicolor is Malassezia furfur, a yeast which is an inhabitant of the skin. Commonly, diagnosis is made by examining skin scales in a KOH mount. In KOH, short thick hyphae can be observed.

TREATMENT

Tinea versicolor can be treated with a 20% sodium hyposulfite solution of karatolytic fungicides.

RECURRENCE

Tinea versicolor can and usually does recur.

2. Tinea Nigra

The disease tinea nigra is characterized by dark discoloration or spots on the palm of the hands. The blotches are usually limited to the palm of the hands.

The causative agents are members of the genus Cladosporium. The fungal infection is superficial. Lesions are flat and not scaly. The spots are brown to black in appearance. Some say the spot resembles a AgNO3 stain on the hand.

The causative agent is Cladosporium (Exophiala) werneckii.

RATE OF GROWTH

Cladosporium werneckii is a relatively slow grower and matures in about 14 days. Dark, shiny greenish black, moist colonies form on cycloheximide agar. The reverse of the colony is black.

MICROSCOPIC APPEARANCE

Microscopic examination reveals single and two-celled budding conidia on a dark mycelium.

FIGURE 5

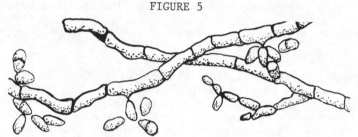

KOH PREPARATION

Cladosporium Conidiophores

KOH mounts show branched brown hyphae measuring approximately 2.5 µm in diameter.

TREATMENT

Usually, keratolytic fungicides are effective in the treatment of tinea nigra. Tinea nigra was discussed considerably because of its having been falsely diagnosed as a malignant melanoma.

Piedra

The disease, piedra, is a hair infection whereby hard nodules form on the distal shaft of the hair. This disease manifests itself in two forms: Black piedra and white piedra.

3. Black Piedra

Piedraia hortae is the etiological agent of Black piedra. Characteristically this agent forms hard brown or black nodules along the shafts of the hair.

GROWTH RATE

Piedraia hortae grows slowly and matures in about 21 days.

COLONY APPEARANCE (morphology)

On SDA, the colonies are small, slightly raised, deep greenish brown to black. The reverse of the colonies is black. The colonies may be either smooth or bear very short hyphae. On cycloheximide agar, green to black raised colonies form.

MICROSCOPIC APPEARANCE

Microscopically, the colonies show dark, thick walled septated hyphae with chlamydospore-like-cells. Occasionally, some workers report the presence of asci in cultures. (See Figure 6)

FIGURE 6

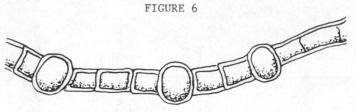

TREATMENT

Termination of this condition consists on shaving off the hair.

White Piedra

Trichosporon cutaneum is the causative agent of White piedra. This differs from Black piedra with respect to both causative agent and nodule formation. Here, the nodules on hair shafts are white and fairly soft. The hairs of the beard or mustache are the prime areas invaded by Trichosporon cutaneum, however, pubic hair and the scalp may also be infected.

GROWTH RATE

Trichosporon cutaneum is a rapid grower that usually matures in 5 days.

COLONY MORPHOLOGY

This fungus is yeast-like in appearance. On SDA, the colonies are moist and creamy in appearance. In older cultures, the center raises and colonies appear grayish. This fungus fails to grow on cycloheximide agar, but grows well in cornmeal agar containg Tween 80.

MICROSCOPIC MORPHOLOGY

T. cutaneum has septated hyphae. Blastospores are present in young cultures. Arthrospores and blastospores are formed by older cultures. The presence of the blastospores on the hyphae aid in the identification of T. cutaneum and differentiates it from Geotrichum spp.

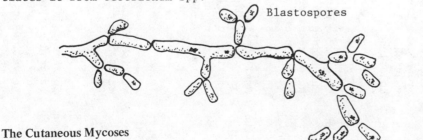

Blastospores

FIGURE 7

The Cutaneous Mycoses

This section will discuss the traits of some of the causative agents of dermatophytoses and the dermal Candidas. The dermatophytes have been classified as imperfect fungi. However, recent data indicate that some of the dermatophytes exhibit a sexual

TABLE 4

CHARACTERISTICS OF SELECTED DERMATOPHYTES

DERMATOPHYTES	MORPHOLOGICAL CHARACTERISTICS COLONY (SDA)	MORPHOLOGICAL CHARACTERISTICS MICROSCOPIC	GROWTH RATE (DAYS)	PATHOGENICITY	DISEASE
Trichophyton tonsurans	Surface color variable --may be whitish, grayish, yellow, pinkish or brownish. Reverse rustish-yellow or colorless.	Septated hyphae, bearing multishaped microconidia --(knobs or balloon shape). Intercalary and terminal chlamydospores. Macroconidia usually not present.	10-12	Ringworm of the scalp; Sometimes infects nails and skin.	Tinea capitis
Trichophyton violaceum	Range from waxy wrinkled and heaped to downy purplish red surface and lavender on bottom.	Irregularly arranged hyphae bearing chlamydospores and granules.	15-21	Primarily infects the scalp but skin and nails may be affected.	Tinea capitis
Trichophyton verrucosum	Small, piled or heaped and shiny; whitish or grayish in color on surface; reverse is yellow to colorless.	Hyphae bearing chlamydospores--finger-like branches often seen.	15-21	Infects beard, scalp and on rare occasions, smooth skin.	Tinea barbae; Tinea capitis
Trichophyton schoenleinii	Colonies are either folded or heaped; whitish surface with tannish or colorless bottom.	Septated hyphae with antler or finger-like tips usually termed "nailheads"; chlamydospores present.	14-15	Causes favus which is a chronic scalp disorder that can cause permanent loss of hair.	Tinea capitis·
Trichophyton rubrum	Surface is white--may be granular or fluffy; reverse, variable: may be yellow-orange, brown or colorless.	Septated hyphae that bear lateral water drop or tear shaped microconidia. Macroconidia may be present. If present, microconidia grow on macroconidia.	10-15	Primarily infects skin and nails and occasionally infects beard, hair, scalp, groin and thighs.	T.corporis T.cruris T.pedis T.manuum T.unguium

TABLE 4 (continued)

DERMATOPHYTES	MORPHOLOGICAL CHARACTERISTICS COLONY (SDA)	MICROSCOPIC	GROWTH RATE (DAYS)	PATHOGENICITY	DISEASE
Trichophyton mentagrophytes	Variable: white and downy or buff and powdery; may turn pink or yellow; reverse dark tan, red, yellow or colorless.	Septated hyphae. Cigar-shaped macroconidia may be present or absent. Microconidia or powdery colonies are round on branched conidiophores. Microconidia are smaller in fluffy cultures.	7-10	Infects smooth skin, groin, thighs, feet, hands and nails. In brief, it infects all body parts. Agent most frequently responsible for "athlete's foot".	T.corporis T.cruris T.pedis T.manuum T.unguium
Microsporum distortum	Flat, hairy buff or cream colored colonies; reverse may be yellow.	Septated hyphae with marcroconidia that are club shaped.	5-10	Occasional agent of ringworm of the scalp.	Tinea capitis
Microsporum canis	White surface; reverse turns yellow; reverse turns brown in older cultures; colonies flully with grooves.	Septated hyphae containing spindle-shaped macroconidia which are "knob-like" and thick walled.	6-12	Infects the skin, feet, hands and scalp.	T.corporis T.pedis T.manuum T.capitis
Microsporum audouini	Flat, silky grayish to buff colonies; reverse is salmon with brownish center.	Septated hyphae. Terminal chlamydospores present and often pointed terminal chlamydospores.	7-10	Causes ringworm of the scalp (especially in children).	Tinea capitis

TABLE 4 (continued)

DERMATOPHYTES	MORPHOLOGICAL CHARACTERISTICS		GROWTH RATE (DAYS)	PATHOGENICITY	DISEASE
	COLONY (SDA)	MICROSCOPIC			
Epidermophyton floccosum	Center of colony has folds; grooves radically from center; surface yellow to odd gray; older cultures are covered by white mycelium. Reverse: off colored yellow; folds obvious.	Septated hyphae. Club-shaped macroconidia; Chlamydospores in older cultures; no microconidia.	6-10	Causes infection of the groin, thighs, feet and hands.	Tinea cruris Tinea pedis Tinea manuum

N.B. Candida albicans is sometimes listed with the dermatophytes, since it causes a clinically similar nail infection as the causative agents of Tinea unguium.

stage and should be classified among the perfect fungi. This classification change resulted in renaming many of the dermatophytes. Consequently, some dermatophytes are listed under two names. Clinically, the dermatophytes are recognized as imperfect fungi and the older taxonomy still prevails, therefore the imperfect classification names will be used here.

The dermatophytes are responsible for the greatest number of fungal infections. The dermatophytes may be differentiated into three genera: Trichophyton, Microsporum and Epidermophyton. The members of the genus Epidermophyton do not invade the hair. The dermatophytes differ structurally from most of the other pathogenic fungi in that:

(1) their cells are multinucleated and usually bear 4 to 6 nuclei;
(2) their chlamydospores and arthrospores are also multinucleated;
(3) cells of the macroaleuriospores are multinucleated, but contain but one nucleus, and
(4) they divide amitotically.

MEDIA AND NUTRITIONAL REQUIREMENT OF DERMATOPHYTES

Glucose enriched cornmeal agar differentiates Trichophyton rubrum from Trichophyton mentagrophytes on the basis of pigment production.

SABOURAUD DEXTROSE AGAR

All dermatophytes grow on SDA with antibiotic.

POTATO DEXTROSE AGAR

This medium stimulates pigment production in Microsporum audouini.

DERMOTOPHYTE TEST MEDIUM (DMT)

Hair, skin and nail specimens may be inoculated into this medium. Dermatophytes cause the medium to turn from yellow to red within 14 days.

Many false positives have been reported due to contaminants. Dermatophyte morphology can be studied from this medium, but pigment production cannot, since the medium turns deep red with positive results.

The structure and characteristics of the macroaleuriospore constitutes the primary differentiation of the dermatophytes. This microscopic distinction for each genus is listed in Table 3. Arthrospore location also plays a role in differentiations (endothrix arthrospores are within the hair; ectothrix arthrospores are on the surface of the hair). T. schoenleinii produces no spores but only "air bubbles" in the shaft of the hair.

Physiological studies also demonstrate that amino acids and vitamins are required for certain dermatophytes to grow properly. These requirements may provide differentiation. Included in these requirements are:

REQUIREMENT	DERMATOPHYTES
Thiamine	Trichophyton violaceum
Thiamine	Trichophyton tonsurans
Inositol/Thiamine	Trichophyton verrucosum
Nicotinic Acid	Trichophyton equinum

Commercially prepared media containing amino acids and vitamins are available. These include:

Trichophyton Agar #1	Casein/Agar Base (Plain)
Trichophyton Agar #2	Casein Agar/Base + Inositol
Trichophyton Agar #3	Casein Agar/Base + Inositol and Thiamine
Trichophyton Agar #4	Casein Agar Base + Thiamine
Trichophyton Agar #5	Casein Agar Base + Nicotinic Acid
Trichophyton Agar #6	Ammonium Nitrate Agar Base
Trichophyton Agar #7	Ammonium Nitrate Agar Base + Histidine

Temperature requirements also help to differentiate the Trichophyton species.

Trichophyton verrucosum grows best at 37°C while the growth of the other dermatophytes is limited or inhibited at this temperature.

MACROALEURIOSPORES

Since the macroaleuriospores play such a major role in the primary isolation of the dermatophytes, the gross characteristics of the three genera are illustrated below.

FIGURE 8

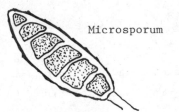 Microsporum

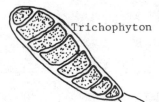 Trichophyton

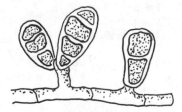

Epidermophyton

The Subcutaneous Mycoses

The subcutaneous fungi invade the skin and subcutaneous tissues, but do not (usually) disseminate to, or invade internal organs. The most clinically important subcutaneous diseases are: Chromomycosis, Sporotrichosis, Lobomycosis, Rhinosporidiosis, and Entomophthoromycosis. Mycetoma is also a subcutaneous mycosis, but its etiologic agent is an actinomycete and will not be discussed in this section.

Chromomycosis

The etiologic agents of Chromomycosis closely resemble the Cladosporium species.

KOH, DMSO and lactophenol cotton blue preparations of these fungi help to reveal their microscopic traits and should be used simultaneously with plating media.

The etiologic agents of chromomycosis are: Fonsecaea pedrosoi, F. compactum, and Phialophora verrucosum. F. pedrosoi has been reported to be responsible for the greatest number of cases. Occasionally, Cladosporium carrioni and Exophiala jeanselmi have been recovered and seem implicated.

Sporotrichosis

Sporothrix schenckii is the causative agent of sporotrichosis. The soil is the natural habitat of this fungus. S. schenckii usually invades humans via a split in the skin made by either a thorn or splinter contaminated with this fungus. Lympho-cutaneous sporotrichosis is the most frequent occurence of the disease. Characteris-tically, nodular lesions of the skin and subcutaneous tissues are observed. The nodules ultimately ulcerate and drain. Bone, lung and joint sporotrichosis may also be caused by S. schenckii. In fact, all tissues are vulnerable to this fungus. Table 4 illustrates the morphological and pathogenic traits of certain subcutaneous fungi.

The Systemic Mycoses

The sytemic fungi can invade any organ of the body as well as the cutaneous, sub-cutaneous and skeletal components of the body. Generally, the etiologic agents of systemic mycoses enter the system via the lungs. The fungal agents implicated in systemic mycoses seem to have an affinity for a particular organ or tissue. The sys-temic fungi consists of two types:

(1) those fungi which can attack healthy individuals, and
(2) the opportunistic pathogens which invade the chronically ill, debilitated or those exposed to immunosuppressive drugs or prolonged use of antibiotics.

The tissue dimorphic or thermal fungi may invade the healthy to cause histoplas-mosis, blastomycosis, coccidioidomycosis and paracoccidiodomycosis. Contrastingly, the opportunistic pathogens are not tissue dimorphic, that is, they do not change morphology in the host. The opportunistic pathogens may cause mucormycosis or aspergillosis.

Histoplasmosis

The dimorphic fungus, Histoplasma capsulatum, is the causative agent of histo-plasmosis.

This fungus is contracted by inhaling or coming in contact with contaminated air or excreta from infested chicken coops, pigeon roosts or bat nooks. Inhalation of the H. capsulatum spores results in a pulmonary infection which usually disseminates. Isolation of this fungus from either bronchial washings, bronchial aspirates, trans-tracheal aspirates or sputum is difficult for few H. capsulatum cells are recovered in respiratory tract specimens.

Consequently, a concentration prodecure is needed to obtain a sufficient number of H. capsulatum for isolation on artificial media.

In tissues, H. capsulatum appears as small, oval yeast-like cells (2 to 4 μm in diameter). The cell wall often appears like a capsule, but no capsule is present. Generally, H. capsulatum is intracellular and can be found in the mononuclear

TABLE 5

CHARACTERISTICS OF SELECTED SUBCUTANEOUS FUNGI

FUNGI	COLONY	MORPHOLOGY MICROSCOPIC	GROWTH RATE (DAYS)	DISEASE	PATOGENICITY
Fonsecaea pedrosoi (Phialophorum pedrosoi)	Gray surface; reverse is dark green; colony is covered with velvety silver mycelium	Brown, branched septated hyphae--three conidia types	15	Chromomycosis	ALL CAUSE CHRONIC SKIN DISEASES WHICH PRODUCE WARTY NODULES: TUMOR-LIKE GROWTHS OR LESIONS
Fonsecaea compactum	Dark green or black surface; reverse is black; colonies look piled and have irregular peripheries; hyphae and conidiophores	Brown, branched septated hyphae; conidiophores produce round conidia	30	Chromomycosis	
Phialophorum verrucosum	Brownish to black surface; reverse is black; gray or olive mycelium; colonies may be granular and heaped or flat and matted	Brown, branched septated hyphae with vase shaped conidiophores	14	Chromomycosis	
Sporotrichum schenckii	Young cultures are white and creamy; older cultures are darker; yeast-like on BHI and cystine blood agar (37°C); dimorphic	Dimorphic--pear shaped at 25°C septated hyphae; conidiophore; at 37°C bears oval cells called "cigar bodies"	4	Sporotrichosis	

leukocytes of the peripheral blood and in the bone marrow and spleen macrophages. Since this fungus is basically intracellular, often this disease is referred to as cytomycosis or reticuloendothelial cytomycosis.

DIAGNOSIS

Microscopic observation of the fungus is suggestive of the disease, but isolation and identification on media are essential for identification. Isolates may be obtained from blood cultures, biopsy specimens and concentrated respiratory tract specimens.

Subouraud dextrose agar and Brain heart infusion agar are not the media of choice to isolate this fungus.

Yeast peptone phosphate (YPP) medium (or Yeast extract phosphate YEP) is recommended for the recovery of H. capsulatum. Blood agar is used a great deal in conjunction with YPP (or YEP). Others prefer Sabhi medium to YPP. Both media provide good results.

DIMORPHIC TRAIT

Demonstrations of the conversion of a mold (suspected to be H. capsulatum) to a yeast confirms the identification of H. capsulatum.

Media used to isolate this fungus are not satisfactory for conversion to the yeast form. Unfortunately, 20-25% of isolates of H. capsulatum will not go into the yeast form in vitro. Animals or special serologic techniques are needed to confirm their identity.

MOLD FORM/PLATE EXAMINATION

Examine plates every 48-72 hours. Although colonies may develop within a week, it usually takes 12 to 21 days before H. capsulatum colonies are seen on isolation media. H. capsulatum isolates vary greatly in their gross morphology. The young colonies are thin and membranous and tufts of aerial hyphae may develop over the surface. As the colonies continue to mature, they may become woolly, velvety, or granular in appearance, or they may remain smooth. Colonies may be white to tan or brown.

As fungal colonies appear on plates, they should be subcultured to Sabouraud dextrose agar without antibiotics.

When subcultures have grown, lactophenol cotton blue preparation should be made to study the conidiophores and conidia. H. capsulatum usually produces two types of conidia (aleurioconidia): a single-celled macroconidium and a microconidium.

The macroconidia are round or slightly pyriform and their average size is 7 to 12 μm in diameter. The cell wall may be tuberculated or have fin-like structures protruding from the wall surface. Occasionally, these cell walls may be smooth.

Microconidia are usually round and measure approximately 2-5 μm in diameter and are smooth walled.

Some isolates of H. capsulatum may produce no conidia or only microconidia or macroconidia. Care must be taken not to confuse the conidia of H. capsulatum with those of some Chrysosporium or Sepedonium species.

MOLD FORM TO YEAST FORM (DIMORPHISM)

Demonstration of conversion of a mold suspected to be H. capsulatum to a yeast form confirms the identity of this fungus. To do this, inoculate 2 to 5 slants of BHI agar containing 5% blood and incubate at 37°C.

Once a week, place a fragment of the growth from the periphery and under surface of the agar into lactophenol cotton blue; tease carefully and mount the preparation with a coverslip. Examine for the presence of yeast cells with buds attached by a narrow neck. The yeast form is sensitive to cycloheximide.

Blastomycosis

The dimorphic fungus, Blastomyces dermatitidis is the causative agent of blastomycosis.

In tissue or in vitro at 37°C, B. dermatitidis appears as a unicellular budding yeast-like form, but appears as a mycelial form in a culture incubated at 25°C. KOH preparations of pus or sputum specimens demonstrate the unicellular yeast-like form which have a single broad-based bud. The cells, which measure approximately 0.9 μm in diameter, are round or oval and multinucleated. This direct microscopic examination of the yeast form is suggestive of blastomycosis, but isolation and identification on media are essential for confirmation.

Sabouraud dextrose agar (containing antibiotics) is the inoculating medium recommended by most workers. YPP (or YEP) plates with chloramphenicol may be used also. The plates should be sealed with parafilm and incubated at 25°C for approximately 28 days. Three to 5 plates should be used.

Negative plates should be kept for at least 6 weeks before discarding.

Plate Reading

Examine plates every three or four days for development of fungal colonies. Subculture colonies to Sabouraud dextrose agar without antibiotics. Although some isolates of B. dermatitidis may appear on isolation media in approximately seven days, usually 10 to 14 days are required for growth to appear.

Colonies of this fungus vary greatly. They may be smooth, developing no aerial mycelium or spores. Some isolates begin as a thin colony gradually developing aerial hyphae over the surface of the colony. Other isolates may develop colonies that are velvety or woolly. Color ranges from a dirty white to tannish. It is not possible to differentiate colonies of B. dermatitidis and H. capsulatum for one another on gross morphology.

Working in a biological hood, lactophenol cotton blue preparations should be made of mature subcultures to determine sporulation. Conidia (aleurioconidia) are small, oval and smooth walled. They are borne on short lateral branches. Occasionally, these conidia may be confused with microconidia of H. capsulatum or with some isolates of Chrysosporium.

CONVERSION TO YEAST FORM

Final identification of B. dermatitidis is made by converting the mold form to the characteristic yeast form.

B. dermatitidis

Several excellent media are available for converting the mold form of this fungus to the yeast form. BHI and cottonseed agars are satisfactory. It is essential that these tubes contain approximately 0.5 ml of moisture at the bottom of the slant. Conversion is poor on any slant that does not contain adequate moisture.

Place several fragments of the mold culture approximately 5 mm above the fluid level of each of several slants of conversion medium. Incubate the cultures at 37°C.

In approximately five days, pick a fragment of the inoculum on a slant and tease it apart in a drop of lactophenol cotton blue. Although hyphal elements will predominate, a few yeast cells may be seen coming directly off of hyphae.

Yeast cells of B. dermatitidis are round and have a very thick wall. Usually one bud is seen attached by a broad neck to the parent cell. These yeasts are diagnostic for B. dermatitidis.

If yeast cells are not found after 5 days of incubation, reincubate the culture for two or three more days. If no conversion is noted within 14 days, the culture should be inoculated into animals or sent to a reference laboratory.

Coccidioidomycosis

Coccidioidomycosis is contracted by inhaling Coccidioides immitis spores. Coccidioides immitis is a dimorphic fungus, but the tissue form is not a yeast. Consequently, unlike other yeast-like fungi, it never reproduces by budding, but rather reproduces in tissues by spore formation. The tissue form is usually referred to as a *spherule* which, when mature, contains many endospores.

ISOLATION

Studies have indicated that C. immitis may survive for 48-72 hours in sputum specimens that are kept at room temperature.

Place 0.05 ml to 0.1 ml of concentrated sediment of contaminated specimens to each of two tissue culture bottles containing Sabouraud dextrose agar with antibiotics.

If the specimen is not from a contaminated site, it is not necessary to concentrate it before inoculation into media.

Streak the inoculum over the agar surface; incubate all cultures at room temperature for 4 weeks before discarding them as negative.

PLATE READING AND IDENTIFICATION

Examine all cultures every 48 hours for fungal colonies. Working in a biological hood, subculture colonies to Sabouraud agar slants. At room temeprature, colonies of C. immitis may appear in 5 to 7 days. Cultures incubated at 37°C may grow more rapidly, often filling the bottle within 4 to 5 days. Colonies of C. immitis isolates vary greatly. Young colonies may appear as a thin smooth sheet on the agar surface and aerial hyphae may develop. The colonies may be dirty white to tan or even blackish.

C. immitis is a rapid grower. Many workers think it is a contaminant and, if careless, end up with a laboratory acquired infection.

C. IMMITIS SUSPENSION/ISOLATION

A culture, thought to be C. immitis, may be worked with as follows: into a 5 ml syringe, draw up approximately 4 ml o sterile distilled water containing 0.05% Tween 80. Place a long needle on the syringe.

Insert the needle into the culture tube by pushing it between the cotton plug and the test tube wall for a depth of 1 cm; then force the needle into the bottom portion of the cotton plug until it has passed completely through. Gently expell the syringe contents down the inside wall of the tube opposite the agar surface. This will wet the fungus culture preventing arthrospores from escaping.

While holding the test tube, needle and syringe, gently agitate the tube.

Withdraw some of the suspension back into the syringe; bring needle out of the fluid remaining in the tube and pull back on the syringe plunger slightly. This will prevent leakage from the needle tip. Pull the needle out of the cotton plug and place the contents into a sterile test tube.

Make lactophenol cotton blue preparation with a drop of the culture suspension. Microscopic examination of the lactophenol cotton blue preparation should demonstrate thin-walled, rectangular or barrel-shaped arthrospores. When they break free of the hypha, the arthrospores may have an empty cell attached.

ANIMAL INOCULATION

If arthrospores are present, the suspension can be inoculated into animals to obtain the tissue form of the fungus. If animals are not available, the suspension can be subcultured onto a Sabouaud agar slant which can be sent to a reference laboratory. Demonstration of spherules in tissue is the confirmatory test for the identity of C. immitis. This confirmatory test requires animal inoculation because these arthrospore may be confused with those of C. immitis, demonstration of spherule production in vivo is required before identifying a fungus as C. immitis.

Experienced technologists usually wet the culture and remove some of the growth to make a teased preparation. Water and Tween 80 can be used to wet the culture.

Opportunistic Fungi

Some fungi are not the direct cause of a disease, but rather invade the host when the host's physiological defenses are lowered. Many opportunistic pathogens are part of the "normal flora" and remain suppressed by the other members of the normal flora. Any drastic reduction in the normal flora can predispose the host to these opportunistic fungi (as well as bacterial and viral infections). A massive intake or prolonged use of antibiotics, impairment of the immune system with immunosuppressive drugs or a debilitated state can predispose the host to these opportunistic fungi. The three fungal genera which constitute the most common opportunistic fungi are: Candida, Aspergillus and Rhizopus.

Candidiasis

Several Candida species are etiologic agents of candidiasis, however Candida albicans is responsible for the greatest number of cases. C. krusei, and C. parapsilosis are also agents of candidiasis. Candida species are not always opportunistic pathogens and are frequently primary agents of infection. Vaginitis, thrush, dermatitis, and nail infections all seem to be primary Candida infections.

Candida species are normal inhabitants of the urogenital, respiratory and alimentary tracts. Massive or prolonged usage of antibiotics immunosuppressive drugs and contraction of certain diseases alter their normal state and permit them to become opportunistic pathogens capable of causing local or systemic infections.

The Candida species are fermentative yeasts that form pseudomycelia on certain media such as cornmeal-Tween 80 agar (CTA) preparations. Cut streaks on CTA preparations enhance the pseudomycelia formation.

Clinical differentiation of the Candida species depends upon carbohydrate fermentation test results.

Aspergillosis

Members of the genus Aspergillus cause aspergillosis, but A. fumigatus is responsible for the majority of the cases. A. fumigatus is an opportunistic fungus induced by immunosuppressive drugs, massive intake of antibiotics or host debilitation, especially due to tuberculosis. Aspergillosis causes a pulmonary disease and lung tissue necrosis. Lung tissue damage by tuberculosis is a prime target for the fungus. Generally, the fungus does not cause a systemic infection, but it can do so on rare occasions.

A. fumigatus morphological traits are readily seen on SDA plates and the fungus may be identified serologically.

Mucormycosis

Members of the genera Rhizopus, Mucor and Absidia are the causative agents of mucormycosis. These fungi proliferate when body tissues abnormally contain high amounts of glucose, acids and ketones. The fungi enter the host via the respiratory tract and the paranasal sinuses are their prime target. The fungi rapidly proliferate in the high glucose, acid and ketone concentrations. The fungi then extend to the eyes, nose, brain and arteries. Arterial blockage and tissue necrosis may occur. Rhinocerebral infections are frequently fatal. Patient recovery depends upon the time exposed prior to diagnosis and treatment

BIBLIOGRAPHY AND RECOMMENDED READINGS

Al-Doory, Yousef. *LABORATORY MEEICAL MYCOLOGY*. 1980. Lea and Febiger Publishers.
   Philadelphia.

Boyd, Robert F. and Bryan G. Hoerl. *BASIC MEDICAL MICROBIOLOGY*. 1977. Little,
   Brown and Company. Boston.

Emmons, C. W., Binford, C. H., UTZ, J. P. and K. J. Kwon-Chung. *MEDICAL MYCOLOGY*.
   Third Edition. 1977. Lea and Febiger Publishers. Philadelphia.

Finegold, M. Sidney, Martin, William J. and Elvyn G. Scott. *BAILEY AND SCOTT'S
   DIAGNOSTIC MICROBIOLOGY*. Fifth Edition. 1978. The C. V. Mosby Company.
   St. Louis.

Freeman, Bob A. *BURROW'S TEXTBOOK OF MICROBIOLOGY*. Twenty-first Edition. 1979.
   W. B. Saunders Company. Philadelphia.

Koneman, Elmer W., Roberts, Glenn D., and Sara E. Wright. *PRACTICAL LABORATORY
   MYCOLOGY*. Second Edition. 1979. The Williams and Wilkins Company. Baltimore

Larone, Davise Honig. *MEDICALLY IMPORTANT FUNGI: A GUIDE TO IDENTIFICATION*.
   1976. Harper and Row Publishers. New York.

Moore, Gary S. and Douglas M. Jaciow. *MYCOLOGY FOR THE CLINICAL LABORATORY*.
   1979. Reston Publishing Company. Reston, VA.

Schuhardt, Vernon T. *PATHOGENIC MICROBIOLOGY*. 1978. J. B. Lippincott Company.
   Philadelphia.

Volk, Wesley A. *ESSENTIALS OF MEDICAL MICROBIOLOGY*. 1978. J. B. Lippincott
   Company. Philadelphia.

Chapter 3

Parasitology

ALBERT E. PACKARD, BS, MT (ASCP)
Instructor of Biology
Natural Science Division
Notre Dame College
Manchester, New Hampshire

```
INTRODUCTION
THE   PROTOZOA
    The Sarcodina
        Intestinal Amebas
            Entamoeba Histolytica
            Entamoeba Hartmani
            Entamoeba Coli
            Endolimax Nana
            Iodamoeba Butschlii
            Dientamoeba Fragilis
        Extraintestinal Amebas
            Naegleria Fowleri
            Acanthamoeba
    The Mastigophora
        The Intestinal Flagellates
            Chilomastix Mesnili
            Trichomonas Hominis
        The Flagellates of the Oral Cavity and Genito Urinary System
            Trichomonas Tenax
            Trichomonas Vaginalis
        Blood and Tissue Flagellates
            Trypanosoma Gambiense
            Trypanosoma Rhodesiense
            Trypanosoma Cruzi
            Leishmania Tropica
            Leishmania Braziliensis
            Leishmania Donovani
    The Ciliata
        The Intestinal Ciliate
            Balantidium Coli
    The Sporozoa
        The Intestinal Sporozoa
            Isospora Belli
        Tissue Sporozoa
            Toxoplasma Gondii
```

INTRODUCTION

Traditionally, the student of Clinical Laboratory Science has been taught clinical parasitology as a minor part of clinical microbiology. Undergraduate courses in Medical Microbiology either offered very little parasitology or none at all. Clinically based Medical Technology programs, for the most part, generally offered little more than two weeks of parasitology as part of a clinical microbiology rotation. Consequently, students of clinical laboratory science, and many practicing clinical laboratory scientists, feel ill-prepared to perform parasitological studies with any degree of certainty.

Though it is true that in many parts of the United States there is a paucity of patients who present with parasitic disorders, it remains that the numbers of parasitic disorders being diagnosed and treated in the United States is on the increase. Recent figures from the World Health Organization indicate that literally millions of the world's population have parasitic disorders. For many years, most of the parasitic disorders that were diagnosed and treated in the United States were seen in members of the armed forces and missionaries returning from foreign bases of opera tion. More recently parasitic disorders are being found in civilian consultants and in construction crews, who have been sent to endemic areas throughout the world. In addition, our relative affluence has provided us with opportunities for foreign travel as students and vacationers. In our age of the SST, it is possible to have breakfast in New York, lunch in London, and dinner in Paris. Our increased mobility has given us the opportunity to travel to exotic places, eat exotic foods, and acquire exotic parasitic diseases.

The purpose of this chapter is two-fold. First, it is intended for use by students of clinical laboratory science as a study tool in preparation for registry and certification examinations, and second, it is intended for use by practicing clinical laboratory scientists to update their knowledge of clinical parasitology. In order to serve these purposes effectively, the information presented is offered in a concise form utilizing tables for the bulk of the differential identification criteria. These tables have been designed to provide a visual image, in the form of line drawings, of the organism, with the identification criteria following the line drawing.

This chapter deals with those parasites that are of greatest clinical significance. The protozoa discussed include the Sarcodia, Mastigophora, Ciliata, and Sporozoa that are most commonly responsible for human disease. The Helminths discussed include the Trematodes, Cestodes, and Nematodes that are most commonly responsible for human disease. The Arthropods discussed are those which are, in fact, human parasites. Discussion of Arthropods as vectors or as stinging and biting organisms has not been included. For this information, the reader is referred to more complete texts on parasitology.

PROTOZOA

Sarcodina

Intestinal Amebas

The organisms of this group are: Entamoeba histolytica, Entamoeba hartmani, Entamoeba coli, Endolimax nana, Iodameoba butschlii, and Dientamoeba fragilis.

Of these organisms, only E. histolytica is considered to be pathogenic. Although the remainder are considered non-pathogenic, they are of clinical importance in that, when they are present, (1) they must be distinguished from E. histolytica, and (2) identification of these organisms is essential since they may be opportunistic organisms or potential pathogens. The differential identification criteria for these organisms may be found in Tables 1 and 2.

ENTAMOEBA HISTOLYTICA   E. histolytica is the causative agent of amebic dysentery or amebiasis.

DISTRIBUTION   Although E. histolytica is most commonly found in the sub-tropics, and tropics, it is cosmopolitan in distribution. However, it is most frequently found in areas of poor sanitation, or where poor personal hygiene is the rule.

EPIDEMIOLOGY   E. histolytica is usually acquired from contaminated food and water. Most often it is the result of fecal contamination of food by food handlers. However, it may be the result of contamination of food or water by mechanical transmission via such organisms as flies and cockroaches. Moreover, even though water treatment facilities may help to reduce the spread of disease, the levels of chlorine commonly used does not kill the cyst stage of the organism, and, water treatment facilities have no control over possible contamination of the water after it leaves the treatment plant.

LIFE CYCLE   E. histolytica has two distinct stages: the trophozoite or active, motile state and the cyst, or inactive stage. The trophozoite stage is a very fragile, delicate stage, and a very invasive stage. The cyst stage is the infective stage. Once the cyst is ingested, the cyst wall is dissolved, releasing a quadranucleate trophozoite which divides by binary fission into four single nucleated trophozoites. The active trophozoites inhabit the large intestine. Some of these trophozoites will ultimately expel their nutritional material and develop into pre-cysts. These pre-cysts will develop a resistant membrane, and will then be known as cysts. Early cysts have only one nucleus, but the nucleus will divide twice producing a quadranucleate mature cyst. The cyst state is resistant to adverse conditions and may survive many days or even weeks in cool water.

PATHOGENESIS   The majority of the cases of human infection with E. histolytica, approximately 90%, are symptomatic. Of the symptomatic cases, some have only vague abdominal symptoms while others have definitive symptoms such as diarrhea, abdominal pain and cramps, weight loss and fatigue. Most often, all symptomatic cases have amebic dysentery. E. histolytica is an extremely invasive organism which may penetrate the muscularis mucosa, the sub-mucosa, and eventually erode into the blood vessels. Extensive ulceration results in diarrhea. In a very small percentage of cases, the ulceration may be severe enough to produce extraintestinal amebiasis involving the liver and lungs.

DIAGNOSTIC CRITERIA   Diagnosis is most commonly based on finding either the cysts or the trophozoites in stool specimens. The cysts are more frequently found in formed stools, while the trophozoites are more frequently found in loose, watery stools. Of primary importance is the ability of the laboratory scientist to distinguish E. histolytica from the non-pathogenic amebas. The definitive criteria for the cyst of E. histolytica include: size, number of nuclei, nuclear structure, and chromatoidal bar structure. The definitive criteria for the trophozoite include: size, nuclear structure, and the possible presence of red blood cells in the cytoplasm. In cases of extraintestinal amebiasis, stool examinations may prove useless, and one must rely on serological procedures such as IHA, IIF, and CEP.

ENTAMOEBA HARTMANI   Entamoeba hartmani is morphologically very similar to E. histolytica, to the extent that until recently it was known as the "small race". However, E. hartmani has been shown to be a non-invasive, non-pathogenic organism. In the case of E. hartmani, the differential criteria lie in the size of the organism and the absence of ingested red blood cells in the trophozoite.

ENTAMOEBA COLI   E. coli, like E. hartmani, is very similar to E. histolytica. This organism is also non-invasive and non-pathogenic. The differential criteria are: the number of nuclei that may be found in the cyst stage, the shape of the chromatoidal bars in the cyst, the karyosomal and peripheral chromatin distribution in the nuclei of both the cyst and the trophozoite, and the absence of ingested red blood cells in the trophozoite stage.

It may be difficult to establish or deny the presence of E. histolytica in the presence of either E. hartmani and for E. coli due to the fact that mixed infections are not uncommon. If E. hartmani or E. coli is seen, one must continue the search for the possibility of E. histolytica, particularly if symptoms are present.

ENDOLIMAX NANA   E. nana is another non-pathogen that, if found, must be differentiated from E. histolytica. The differential criteria are: the distribution of the karyosomal and peripheral chromatin in both the cyst and trophozoite, the vacuolated cytoplasm of the trophozoite, and the absence of ingested red blood cells.

IODAMOEBA BUTSCHLII   This organism is also considered to be a non-pathogen, although recently it has been seen in at least one pathogenic situation and ought to be considered a potential pathogen or at least an opportunistic organism. The differential criteria are: the karyosomal and peripheral chromatin distribution in both the cyst and trophozoite, the prominent glycogen mass in both the cyst and trophozoite, the number of nuclei in the cyst, and the absence of ingested red blood cells in the trophozoite.

DIANTAMOEBA FRAGILIS   This organism has only a trophozoite stage. The differential criteria are: the distribution of the karyosomal and peripheral chromatin, the presence of two nuclei in the trophozoite, and the absence of ingested red blood cells in the trophozoite.

Extraintestinal Amebas

The organisms of this group are: Naegleria fowleri and Acanthamoeba.

NAEGLERIA FOWLERI   Naegleria fowleri has been shown to be the causative agent of an acute meningoencephalitis.

DISTRIBUTION   The initial cases were reported from Australia and Florida. Since then, cases have been reported from Europe, New Zealand, Africa, India, and the United

States. In the United States, cases have been reported in Virginia, Georgia, Texas, and California.

EPIDEMIOLOGY   The source of infection is warm, fresh, or brackish water in swimming pools, ponds and streams. Naegleria trophozoites gain entry into humans via the nasal mucosa.

LIFE CYCLE   Naegleria belongs to a group of amoeboflagellates which have an amoeboid phase and a flagellar phase.

PATHOGENESIS   Naegleria has been reported in approximately 60 cases (all fatal) of an acute amebic meningoencephalitis.   The onset and course of the disease is rapid and dramatic resulting in death in 3-6 days.

DIAGNOSTIC CRITERIA   Diagnosis is made upon finding the characteristic organisms in the cerebrospinal fluid (CSF) of infected patients. When stained with iron hematoxylin, these amoeba characteristically display a nucleus having a large central karyosomal chromatin mass. The organisms, when found in CSF, will be active. The cytoplasm of naegleria may contain red blood cells. The organisms will develop pseudopods. The formation of pseudopods may be enhanced by warming the slide.

ACANTHAMOEBA   Organisms of the genus Acanthamoeba have been reported in a number of non-fatal cases of cerebral infection, and in cases of corneal ulcerations. In these cases, diagnosis is made by finding the characteristic cysts in tissue specimens. It is of major importance to distinguish Acanthamoeba from Naegleria. There are two definitive criteria for distinguishing Acanthamoeba from Naegleria: (1) the Acanthamoeba does not have a flagellar phase while Naegleria does have a flagellar phase, and (2) Acanthamoeba infections are diagnosed by the findings of the characteristic cysts, while Naegleria infections will be diagnosed by the finding of the characteristic trophozoites.

The Mastigophora

The Intestinal Flagellates

     The differential identification criteria for these organisms may be found in Table 3.

GIARDIA LAMBLIA   Giardia lamblia is the only one of the intestinal flagellates that is considered to be pathogenic. It is the causative agent of "giardiasis".

DISTRIBUTION   Giardia lamblia is world-wide in distribution. As in the case of E. histolytica, it is most prevalent in areas where poor hygiene and poor sanitation prevail. Although not often seen in epidemic outbreaks, more and more cases are being reported, most of which have been traced to contaminated drinking water.

EPIDEMIOLOGY   Human infection with Giardia is usually acquired by means of food and water contamination in much the same way as E. histolytica infection.

LIFE CYCLE   Giardia lamblia has two distinct stages: the cyst stage and the trophozoite stage. The cyst is the infective stage. Once ingested, the cyst will break down in the duodenum. The trophozoite will then attach on the epithelial cells of the intestine by means of their sucking discs. Cysts will develop as the trophozoites descend the intestinal tract.

PATHOGENESIS   Children are more frequently affected by G. lamblia than are adults. The most frequent symptoms include diarrhea, abdominal cramps and pains, epigastric tenderness, and large amounts of fatty stools. In severe cases, fat soluble vitamin deficiencies, hypoproteinemia, and folic acid deficiency may develop.

DIAGNOSTIC CRITERIA   The diagnosis is primarily made upon finding characteristic cysts or trophozoites in stool specimens. Giardia lamblia is probably the easiest of all the intestinal protozoa to identify. The specific diagnostic and identification criteria are shown on Table 2. The definitive criteria include: (a) in the cyst: the number, location, and karyosomal chromatin mass of the nuclei, and the presence of an axostyle; (b) in the trophozoite the shape of the organism: the number, location, and karysomal chromatin pattern of the nuclei, the organism's bilateral symmetry, motility, and the sucking disc.

CHILOMASTIX MESNILI   This organism is considered non-pathogenic. It is of clinical importance in that it must be distinguished from the pathogenic Giardia lamblia. The cysts of Chilomastix may be distinguished from those of Giardia by their shape, the presence of a knob-like projection on the cyst, and the nuclear structure. The trophozoites of Chilomastix may be distinguished from those of Giardia by the shape of the trophozoite, the presence of a spiral groove, by the cytostome, and by the nuclear structure.

TRICHOMONAS HOMINIS   This organism is considered to be non-pathogenic. It is of clinical importance for two reasons: (1) T. hominis must be distinguished from the pathogenic Giardia lamblia, and (2) since T. hominis is the only intestinal flagellate that does not have a cyst stage, the finding of T. hominis in stool specimens is indicative of direct fecal contamination. The specific diagnostic criteria include: the organisms jerky motility, the presence of an undulating membrane, and the size and length of the organisms axostyle.

Flagellates of the Oral Cavity and the Genito-Urinary System

The organisms of this group are: Trichomonas tenax and Trichomonas vaginalis. These two species of Trichomonas are closely related to T. hominis. One is a commensal organism found in the oral cavity, while the other is a pathogenic organism of the genito-urinary system. While it might be an academic adventure to try to distinguish these morphologically, it is not necessary for the clinical laboratory scientist to attempt to do so since the trichomonads are site specific.

TRICHOMONAS TENAX   This organism is a commensal organism found in the oral cavity. T. tenax is usually found in individuals having unclean or diseased oral cavities and it is usually transmitted by direct contact.

TRICHOMONAS VAGINALIS   This organism is considered pathogenic. It appears more frequently in females than in males.

DISTRIBUTION   T. vaginalis is cosmopolitan in distribution.

EPIDEMIOLOGY   Since there is no cyst stage to the trichomonads, the most probable mode of transmission is probably through sexual contact, while the secondary mode is probably via contaminated clothing and towels.

PATHOGENESIS   T. vaginalis produces a profuse vaginal discharge, itching and burning sensations, frequency of urination, dysuria, and possible urethritis.

DIAGNOSTIC CRITERIA   Diagnosis of T. vaginalis is most commonly made upon finding the characteristic trophozoites in vaginal and urethral discharges. Definitive criteria include: site of infection, shape, mobility, and the undulating membrane.

Blood and Tissue Flagellates

The organisms of this group are: Trypanosoma gambiense, Trypanosoma rhodesiense, Trypanosoma crizi, Leishmania tropica, Leishmania braziliensis and Leishmandia donovani.

TRYPANOSOMA GAMBIENSE   T. gambiense is the causitive agent of West African or Gambian sleeping sickness.

DISTRIBUTION   T. gambiense is widely distributed in central western Africa.

EPIDEMIOLOGY   T. gambiense is transmitted to humans via a certain species of Glossina (tsetse fly).

LIFE CYCLE   The life cycle in the tsetse fly takes about 20-22 days. The trypanosomal form is ingested by the tsetse, and divides in the stomach. The crithidial form of the organism migrates to the salivary glands where further multiplication takes place. Further development leads to formation of the trypanosomal form which is now ready for transmission to the vertebrate host at the next feeding.

PATHOGENESIS   Following the infecting bite of the tsetse, a local reaction in the form of a nodule, appears in about 1 week. Ten days to four years later, additional symptoms follow, including: fever, night sweats, headache, and lymphadenopathy. Within 6 months to a year, CNS symptoms appear. These symptoms include: lethargy, apathy, irritability, character changes, headache, motor and sensory changes, convulsions, hemiplegia or paraplegia, tremors, and slurred speach. These CNS symptoms may be intermittent or progressive. The patient eventually becomes comatose, and dies due to malnutrition or infection.

DIAGNOSTIC CRITERIA   Diagnosis of T. gambiense is made upon finding the characteristic organisms in blood, or nodule aspirates. Thick film blood preparations stained with one of the Romanowsky stains yields the best results.

TRYPANOSOMA RHODESIENSE   T. rhodesiense is the causative agent of East African or Rhodesian sleeping sickness.

DISTRIBUTION   T. rhodesiense is found in a smaller area of Africa than T. gambinese. T. rhodesiense is found in Eastern Africa, although there is some overlap, primarily in Uganda.

EPIDEMIOLOGY   T. rhodesiense, like T. gambinese is transmitted via a species of Glossina (tsetse fly).

LIFE CYCLE   The life cycle of T. rhodesiense is similar to that of T. gambiense.

PATHOGENSIS   The most significant difference between T. rhodesiense and T. gambiense is found in the course of the disease. T. rhodesiense is similar to T. gambiense, however, the progression of symptoms is much more acute with T. rhodesiense. The incubation period is much shorter. CNS involvement may appear as early as 1 month after infection.

DIAGNOSTIC CRITERIA   Diagnosis of T. rhodesiense is made upon finding the characteristic organisms in blood, or nodule aspirates. Thick film blood preparations stained with one of the Romanowsky stains yields the best results.

TRYPANOSOMA CRUZI   This organism is the causative agent of Chagas' disease of South American trypanosomiasis.

DISTRIBUTION   T. cruzi is found in Mexico, Central America, South America, and some southern parts of the United States.

EPIDEMIOLOGY   T. cruzi is transmitted to man by the bite of the reduviid bug (Panstrongylus megistus) a species of triatomid bugs, also known as kissing bugs. When the reduviid bug bites, then deficates, the infective organisms in the feces of the bug migrate into the open wound of the bite.

MORPHOLOGY   The trypanomastigote (trypanosomal form) of the organism measures approximately 20 microns in length. It has a centrally located nucleus and a large, prominent, oval kinetoplast. In peripheral blood films, T. cruzi characteristically is found in C or U forms.

PATHOGENESIS   The acute form of the disease is most commonly found in children under 5 years of age. The subacute and chronic forms are more commonly found in older children and adults. The initial reaction to the bite results in the formation of an erythematous lesion known as a chagoma. Chagomas are most frequently found on the face, but many also are found elsewhere. The chagoma may become quite large and very painful. These lesions will subside over a period of 2-3 months. Enlargement of lymph nodes, and facial edema follow. In about 10 days, the organisms may be found in the blood stream. In the acute stage, chills, fever, muscular aches, and exhaustion are characteristic. Young children may exhibit CNS signs within a few days. Older children and adults may not have or exhibit CNS involvement. Severe cases may end fatally or may continue as a chronic case. Chronic cases may display a variety of cardiac arrhythmias and/or cardiac failure.

Unlike African trypanosomiasis, Chagas' disease characteristically shows development of the amastigotes (leishmanial forms) in cells of many of the body's tissues, most often cardiac tissue.

DIAGNOSTIC CRITERIA   Diagnosis is generally based on finding the characteristic trypanomastigotes in peripheral blood films or finding the amastigotes in biopsies of affected lymph nodes and other body tissues. A complement fixation test, the Machado-Guerreiro test, which utilizes T. cruzi antigen is very specific. Indirect hemagglatination and indirect fluorescent antibody tests are also available.

LEISHMANIAS   Three species of Leishmanias are recognized pathogens in man. The life cycles and morphology of the Leishmanias are identical, and speciation is usually based on clinical findings.

LEISHMANIA TROPICA   Leishmania tropica is the causative agent of cutaneous leishmaniasis or oriental sore.

DISTRIBUTION   Leishmania tropica is endemic in the countries bordering the Mediterranean Sea, Central Africa, Central and Northern India and Turkestan.

EPIDEMIOLOGY   Transmission of the disease is most frequently through the bite of sandflies of the genus Phlebotomus, although it may occur by way of other reservoirs such as gerbils, dogs, cats, cattle, and sheep. Contact infection is also possible. When the sandfly bites, it regurgitates the promastigote (leptomonal form) into the wound. The promastigotes invade local tissues and become amastigotes which are obligate intracellular parasitic organisms. Multiplication of the amastigotes takes place in tissue cells, ultimately causing rupture of the host cells.

The organisms released then invade more cells producing lesions that are characteristic of the species.

MORPHOLOGY   The amastigotes of all three species are identical in morphology. In size, the amastigotes are similar to normal platelets, measuring 1.5-4.0 microns. They are ovoid to spherical intracellular organisms with a rounded nucleus and elongated parabasal body. They are found parasitizing endothelial cells, monocytes, and polymorphonuclear leukocytes.

PATHOGENESIS   After an incubation period, which averages between 2-6 months, a small red papule appears at the site of inoculation. The lesion grows and eventually ulcerates. Once ulcerated, the lesion enlarges centrifugally forming a crateriform ulcer with raised erythematous edges. The ulcers almost always become secondarily infected by bacteria. Regional lymph nodes may become enlarged. Untreated infections usually heal within a year leaving a depressed scar.

DIAGNOSTIC CRITERIA   Diagnosis of L. tropica is made upon finding the characteristic organisms in skin scrapings or cultures. The Montenegro skin test will be positive in L. tropica infections.

LEISHMANIA BRAZILIENSIS   L. braziliensis is the causative agent of mucocutaneous leishmaniasis.

DISTRIBUTION   This form of leishmaniasis is seen in the Western hemisphere, primarily in Mexico, Central America, and South America.

EPIDEMIOLOGY   The epidemiology of L. braziliensis is identical to that of L. tropica.

MORPHOLOGY   The morphology of L. braziliensis is identical to that of L. tropica.

PATHOGENESIS   There is an incubation period of 10 days to several months following the inoculation of the organisms. The initial lesion is usually a papule that may burn and itch. The papule then becomes a nodule. The lesions then assume characteristics peculiar to the geographic location. These characteristic lesions range from cauliflower masses found on infected people in parts of South America, to the chiclero ulcer found on the chicle-plantation workers of Mexico and Guatemala. The lesions are painful, may invade the mucous membranes, and are often subject to secondary bacterial infection. The lesions may heal spontaneously, may be secondarily infected by bacteria, or may result in death due to complicating infection.

DIAGNOSTIC CRITERIA   The diagnosis is based on the finding of the parasite from skin scrapings, culturing, and the Montenegro skin test.

LEISHMANIA DONOVANI L. donovani is the causative agent of visceral leishmaniasis or kala-azar.

DISTRIBUTION   L. donovani is endemic in parts of India, China, USSR, South America, and countries bordering the Mediterranean Sea.

EPIDEMIOLOGY   Transmission of L. donovani is the same as that of L. tropica and L. braziliensis, that is, primarily through the bite of sandflies of the genus Phlebotomus.

MORPHOLOGY   The morphology of the parasites of L. donovani is the same as that of L. tropica and L. braziliensis.

PATHOGENESIS   An incubation period ranging from several months to many years follows the bite of the sandfly. The incubation period is sometimes followed by the appearance of small papules. There is often a chill and fever that may be confused with malaria, but may be distinguished by a common finding of two fever spikes in a day. There may be marked hepatosplenomegally resulting in a swollen abdomen. Dysentery may be produced by invasion of the intestinal tract, and secondary bacterial infection may follow a complicating leukopenia.

DIAGNOSTIC CRITERIA   Diagnosis is made on finding the characteristic organisms from biopsies of tissues, blood smears, or from culture. The Montenegro skin test is positive *after* successful treatment.

Ciliata

BALANTIDIUM COLI   Balantidium coli is the only ciliate currently recognized as being parasitic to humans.

DISTRIBUTION   Although B. coli is cosmopolitan in distribution, it is rarely found in most areas, and is rarely encountered in humans.

EPIDEMIOLOGY   Infection is primarily due to contamination of food by fecal material containing the cysts of the organism. Epidemic outbreaks in the U. S. have been reported in mental hospitals, but rarely in the general population.

MORPHOLOGY   B. coli like most amebas, has two stages, a trophozoite state and a cyst stage.

PATHOGENESIS   After ingestion, the organisms usually inhabit the large intestine. The organisms are most frequently found in the cecum, but may be found elsewhere in the colon. The organisms may invade the intestinal mucosa producing ulceration of the bowel and colitis and/or dysentery closely resembling amebiasis. Ulceration through the muscularis mucosa may occur resulting in peritonitis, but this is rare.

DIAGNOSTIC CRITERIA   Diagnosis is made on finding the characteristic cysts in fecal specimens.

Sporozoa

Intestinal Sporozoa

ISOSPORA BELLI   Isopora belli is a parasite of the intestines.

DISTRIBUTION   Infections with Isospora belli have been reported from all parts of the world.

LIFE CYCLE   There is very little information available concerning the life cycle of Isospora. Both asexual and sexual development take place in man's intestine. Asexual development takes place in the intestinal wall. Eventually, the gametocytes are formed, and produce oocysts. These oocysts are oval or elliptical, measuring 30 microns X 10 microns. Soon after the oocyst formation, two sporablasts are formed within the oocyst. The sporoblasts develop heavy cyst walls becoming sporocysts. Within each sporocyst, four sporozoites develop. All states of oocysts and sporocysts may be found in stool specimens.

PATHOGENESIS   Infection with Isospora, for the most part, is asymptomatic. Those infections that do produce symptoms have symptoms that may include: nausea, abdominal pain or diarrhea. There are further indications that infection with Isospora may produce intestinal malabsorption.

DIAGNOSTIC CRITERIA   Diagnosis is made on the basis of finding the characteristic oocysts or sporocysts in stool specimens. These organisms are very often missed, and special care should be taken when these organisms are suspected.

Tissue Sporozoa

TOXOPLASMA GONDII   Toxoplasma gondii is the causative agent of toxoplasmosis.

DISTRIBUTION   Toxoplasma is cosmopolitan is distribution.

EPIDEMIOLOGY   Human infection with Toxoplasma occurs in a variety of ways. It occurs most commonly through the soiled hands-to-mouth route, through contaminated food, and transplacentally. The soiled hands-to-mouth route is commonly the result of handling contaminated cat feces, litterpans, or soil. Contamination of food is usually the result of handling infected meat. Infection from ingestion of contaminated meat is usually due to insufficient cooking. Transplacental transmission usually occurs in acute maternal infections and may lead to severe problems for the unborn or newborn child.

LIFE CYCLE   The complete life cycle of Toxoplasma is best seen in the cat. There are both asexual and sexual stages of development. In humans, tachyzoites, rapidly multiplying and spreading infections, and bradyzoites, slowly developing chronic infections, are the only phases of development. These are known as the tissue stages. The organisms have been described as crescent shaped with one end more pointed than the other, containing a round nucleus located closer to the rounded end. They measure approximately 5 microns X 2 microns.

PATHOGENESIS   Most infections in adults and older children are asymptomatic. Mild to severe infections most often have symptoms similar to those of infectious mononucleosis. These are chills, fever, headache, lymphadenitis and exhaustion. However, in intra-uterine and neonatal infections, the infection is much more serious. Most of these infections are severe infections which may result in chorioretinitis leading to blindness, or may produce hydrocephalus, microcephaly, cerebral calcification, convulsions, and mental retardation.

DIAGNOSTIC CRITERIA   Diagnosis of toxoplasmosis is often based on positive Sabin-Feldman dye tests, indirect fluroscent antibody tests, or indirect hemagglulination tests.

PNEUMOCYSTIS CARINII   Pneumocystis carinii has traditionally been associated with plasma cell pneumonia in infants, and more recently, as a cause of penumonia in patients having immune paresis due to immunologic disorders and immunosuppresion.

DISTRIBUTION   Pneumocystis carinii is cosmopolitan in distribution.

EPIDEMIOLOGY   Pneumocystis is primarily an air-borne infection.

LIFE CYCLE   Very little information is available about the life cycle of Pneumocystis carinii.

PATHOGENESIS   Pneumocystis carinii produces a pneumonia that is usually severe and fatal in neonates. This is most often a pneumonia without fever or cough.

DIAGNOSTIC CRITERIA   Diagnosis of infection with Pneumocystis carinii is based on the findings of the parasites or cysts in smears from the lungs and sputum.

Blood Sporozoa

The differential identification criteria for these organisms may be found in Table 4.

The organisms of this group are: Plasmodium vivax, Plasmodium ovale, Plasmodium malariae, Plasmodium falciparum, and Babesia bigemina.

PLASMODIUM VIVAX   Plasmodium vivax is the causative agent of benign tertian or vivax malaria.

DISTRIBUTION   Plasmodium vivax is found in all of the geographic areas in which malaria is endemic.

EPIDEMIOLOGY   Plasmodium vivax is spread via the bite of the appropriate species of Anopheles mosquitoes. There are two requisites for transmission: (1) the anopheles mosquito, and (2) infected humans.

LIFE CYCLE   (A) In the mosquito: when the female Anopheles mosquito bites a game-tocyte bearing human, and ingests both male and female gametocytes, sporogeny may commence. Fertilization of the female macrogametocyte by a male microgametocyte results in the formation of a zygote. The zygote develops into an ookinete which penetrates the mosquito's stomach and becomes an oocyst. Maturation of the oocyst results in the production of many sporozoites which break out of the stomach wall. The sporozoites that migrate to the salivary glands of the mosquito are now capable of being injected into a human the next time the mosquito bites. (B) In humans: when the mosquito bites and injects the sporozoites into the blood stream, the sporozoites leave the blood stream very quickly, and enter the parenchymal cells of the liver. It is here in the liver parenchymal cells that schizogony (asexual reproduction) begins. This is known as the pre-erythrocytic or exoerythrocytic phase of development. The asexual development produces merozoites. When the merozoites are released from the liver cells, some of them will infect other parenchymal liver cells, while others will invade red blood cells. The merozoites in the liver cells remain as a reserve or reservoir for probable later release. Those merozoites that enter the red blood cells begin their asexual development in what is referred to as the erythrocytic phase. In the red blood cells, the developing organisms start out as ring shaped trophozoites, which, as they mature will form either schizonts that will produce more merozoites to continue the erythocytic process, or gametocytes which the mosquito will pick up to continue the cycle.

MORPHOLOGY   The morphology of Plasmodium vivax in red blood cells proceeds as follows: when the red blood cell is first infected, the parasites will be found in the form of early trophozoites as small discs. In P. vivax, the early trophozoites may also be found in the form of crescent shapes at the very border of the red cell in what is sometimes referred to as the applique form. The next stage is the signet ring stage, in which the trophozoite will have developed into a ring form that is approximately 1/3 the diameter of the infected cell. As this ring form develops, there may be basophilic strippling of the red cell. The ring form will ultimately give way to a very ameboid form with many irregular shapes. As this occurs, the red blood cell will become enlarged, and Schuffner's dots may be seen in the red cell. The mature trophozoite will develop into what is known as a schizont. As the schizont matures, the nucleus will divide producing from 12-24 nuclear masses, each of which will become enveloped in cytoplasm resulting in the formation of merozoites. Ultimately the red blood cell ruptures, releasing the merozoites which will then infect other red blood cells. Those organisms that do not develop into merozoites will develop into gametocytes. The macro and micro gametocytes may be distinguished by the density of their nucleii.

PATHOGENESIS   The incubation period following the bite of the mosquito ranges from 1-3 weeks, during which time the organisms are developing in the liver cells. Towards the end of this incubation period, the patient may suffer prodromal symptoms that include: headache, myalgia, nausea and vomiting. The primary attack is rarely a typical paroxysm of vivax malaria because the organisms are not in cycle. Eventually, one particular group of organisms tends to dominate, and typical paroxyms occur. A typical paroxysm of vivax malaria usually follows this pattern: the paroxysm starts with sudden, shaking chills which may last for hours; this is followed by the "hot" stage, with fevers as high as 104° - 105°F, headache, nausea, and myalgia; this is followed by the "sweating" or wet stage where the patient sweats profusely for a period of 2 - 6 hours. The entire paroxysm may last 10 - 12 hours or longer. These paroxysms will continue, every 48 hours, for approximately 2 weeks, each one somewhat less intense that the previous. Following this primary attack, there is a latent period, after which a second attack may occur. These attacks may continue for as long as 2 months. Recurrences of this cycle may take place periodically for 2 - 5 years, until the exoerythrocytic cycle is spent. In addition to the symptoms of the paroxysm, the patient usually exhibits hepatosplenomegally, anemia, and iron deficiency due to increased red cell destruction, formation of malarial pigment from the infected cells' hemoglobin, and depletes iron stores. Since Plasmodium vivax has an affinity for newly formed red blood cells (reticulocytes) there is rarely more than 2% of the circulating red blood cells that are affected.

DIAGNOSTIC CRITERIA   Diagnosis of vivax malaria is based on: (1) clinical findings; (2) finding the characteristic parasites in thick and think blood smears; and (3) indirect fluorescent antibody (IFA) tests.

PLASMODIUM OVALE   Plasmodium ovale is the causative agent of benign tertian or ovale malaria.

DISTRIBUTION   Plasmodium ovale is found in West Africa, South America, and Asia.

EPIDEMIOLOGY   The epidemiology of P. ovale is similar to that of P. vivax.

LIFE CYCLE   The life cycle of P. ovale is similar to that of P. vivax.

MORPHOLOGY   The morphology of P. ovale is similar to that of P. vivax, with certain specific differences. These differences are: (1) the applique form is not usually seen in P. ovale; (2) while the cell is enlarged, and contains Schuffner's dots or granules, it usually results in the production of red cells that are ovoid or irregularly shaped; (3) the red cells infected with P. ovale often have fimbrinated edges; and (4) the number of merozoites produced averages about 8, and on rare occasions up to 18.

PATHOGENESIS   The pathogenesis of P. ovale is similar to that of P. vivax, but usually is milder.

DIAGNOSTIC CRITERIA   Diagnosis of ovale malaria is based on finding the characteristic organisms on thick and thin blood smears.

PLASMODIUM MALARIAE   Plasmodium malariae is the causative agent of benign quartan or malariae malaria.

DISTRIBUTION   Plasmodium malariae is predominantly found in those endemic areas that are subtropical or temperate in climate.

EPIDEMIOLOGY   The epidemiology of P. malariae is similar to that of P. vivax.

LIFE CYCLE   The life cycle of P. malariae is similar to that of P. vivax except that there is probably one cycle of schizogony in the liver, and the erythrocytic phase takes 72 hours instead of 48 hours.

MORPHOLOGY   The intracellular morphology of Plasmodium malariae is similar to that of Plasmodium vivax with specific differences that include: (1) the lack of the applique form; (2) there is no enlargement of the red blood cells; (3) the amoeboid activity of the trophozoite often produces band or ribbon like structures in the red cells; (4) there is significantly more malarial pigment formed and found in the cells; and (5) the number of merozoites formed is usually 8, and sometimes found encircling a rather large mass of malarial pigment.

PATHOGENESIS   The pathogenesis of P. Malariae is similar to that of P. vivax with three exceptions: (1) the incubation period is longer; (2) there is a 72-hour cycle instead of 48 hours; and (3) nephrotic syndrome is a complication that seems to be peculiar to P. malariae. In addition, P. malariae has an affinity for older red blood cells.

PLASMODIUM FALCIPARUM   Plasmodium falciparum is the causative agent of malignant tertian, sub-tertian, estivoautumnal, or falciparum malaria.

EPIDEMIOLOGY   The epidemiology of Plasmodium falciparum is similar to that of Plasmodium vivax with the exception that transmission and infection with P. falciparum takes place during the hot summer and early autumn weather.

LIFE CYCLE   The life cycle of Plasmodium falciparum is similar to that of Plasmodium vivax except that there is only one exoerythrocytic cycle in the liver.

MORPHOLOGY   The morphology of Plasmodium falciparum is essentially the same as that of Plasmodium vivax with the following exceptions: (1) applique forms are found; (2) multiple infection of individual red blood cells is common; (3) whereas P. vivax and P. ovale have an affinity for young red cells, and P. malariae has an affinity for older red cells, P. falciparum will attack any red blood cell; (4) Maurer's dots may be found; (5) the mature schizont produces an average of 24 merozoites; and (6) the gametocytes of Plasmodium falciparum are elongated or sausage shaped.

PATHOGENESIS   The pathogenesis of Plasmodium falciparum is significantly different from other forms of malaria in that the other forms are not usually fatal and Plasmodium falciparum can cause death. The paroxysm differs in that the chill state is mild, and often undetectable, the fever or hot stage, is prolonged with very high temperatures, and the wet or sweating period is short. The paroxysm may last as long as 36 hours. There may be continual paroxysms due to the fact that one paroxysm may be subsiding as the next is starting. Complications of Plasmodium falciparum infection include: (1) hyperpyrexia, where the temperature may exceed 108° F resulting in delirium, coma, and death; (2) algid malaria is another complication where the external temperature may be cool, while the internal temperature may be extremely high; (3) complications resembling cholera with the patient having loose, numerous stools, severe hydration and death; (4) acute hemolytic crisis may occur known as black-water fever, so called because of a very severe hemoglobinuria, which results in anemia and renal failure; and (5) red cells that are parasitized with Plasmodium falciparum have a tendency to stick to the walls of capillaries and other small blood vessels resulting in impared blood flow, hemostasis, and the production of thrombi.

DIAGNOSTIC CRITERIA   Diagnosis is based upon finding the appropriate morphological forms in thin and thick blood smears, and indirect fluorescent antibody (IFA) tests.

BABESIA BIGEMINA   This is the causative agent of Babesiosis in humans, and Texas cattle fever in bovines.

DISTRIBUTION   Human infection has been reported from Nantucket Island in Massachusetts.

EPIDEMIOLOGY   Infection with Babesia is by the appropriate species of ticks.

MORPHOLOGY   The organisms are intracellular organisms found in human red blood cells.   They are pleomorphic ringlike structures that appear, usually, as rabbit ear-like structures.   These organisms must be distinguished from malarial parasites and this may be accomplished by the fact that Babesia does not display the typical red staining chromatin mass.

PATHOGENESIS   Babesia predominantly presents with flu-like symptoms of malaise, fever, chills, sweats, body aches, and weakness.   The symptoms last for several weeks.

DIAGNOSTIC CRITERIA   Diagnosis of Babesiosis is based on finding the characteristic organisms on blood smears, physical findings, and history of travel to an endemic area.

HELMINTHS

Trematodes

The trematodes are commonly referred to as flukes.   These are organisms that are capable of self-fertilization, are flattened, have complex life-cycles, and have one or more intermediate hosts.   The differential identification criteria for these organisms may be found in Table 5.

Intestinal Flukes

The organisms of this group are: Fasciolopsis buski, Heterophyes heterophyes, and Metagonimus yokogawi.

FASCIOLOPSIS BUSKI   This organism is also known as the giant intestinal fluke.

DISTRIBUTION   Fasciolopsis buski is endemic in China, Thailand, Vietnam, and other parts of Southeast Asia.

EPIDEMIOLOGY   Infection with Fasciolopsis buski is acquired by the ingestion of the infective metacercariae which are found encysted on fresh water vegetation.

LIFE CYCLE   The life cycle of Fasciolopsis buski is a typical fluke life cycle. Eggs, which are deposited in the water, hatch releasing a miracidium.   The miracidium is ingested by the appropriate snail (intermediate host).   Development of the miracidium results in the production of cercariae.   These cercariae develop into metacercariae which then encyst on fresh water vegetation such as bamboo shoots and water chestnuts.   The fresh water vegetation are either ingested raw, or peeled with the teeth.   The metacercariae, once ingested, develop   into   the adult worm in the human intestinal tract.

MORPHOLOGY   Fasciolopsis buski is the largest trematode that is parasitic to humans.   The adult worm measures approximately 7.5 cm in length.   The ova measure 130-140 microns X 80-85 microns.

PATHOGENESIS   The adult worm attaches to the mucosa of the small intestine. Light infections may not produce symptoms. In heavy infections, symptoms may include: diarrhea, abdominal pain, intestinal obstruction, edema, and ascites.

DIAGNOSTIC CRITERIA   Diagnosis is based on finding the characteristic ova in the patient's stool specimens.

HETEROPHYIDS   There are two minute flukes that belong to this family; Metagonimus yokogawi, and Heterophyes heterophyes. These two organisms are quite similar and will be discussed together.

DISTRIBUTION   Both of these organisms are found throughout Asia. In addition, Heterophyes has been found in parts of Northern Africa, and Metagonimus has been found in parts of Europe and Russia.

EPIDEMIOLOGY   Infections with both of the organisms are acquired by the ingestion of raw, pickled, or improperly cooked fresh water fish containing the encysted metacercariae.

LIFE CYCLE   The life cycles of these organisms are identical. Ova of these worms are deposited into the water from the stools of infected individuals, infected cats, or infected dogs. The ova hatch, releasing miracidiae. The miracidiae are ingested by the appropriate snails. Development within the snail produces cercariae. The cercariae further develop into metocercariae which will encyst in the fish.

MORPHOLOGY   The adult worms of these two organisms are quite similar. Both are very small worms, measuring approximately 2mm in length by 0.5-0.75mm in width, Metagonimus being slightly larger than Heterophyes. One distinguishing difference is that Heterophyes has a third sucker around the genital pore, which is not found in Metagonimus. Morphology of the ova are also similar, measuring approximately 28 microns in length by 16 microns in width, operculated, yellow-brown in color, and have prominent opercular shoulders.

PATHOGENESIS   Patients infected with these organisms are usually asymptomatic; however, when heavily infected, patients may experience diarrhea, nausea, and abdominal discomfort.

DIAGNOSTIC CRITERIA   Diagnosis is based on finding the characteristic ova in the patient's stool specimens.

Liver Flukes

The two most important organisms in this group that parasitize humans are: Opistorchis (clonorchis) sinensis and Fasciola hepatica. These organisms invade the biliary tree and gall bladder.

OPISTORCHIS (CLONORCHIS) SINENSIS   This organism is also known as the Chinese Liver Fluke.

DISTRIBUTION   Opistorchis sinensis is found in areas of China, Japan, and Southeast Asia.

EPIDEMIOLOGY   Infection with Opistorchis is acquired by the ingestion of raw pickled, or improperly cooked fish containing the encysted metacercaria.

LIFE CYCLE   The life cycle of Opistorchis sinensis is similar to that of Heterophyes and Metagonimus.

MORPHOLOGY   The adult worms are flat, elongated, and narrow, measuring approximately 2 cm in length by approximately 0.5 cm in width. The ova are quite similar to those of Heterophyes and Metagonimus, with one distinguishing characteristic; opposite to the opercular end of the ovum is a knob or comma-like structure.

PATHOGENESIS   Humans that are heavily infected with Opistorchis may have fever, diarrhea, abdominal pain, hepatomegally, biliary obstruction, cholecystitis, cholelithiasis, and in some cases, portal cirrhosis.

DIAGNOSTIC CRITERIA   Diagnosis of infection with Opistorchis sinensis is based on finding the characteristic ova in the patient's stool specimens or bile aspirates.

FASCIOLA HEPATICA   This organism is also known as the sheep liver fluke.

DISTRIBUTION   Fasciola hepatica is cosmopolitan in distribution.

EPIDEMIOLOGY   Infection with Fasciola hepatica usually occurs after ingestion of aquatic vegetation, such as water cress, containing the infective metacercariae.

LIFE CYCLE   The life cycle of Fasciola hepatica is similar to that of Fasciolopsis buski.

MORPHOLOGY   The adult worm measures approximately 3 cm by 1.5 cm and has a characteristic shape. At the anterior end of the organism is a projection that is referred to as the "cephalic cone". The ova measure approximately 140 microns by 70 microns. They are difficult to distinguish from those of Fasciolopsis buski.

PATHOGENESIS   Light infections with Fasciola hepatica may be totally asymptomatic. Heavy infections may lead to hepatomegally, hepatitis, cirrhosis, and peritonitis.

DIAGNOSTIC CRITERIA   Diagnosis is made on finding the characteristic ova in stool specimens of infected patients. The major problem in the diagnosis of infection with Fasciola hepatica is the ability of the laboratory scientist to distinguish between the ova of Fasciola hepatica and those of Fasciolopsis buski for their ova are practically identical. Definitive diagnosis must include a history of travel and eating habits.

Blood Flukes

The organisms in this group are: Schistosoma mansoni, Schistosoma japonicum, and Schistosoma haematobium. The schistosomes, as a group, are significantly different from other trematodes because they have two sexes which are morphologically different.

SCHISTOSOMA MANSONI   Schistosoma mansoni is one of the causative agents of schistosomiasis or bilharzia.

DISTRIBUTION   Schistosoma mansoni is found in Africa, Brazil, Venezuela, the Guianas, parts of the West Indies, and Puerto Rico. In the United States, schistosomiasis due to Schistosoma mansoni is seen primarily in areas where there is a large number of people who have moved to the United States from Puerto Rico.

EPIDEMIOLOGY   Infection of humans occurs when the cercariae of Schistosoma penetrate skin which has been exposed to water containing the infective cercariae.

LIFE CYCLE   The life cycle of Schistosoma mansoni is typical of that of all of the schistosomes that parasitize humans. The eggs of Schistosoma mansoni are deposited in fresh water, where they hatch, releasing miracidiae. The miracidiae then penetrate the appropriate snail (intermediate host) and develop into many cercariae. The infective cercariae are then liberated from the snail into the water. When human skin is exposed to the water containing these cercariae, the cercariae penetrate the skin and invade the circulatory system. Once the young schistosomes are in the blood stream, they are carried to the liver. In the liver, further development to the adult stage takes place. The schistosomes then migrate through the portal system, against the blood flow, to the inferior mesenteric vein. Once in the inferior mesenteric vein, the schistosomes migrate to the small venules of the large intestine. In the venules of the large intestine the schistosomes deposit large numbers of ova which then break out into the lumen and are passed out of the body in the feces.

MORPHOLOGY   The schistosomes differ from other nematodes that parasitize humans because they have two distinct sexual types. The male adult schistosome measures approximately 1 cm in length with a flattened, incurved body giving it a cylindrical appearance. The female adult schistosome is significantly longer and more slender, measuring approximately 1.5 - 2.0 cm in length with an almost cylindrical body. The incurved body of the male adult schistosome forms a gynecophoral canal in which the female lies. The ova of Schistosoma mansoni measure 115-180 microns in length by 45-70 microns in width. These ova are ovoid, yellow-brown in color, and have a prominent lateral spine. The lateral spine is the distinguishing feature of the ova of Schistosoma mansoni.

PATHOGENESIS   The penetration of the infective cercariae of Schistosoma mansoni is, for the most part, asymptomatic. Adult development is likewise essentially asymptomatic. Symptoms usually appear with egg deposition. Egg deposition is usually accompanied by symptoms ranging from fever, chills, and gastrointestinal complaints to hepatic and pulmonary disorders. Eggs may be swept back to the liver by the portal blood flow and lodge in portal systems. This back flow of eggs is often accompanied by a tissue reaction. The tissue reaction results in the formulation of granulomas which may result in cirrhosis, portal hypertension and splenomegally. The complicating pulmonary or CNS disorders are usually the result of eggs that have been swept to those respective organs.

DIAGNOSTIC CRITERIA   Diagnosis of infection with Schistosoma mansoni is made by: (1) finding the characteristic ova in stool specimens; (2) finding the characteristic ova in tissue specimens; and (3) immunodiagnostic tests such as intradermal tests, complement fixation tests, and indirect hemagglutination tests.

SCHISTOSOMA JAPONICUM   This organism is also known as the Oriental blood fluke.

DISTRIBUTION   Schistosoma japonicum is confined to the Far East. It is found in the Yangtze river area of China, Japan, the Philippines, Laos, and Cambodia.

EPIDEMIOLOGY   The epidemiology of Schistosoma japonicum is similar to that of Schistosoma mansoni.

LIFE CYCLE   The life cycle of Schistosoma japonicum is similar to that of Schistosoma mansoni; however, there is one exception. The adults of Schistosoma japonicum inhabit the superior mesenterics.

MORPHOLOGY   The adult worms of Schistosoma japonicum tend to be larger than those of Schistosoma mansoni. The adult male worms measure approximately 2 cm in length while the females measure approximately 2.5 cm in length. The ova of Schistosoma japonicum are smaller than those of Schistosoma mansoni, measuring approximately

75-105 microns in length by approximately 50-80 microns in width. They are more round than oval, and do not exhibit a prominent spine. The ova of Schistosoma japonicum have a rudimentary lateral spine that is usually difficult to observe.

PATHOGENESIS   The course of this disease differs from that of Schistosoma mansoni in that the early course of the disease is more severe. This early stage is also known as Katayama disease or Yangtze River Fever.

DIAGNOSTIC CRITERIA   Diagnosis of Oriental schistosomiasis is made by: (1) finding the characteristic ova in stool specimens; (2) finding the characteristic ova in tissue specimens; and (3) immunodiagnostic tests such as intradermal tests, complement fixation tests and indirect hemagglutination tests.

SCHISTOSOMA HAEMATOBIUM   Schistosoma haematobium is the causative agent of urinary schistosomiasis.

DISTRIBUTION   Schistosoma haematobium is found throughout Africa, most abundantly in the Nile Valley.

EPIDEMIOLOGY   The epidemiology of Schistosoma haematobium is similar to that of Schistosoma mansoni.

LIFE CYCLE   The life cycle of Schistosoma haematobium is similar to that of Schistosoma mansoni. However, the adult worms migrate to the vesicle plexus. Schistosoma haematobium deposits its eggs in the walls of the urinary bladder. Those eggs deposited in the bladder wall may then break into the lumen of the bladder and be expelled in the urine.

MORPHOLOGY   The adult worms of Schistosoma haematobium are larger than those of Schistosoma mansoni. The adult male worm measures approximately 1.5 cm while the adult female measures approximately 2 cm. The ova of Schistosoma haematobium are the same size as those of Schistosoma mansoni. The differential characteristic of the ova of Schistosoma haematobium is the position of the spine on the ova. The spine is terminal on the ova of Schistosoma haematobium.

PATHOGENESIS   The initial reaction to the invasion of Schistosoma haematobium is similar to that of the other schistosomes. However, hepatic involvement is rare in urinary schistosomiasis. Urinary symptoms range from hematuria, cystitis, and fibrosis of the urinary bladder to hydronephrosis, ureter obstruction, and renal failure.

DIAGNOSTIC CRITERIA   Diagnosis of infection with Schistosoma haematobium is made by: (1) finding the characteristic ova in urine specimens; (2) finding the characteristic ova in tissue specimens; and (3) immunodiagnostic tests such as intradermal tests, complement fixation tests and indirect hemagglutination tests.

Lung Fluke

PARAGONIMUS WESTERMANI

DISTRIBUTION   Paragonimus westermani is found in the Far East, parts of South America and parts of Africa.

EPIDEMIOLOGY   Infection with Paragonimus westermani is acquired by the ingestion of raw, pickled, or improperly cooked fresh water crabs and crayfish containing the encysted metacercariae.

LIFE CYCLE   Eggs which are deposited in water will hatch releasing miracidiae.   The miracidiae then swim to the appropriate snail host, penetrate the snail, and undergo asexual development.   The asexual development results in the production of cercariae. When the cercariae escape they invade the appropriate fresh water crabs and crayfish and continue development which results in encysted metacercariae.   When humans ingest the raw, pickled, or improperly cooked infected crabs and crayfish the metacercariae excyst and penetrate the intestinal wall.   The young worms then wander in the abdominal cavity.   In approximately three weeks they penetrate the diaphragm, enter the lungs and become encapsulated.   Rupture of the capsule into a bronchiole results in large numbers of eggs being released.   Sputum containing these eggs is then expectorated or swallowed.

MORPHOLOGY   The adult worm of Paragonimus westermani is reddish-brown in color, and measures approximately 5mm-12mm in length.   The ova of Paragonimus westermani are brown, ovoid, operculated with raised opercular shoulders, and measure approximately 90 microns in length by 50 microns in width.

PATHOGENESIS   Infection with Paragonimus westermani produces few, if any symptoms, until the worm reaches maturity.   The adult worm, in the lungs, produces a variety of symptoms ranging from fever, cough, hemoptysis and bronchitis to bronchiectasis and progressive fibrosis of the lung.   Those worms that do not penetrate the diaphragm produce symptoms that vary with their location, such as, peritonitis, hepatitis, enteritis and brain lesions.

DIAGNOSTIC CRITERIA   Diagnosis of paragonimiasis is based on finding the characteristic ova in sputum or stool specimens.

The Cestodes

Intestinal Cestodes

   The organisms of this group are: Diphyllobothrium latum, Taenia solium, Taenia saginata, Dipylidium caninum, Hymenolepsis nana, and Hymenolepsis diminuta.   The differential identification criteria for these organisms may be found in Table 6.

DIPHYLLOBOTHRIUM LATUM   This organism is also known as the fish tapeworm and the broad tapeworm.

DISTRIBUTION   Diphyllobothrium latum is world-wide in distribution.   It is most frequently found in temperate regions.

EPIDEMIOLOGY   Human infection with Diphyllobothrium latum is acquired by the ingestion of raw, pickled, smoked, or improperly cooked fresh water fish containing the infective larval stage (sparganum).

LIFE CYCLE   The eggs of Diphyllobothrium latum hatch releasing a ciliated embryo called a coracidium.   The coracidium is then ingested by a copepod.   Within the copepod, the hexacanth ova will develop, becoming a larva.   When the copepod is eaten by the appropriate fresh water fish, the liberated larva will burrow into the flesh of the fish, developing into the next larval stage, the sparganum.   When humans eat the raw, pickled, smoked, or improperly cooked fish containing the sparaganum, the larva will degenerate leaving just the scolex which attaches to the mucosa.   Once attached, the scolex will develop a strobila.   Gravid proglottids produce ova which are passed in the feces.

MORPHOLOGY   The adult worm of Diphyllobothrium latum may grow to a length of 9 meters or more. The scolex of Diphyllobothrium latum is elongated, spoon shaped, and has two longtitudinal grooves. The proglottids are characteristically wider than long. The fact that the proglottids are wider than they are in length is the source of D. latum's name "the broad tapeworm". The gravid proglottids display a coiled uterus with a central uterine pore through which the eggs are released. The ova of Diphyllobothrium latum measure approximately 65 microns X 45 microns, are operculated, and at the end opposite the operculum there is a small knob-like projection.

PATHOGENESIS   Most infections with Diphyllobothrium latum are single worm infections. Most infected individuals exhibit no symptoms. Those infected people who do exhibit symptoms complain of abdominal discomfort, loss of appetite and weakness. A very small percentage of infected people have a megaloblastic anemia similar to pernicious anemia. The anemia that is associated with Diphyllobothrium latum infection appears to be the result of the location of the attachment of the adult worm. If the adult worm is attached to the small intestine, near the duodenum, it competes with the body for Vitamin B-12. Diphyllobothrium latum selectively absorbs Vitamin B-12 in large amounts, thereby producing a Vitamin B-12 deficiency and subsequent megaloblastic anemia.

DIAGNOSTIC CRITERIA   Diagnosis of human infection with Diphyllobothrium latum is made by finding the characteristic ova in stool specimens or finding the spent, atrophied proglottids. Of particular importance, is the differentiation between the ova of Diphyllobothrium latum and those of Paragonimus westermami. The terminal knob-like projection, when seen, provides the basis for this differentiation.

TAENIA SOLIUM   This organism is also known as the pork tapeworm.

DISTRIBUTION   Taenia solium is cosmopolitan in distribution. It is most commonly found in groups of people who eat pork.

EPIDEMIOLOGY   Infection with Taenia solium is acquired after ingestion of infected pork containing the infective larva.

LIFE CYCLE   When the gravid proglottids of Taenia solium are passed into the soil or upon vegetation, they are then ingested by a pig. After ingestion, the hexacanth ova are liberated and they penetrate the mucosal wall. After penetrating the mucosa, they enter the lymphatic system or the circulatory system and are carried throughout the body of the pig. They finally embed in the muscles of the pig, in the form of cysticerci. When humans ingest the infected pork, the scolex is liberated and attaches to the human intestinal mucosa. The attached scolex then develops a strobila. Gravid proglottids eventually are shed onto the soil and vegetation.

MORPHOLOGY   The adult worm of Taenia solium may reach a length of 3 meters. The scolex has four suckers and a double crown of hooks that are used for attachment to the mucosa. The proglottids are characteristically longer than wide. The mature proglottids have seven to ten lateral branches of the organisms uterus. The ova of Taenia solium measure approximately 35 microns in diameter and bear a hexacanth embryo.

PATHOGENESIS   Human infection with Taenia solium is usually asymptomatic.

DIAGNOSTIC CRITERIA   Diagnosis of Taenia solium infection is made upon find the characteristic gravid proglottids in stool specimens. Recovery of the scolex will also aid in diagnosis. Diagnosis cannot be based on finding the ova because the ova of Taenia solium cannot be distinguished from those of Taenia saginata.

TAENIA SAGINATA   This organism is also known as the beef tapeworm.

DISTRIBUTION   Taenia saginata is cosmopolitan in distribution and is found wherever raw or insufficiently cooked beef is consumed. Taenia saginata infection is more common in the United States than Taenia solium infection, because of the large number of people in the United States who prefer to eat rare steaks and rare roast beef.

EPIDEMIOLOGY   Human infection with Taenia saginata is acquired after the ingestion of raw or insufficiently cooked beef containing the infective larva.

LIFE CYCLE   The gravid proglottids of Taenia saginata are deposited into the soil or onto vegetation, and are eaten by cattle. After ingestion, the hexacanth ova are liberated and they penetrate the mucosa wall. After penetrating the musosa, the embryos enter the lymphatic system or the circulatory system and are carried throughout the body of the animal. They ultimately embed in the muscles of the animal in the larval form known as cysticerci. When humans ingest the infected beef, the scolex is liberated and attaches to the human intestinal mucosa. The attached scolex then develops a strobila. Gravid proglottids eventually are shed onto the soil and vegetation.

MORPHOLOGY   The adult worm of Taenia saginata may reach a length of 8 meters. The scolex has four suckers, but, unlike Taenia solium, it does not have hooks. The proglottids are characteristically longer than wide. The mature proglottids have approximately 15-20 lateral branches of the organisms uterus. The ova of Taenia saginata measure approximately 35 microns in diameter and bear a hexacanth embryo.

PATHOGENESIS   Human infection with Taenia saginata is usually asymptomatic.

DIAGNOSTIC CRITERIA   Diagnosis of Taenia saginata infection is made upon finding the characteristic gravid proglottids in the stool specimens. Recovery of the scolex will also aid in the diagnosis. Diagnosis cannot be based on the ova of Taenia saginata because the ova of Taenia saginata cannot be distinguished from those of Taenia solium.

DIPYLIDIUM CANINUM   This organism is also known as the dog tapeworm.

DISTRIBUTION   Dipylidium caninum is found world-wide in dogs and cats. It is occasionally found in man.

EPIDEMIOLOGY   Human infection with Dipylidium caninum is usually acquired by intimate contact with pets. This contact, usually in the form of kissing or hugging cats and dogs, usually occurs in children.

LIFE CYCLE   Ova of Dipylidium caninum are ingested by the fleas of the dog or cat. Development of cysticercoid larva takes place in the flea. Accidental ingestion of the fleas by the dog or cat results in infection of the dog or cat. The gravid proglottids of the adult worm are extremely motile, and migrate out of the anus of the dog or cat. Ultimately the ova of Dipylidium caninum are liberated from the gravid proglottids, and these are ingested by the flea, or accidentally by humans.

MORPHOLOGY   The adult worm of Dipylidium caninum is small, measuring approximately 20 cm in length. The scolex of Dipylidium caninum is conical, bears four suckers, and is "armed" with circles of hooks. The mature and gravid proglottids are characteristically longer than they are wide, often being referred to as barrel shaped. The ova of Dipylidium caninum are usually found in "packets". These egg packets contain anywhere from 5-30 ova per packet.

PATHOGENESIS   Human infection with Dipylidium caninum produces symptoms such as diarrhea and abdominal discomfort.

DIAGNOSTIC CRITERIA   Diagnosis of human infection with Dipylidium caninum is made upon finding the characteristic gravid proglottids in stool specimens. Occasionally, the diagnosis may be made by finding the egg packets in stool specimens.

HYMENOLEPSIS NANA   This organism is also known as the dwarf tapeworm.

DISTRIBUTION   Hymenolepsis nana is cosmopolitan in distribution.

EPIDEMIOLOGY   Human infection of Hymenolepsis nana is acquired via the hand-to-mouth route or by accidental ingestion of mouse feces.

LIFE CYCLE   When eggs of Hymenolepsis nana are ingested by rat or mice fleas, they develop into cyctercercoid larvae. These intermediate hosts may then be ingested by humans or rodents. When humans ingest the ova, the embryos are released. The hexacanth embryo invades the villi of the intestine and develops into the cysticercoid larva. The larvae then attach themselves to the intestinal mucosa and develop a strobila. The eggs of Hymenolepsis nana are released from the gravid proglottids and are either passed in the feces, or develop in the intestine.

MORPHOLOGY   The adult worm of Hymenolepsis nana is extremely small, measuring approximately 25mm in length. The scolex has four suckers and is "armed" with a single circle of hooks. The mature and gravid proglottids are characteristically wider than they are long. The ova of Hymenolepsis nana measure 35-45 microns in diameter, and consist of a hexacanth embryo surrounded by an inner shell. This oncosphere is oval, has polar knobs, and four to eight filaments projecting from the polar knobs.

PATHOGENESIS   Infection of humans with Hymenolepsis nana is most frequently seen in children. Light infections are generally asymptomatic. Heavy infections may occur as the result of the ova of a single worm developing in the intestine. Heavy infections result in the patient having symptoms that include abdominal pain, nausea, vomiting, diarrhea, and weight loss.

DIAGNOSTIC CRITERIA   Diagnosis of infection with Hymenolepsis nana is made upon finding the characteristic ova in stool specimens.

HYMENOLEPSIS DIMINUTA   This organism is also known as the rat tapeworm.

DISTRIBUTION   Hymenolepsis diminuta is cosmopolitan in distribution.

EPIDEMIOLOGY   Human infection with Hymenolepsis diminuta is usually the result of ingestion of infected insects from flour contaminated with rat droppings.

LIFE CYCLE   The life cycle of Hymenolepsis diminuta is dependent upon an intermediate arthropod host. The ova of Hymenolepsis diminuta are ingested by an insect, most importantly by flour moths and flour beetles, where they develop into a cysticercoid larvae. Ingestion of the infective larva by humans or rodents results in the development of the adult worm. Ingestion of the infected arthropod or rat droppings in flour is the usual source of infection in humans.

MORPHOLOGY   The adult worm of Hymenolepsis diminuta measures approximately 35 cm in length. The scolex has four suckers and a rostellum that does not have hooks. The mature and gravid proglottids are characteristically wider than they are long. The ova are similar to those of Hymenolepsis nana, having a thick outer shell and a hexacanth ova surrounded by an inner shell. The inner shell has polar thickenings but does not have polar filaments.

PATHOGENESIS   Humans infected with Hymenolepsis diminuta usually display no symptoms.

DIAGNOSTIC CRITERIA   Diagnosis of human infection with Hymenolepsis diminuta is made upon finding the characteristic ova in stool specimens of infected individuals.

Extraintestinal Cestodes

SPARGANOSIS

ETIOLOGY   Sparganosis is caused by worms of the genus Diphyllobothrium that normally grow to adulthood in other animals.

EPIDEMIOLOGY   Sparganosis is cosmopolitan in distribution. Human infection is the result of the accidental ingestion of the intermediate hosts.

PATHOGENESIS   When humans ingest the larva of these Diphyllobothrium worms the larva penetrate the gut and migrate to various tissues in the body. Once in the tissues, the larva will develop into the sparganum larval stage. The penetration and migration of the larva are asymptomatic. As the larva grows it produces local inflammatory reactions.

DIAGNOSTIC CRITERIA   Diagnosis of Sparganosis is made by finding the cestode tissue in surgically removed lesions.

CYSTICERCOSIS

ETIOLOGY   Cysticercosis is caused by the larva of Taenia solium.

EPIDEMIOLOGY   Cysticercosis is cosmopolitan in distribution and is the result of the ingestion of the ova of Taenia solium.

PATHOGENESIS   When humans ingest the ova of Taenia solium, either by the hand-to-mouth route or by contaminated food or drink, the oncosphere is liberated and penetrates the intestine. Penetration of the intestinal wall is followed by penetration of a blood vessel. Once in the blood stream, the larva may be carried to any organ. The penetration and migration of the larva is asymptomatic. Light infections are usually asymptomatic. Heavy infections, particularly those in the central nervous system, do produce symptoms. Heavy infections in muscle tissue appear to produce few, if any, symptoms. Heavy infection of visceral organs produce local inflammatory reactions after the death of the organism. Heavy infection in the central nervous system may produce epilepsy, hydrocephalus, and death.

DIAGNOSTIC CRITERIA   Diagnosis of cysticercosis is made by finding the cestode tissue in surgically removed lesions.

ECHINOCOCCUS GRANULOSUS   Echinococcus granulosus is the causative agent of Hydatid disease.

DISTRIBUTION   Echinococcus granulosus is cosmopolitan in distribution.

EPIDEMIOLOGY   Human infection with Echinococcus granulosus is accidental. Infection is usually the result of intimate association with infected dogs. Human infection occurs when man ingests the ova of Echinococcus granulosus.

LIFE CYCLE   The adult worm of Echinococcus granulosus is usually found in the intestine of the dog. The eggs, which are released, and subsequently ingested by humans, contain a hexacanth embryo. When humans ingest the ova of Echinococcus granulosus, the liberated oncosphere penetrates the intestinal wall and is carried to the liver. Development in the liver results in the formation of a cyst. As the cyst grows, brood capsules develop. The brood capsules contain scoleces which develop from the inner wall of the brood capsule. Occasionally daughter cysts will develop within the cyst. The cyst is known as a hydatid cyst, and free floating scoleces and bits of the inner wall are known as hydatid sand.

MORPHOLOGY   The adult worm of Echinococcus granulosus is very small, measuring approximately 6-7mm in length. The adult worm has an armed scolex, and usually three proglottids, one immature, one mature, and one gravid. The ova of Echinococcus granulosus are similar to those of Taenia solium and Taenia saginata. The hydatid cyst has a fibrous connective tissue outer wall and an inner wall of germinal epithelium. The cysts may grow to several centimeters in diameter, and contain liters of fluid.

PATHOGENESIS   Initially, humans with the hydatid cyst are usually asymptomatic. Over a period of years, the cyst will continue to grow. Symptoms will develop as the cyst increases pressure on the surrounding tissue. The majority of the cysts in humans are found in the liver. As the cyst grows, liver tissue may be damaged, resulting in impaired liver function. If the cyst is ruptured, there will be allergic reactions possibly resulting in anaphylactic shock.

DIAGNOSTIC CRITERIA   Diagnosis of Hydatid disease is based on immunodiagnostic procedures such as intradermal tests, complement fixation tests, bentonite-flocculation tests, indirect hemagglutination tests, and indirect fluorescent antibody tests. Confirmation of the diagnosis is made on finding the characteristic scoleces in surgically removed cysts.

MULTICEPS MULTICEPS   Multiceps multiceps is the causative agent of cenurosis.

ETIOLOGY   Cenurosis is the result of human infection with the larva of Multiceps multiceps, a dog tapeworm.

EPIDEMIOLOGY   Human infection with Multiceps multiceps occurs as the result of the accidental ingestion of Multiceps multiceps ova.

PATHOGENESIS   The invasion and migration of the larva of Multiceps multiceps is asymptomatic. Most developing larva in human infections occur in the central nervous system. As the cyst of Multiceps grows, neurological symptoms similar to those seen in brain tumors may develop. Prognosis in these cases of brain infection is poor.

The Nematodes

The Intestinal Nematodes

The organisms in this group are: Ascaris lumbricoides, Enterobius vermicularis, Ancylostoma duodenale, Necator americanus, Strongyloides stercoralis, Trichuris trichiura, and Trichostrongylus. The differential identification criteria for these organisms may be found in Table 7.

ASCARIS LUMBRICOIDES   Ascaris lumbricoides is the causative agent of ascariasis.

DISTRIBUTION   Ascaris lumbricoides is found throughout the world in the tropic, subtropic, and temperate areas.

EPIDEMIOLOGY   Human infection with Ascaris lumbricoides is acquired by the hand-to-mouth route, ingestion of contaminated raw vegetables, or consumption of infected drinking water.   The hand-to-mouth route is usually the manner in which children become infected, since they frequently play in soil which may be contaminated with Ascaris ova.   Contamination of raw vegetables is most frequently seen in areas where the use of night soil as a fertilizer is common.   Infection of drinking water is usually the result of crossed plumbing or pollution of wells with egg bearing top soil.

LIFE CYCLE   Human ingestion of infective ova results in the hatching of the ova, in the small intestine, and liberation of the infective larvae.   The infective larvae penetrate the mucosa and enter the circulatory system.   The larvae are carried to the lungs where they enter the alveoli.   In the alveoli the larvae will continue to grow, and molt.   The larvae then migrate up the respiratory tract to the pharynx.   The larvae are then swallowed and re-enter the intestinal tract where development of the adult takes place.   Approximately three months after the initial ingestion of the infective ova, the now adult female Ascaris, will begin producing eggs.   A mature female Ascaris may produce up to 200,000 ova per day.   These ova, when passed in the feces, are unsegmented.   Three weeks of incubation in moist soil will result in eggs containing infective larvae.

MORPHOLOGY   The adult worms of Ascaris lumbricoides are the largest intestinal roundworms found in humans.   The female worms measure approximately 30cm in length by 0.5 cm in diameter, while the male worms measure approximately 20 cm in length and are significantly thinner than the females.   They are white-pink in color and have a cuticle with circular striations.   Grossly, the adult Ascaris closely resembles the common earthworm.   The eggs of Ascaris lumbricoides are round or oval, measure approximately 45-70 microns in length by 40-60 microns in width, and have a distinctive albuminoid outer coating and thick inner shell.   The albuminoid coating is usually bile stained giving it a yellow to brown color.   Occasionally the Ascaris ova will have lost their albuminoid coating, these ova are referred to as decorticated ova.   Infertile ova may also be found, either due to faulty fertilization or the absence of male worms.   The infertile ova are usually longer than fertile ova measuring approximately 85 microns in length, giving the ova a more barrel shaped appearance.

PATHOGENESIS   Migration of the larvae through the lungs may produce a fever, cough, and pneumonitis.   Heavy infections of Ascaris lumbricoides in humans usually produce symptoms such as malnutrition, intestinal obstruction, blockage of the common bile duct, and penetration of the intestine.

DIAGNOSTIC CRITERIA   Diagnosis of infection with Ascaris lumbricoides is made by finding the characteristic ova in stool specimens.   Adults of Ascaris lumbricoides may be recovered in stool specimens, and occasionally in sputum and vomitus.   Immunodiagnostic tests that are employed in the diagnosis of ascariasis include bentonite flocculation tests and indirect hemagglutination tests.

ENTEROBIUS VERMICULARIS   This organism is more commonly known as the pinworm.

DISTRIBUTION   Enterobius vermicularis is cosmopolitan in distribution.   However, Enterobius is most frequently found in temperate regions of the world.

EPIDEMIOLOGY   Human infection with Enterobius vermicularis may occur through a variety of routes including: hand-to-mouth, contaminated food and drink, inhalation, or contact with contaminated clothing, towels, or bed linen.

LIFE CYCLE   When humans ingest the larvae bearing ova, the ova hatch, and the larvae continue development to adulthood in the small intestine. The worms migrate to the large intestine. In the colon, the adult worms mate. The gravid females then migrate to the anus. The females then, nocturnally, migrate out of the anus and oviposit as they die, liberating as many as 10,000 ova. The ova that are deposited are in the embryonic stage, and are not infective. However, within six hours the larvae in the eggs will be developed, and consequently the ova will be infective. In cool, moist, air, these infective ova will remain viable for approximately one week.

MORPHOLOGY   The adult worms of Enterobius vermicularis are very small. The males measure approximately 2.5mm while the female measure approximately 10mm. The male worms may be distinguished from the females in that the male worms have a curled tail, while the females have a sharply pointed tail. The ova of Enterobius vermicularis are ovoid, measure approximately 55 microns in length by 25 microns in width and are characteristically flattened on one side. These ova are clear, colorless, and usually contain a distinctive larva.

PATHOGENESIS   Infection with Enterobius vermicularis usually produces only one major sympton, namely puritis ani. This rectal itching may cause loss of sleep producing irritability and nervousness. The itching, with resulting scratching, is also a common source of reinfection.

DIAGNOSTIC CRITERIA   Diagnosis of human infection with Enterobius vermicularis is made on finding the characteristic ova in stool specimens or by using the Graham technique. The Graham technique is also known as the Scotch tape test. In the Scotch tape test, someone must apply the sticky side of some Scotch tape to the perianal region of the suspected infected person. The Scotch tape is then examined for the presence of the ova of Enterobius vermicularis. This procedure should be carried out for seven consecutive days.

ANCYLOSTOMA DUODENALE   Ancylostoma duodenale is also known as the Old World hookworm.

DISTRIBUTION   Ancylostoma duodenale is found in tropical and subtropical regions of Europe, Asia, Africa, South America and North America. This organism is also found in the temperate regions of Europe and North America for these areas have conditions favoring the organism's growth and development.

LIFE CYCLE   The eggs of Ancylostoma duodenale will develop in moist sandy soil resulting in the formation of larvae. The young larvae are known as rhabditiform larvae. The rhabditiform larvae grow and develop in the soil. When the rhabditiform larvae molt the second time, the larvae are transformed into filariform larvae. The filariform larvae are the infective form. The filariform larvae extend themselves into the air. When human skin comes in contact with the filariform larvae, the larvae penetrate the skin. After penetrating the skin, the larvae are carried by the circulatory system to the lungs. In the lungs, the larvae break into the alveolar spaces, migrate up the respiratory tract to the pharynx, and are swallowed. The larvae then undergo further development to adulthood in the small intestine. In the small intestine, mating and fertilization take place, and eggs are released which are passed in the feces.

EPIDEMIOLOGY   Human infection with Ancylostoma duodenale is acquired when human skin comes in contact with the infective larvae found in moist, sandy soil.

MORPHOLOGY   The adult worms of Ancylostoma duodenale measure approximately 1 cm in length. The females are slightly larger. The adult worms are whiteish in color. The mouth has three pair of teeth, two on either side of the median line and one further back in the buccal cavity. The males have a distinctive copulatory bursa at the posterior end of their body. The ova of Ancylostoma duodenale are oval, have a thin, colorless shell wall, and measure approximately 60 microns in length by 45 microns in width. The embryo within the ova normally have stages of development ranging from 2 cells to 8 cells.

PATHOGENESIS   Penetration of the skin by the filariform larvae of Ancylostoma duodenale may result in an allergic reaction in the form of a puritic dermatitis that is often referred to as ground itch, miner's itch, or water itch. Large numbers of larvae penetrating the alveoli may produce a pneumonitis. Heavily infected people may have diarrhea and abdominal pain. Since the adult worms attach themselves to the intestinal mucosa and ingest red blood cells, heavy chronic infections may lead to anemia due to the amount of blood lost.

DIAGNOSTIC CRITERIA   Diagnosis of infection with Ancylostoma duodenale is primarily made on finding the characteristic hookworm ova in stool specimens of infected individuals. The ova of Ancylostoma duodenale cannot be distinguished from those of Necator americanus. Occasionally, stool specimens may be examined after the specimens have been standing for long periods. When the specimens have been standing for long periods, the ova of Ancylostoma duodenale may hatch, releasing the rhabditiform larvae which would have to be distinguished from the larvae of Strongyloides stercoralis. The differentiation of these larvae may be accomplished by examining the buccal cavity and esophagus of the two organisms. The buccal cavity of the rhabditiform larva of Ancylostoma duodinale is much longer than that of Strongyloides stercolaris. The esophagus of the rhabditiform larvae of Ancylostoma is somewhat shorter and stouter than that of Strongyloides stercoralis.

NECATOR AMERICANUS   Necator americanus is also known as the New World hookworm.

DISTRIBUTION   The geographical distribution of Necator americanus is worldwide. However, it is the only hookworm found in large areas of North and South America.

EPIDEMIOLOGY   Infection with Necator americanus is acquired by humans in much the same way as infection with Ancylostoma duodenale.

LIFE CYCLE   The life cycle of Necator americanus is similar to that of Ancylostoma duodenale.

MORPHOLOGY   The morphology of Necator americanus is similar to that of Ancylostoma duodenale. However, there is one distinct difference in that Necator americanus has cutting plates in the buccal cavity instead of teeth as in the case of Ancylostoma duodenale.

PATHOGENESIS   The pathogenesis of Necator americanus is similar to that of Ancylostoma duodenale. However, the initial allergic reaction, that accompanies the skin penetration, is more common in humans infected with Necator americanus.

DIAGNOSTIC CRITERIA   Diagnosis of human infection with Necator americanus is similar to that of Ancylostoma duodenale.

STRONGYLOIDES STERCORALIS

DISTRIBUTION   The geographical distribution of Strongyloides stercoralis is similar to that of the hookworms Ancylostoma duodenale and Necator americanus.

EPIDEMIOLOGY   Human infection with Strongyloides stercoralis is acquired in the same way as the hookworms are acquired. There is one exception, namely that humans infected with Strongyloides stercoralis are capable of self re-infection. Re-infection is due to the fact that the ova of Strongyloides are hatched in the mucosa of the small intestine, and may transform into the infective filariform larvae.

LIFE CYCLE   The life cycle of Strongyloides stercoralis is similar to that of the hookworms with the following exceptions: (1) Strongyloides stercoralis may exist as a free-living organism; (2) the ova are deposited in the mucosa and are hatched there; and, (3) the filariform larvae may be developed in the intestine.

MORPHOLOGY   The adults of Strongyloides stercoralis are small, measuring approximately 1mm in length, with females being larger, reaching as much as 2mm in length. The larvae must be distinguished from those of the hookworms. In the manner previously discussed the rhabditiform larvae of Strongyloides stercoralis can be distinguished from the rhabditiform larvae of the hookworm. The filariform larvae of Strongyloides may be distinguished from those of the hookworm by the fact that the larvae of Strongyloides have a notched tail while the tail of the hookworm is not notched.

PATHOGENESIS   The pathogenesis of Strongyloides stercoralis is similar to that of the hookworms.

DIAGNOSTIC CRITERIA   The diagnosis of human infection with Strongyloides stercoralis is made on the same criteria that are used for the hookworms. However, finding the ova of Strongyloides is rather uncommon.

TRICHURIS TRICHIURA   Trichuris trichiura is more commonly referred to as the whipworm.

DISTRIBUTION   Trichuris trichiura is world-wide in distribution, particularly in tropical regions.

EPIDEMIOLOGY   Human infection with Trichuris trichiura is acquired by the ingestion of the fully embryonated ova. The ingestion of the infective ova may occur by way of the hand-to-mouth route, or by contaminated food and drink.

LIFE CYCLE   Once the embryonated eggs of Trichuris trichiura are ingested, they hatch and liberate a larva. The larva penetrates the intestinal villi where it undergoes development into adulthood. The adult worms migrate to the colon. In the colon, egg deposition takes place.

MORPHOLOGY   The adult worms of Trichuris trichiura measure approximately 4 cm in length. They are characteristically narrow at the anterior end, and fatter at the posterior end thus resembling a whip. Adult males may be distinguished from adult females in that the males have a curled posterior. The ova are characteristically oval, measuring approximately 50 microns by 20 microns, have a double shell membrane, are usually bile stained, and have polar plugs.

PATHOGENESIS   Humans infected with Trichuris trichiura are usually asymptomatic. However, patients have complained of fever, headache, diarrhea, vomiting, and constipation. Patients that are heavily infected may have bloody diarrhea.

DIAGNOSTIC CRITERIA   Diagnosis of human infection with Trichuris trichiura is made upon finding the characteristic ova in stool specimens.

TRICHOSTRONGYLUS

DISTRIBUTION   Trichostrongylus is most commonly found in the Far East and Middle East.

EPIDEMIOLOGY   Human infection with Trichostrongylus is accidental and usually occurs through the ingestion of contaminated vegetation.

MORPHOLOGY   The adult worms of Trichostrongylus resemble those of the hookworms. The ova resemble those of the hookworms but may be readily distinguished by the fact that they are different in size. The ova range from 75 microns to 95 microns in length by 45 microns in width, and are more pointed at one end.

PATHOGENESIS   Human infection with Trichostrongylus are usually asymptomatic, though some patients have blood loss due to heavy infection.

DIAGNOSTIC CRITERIA   Diagnosis of human infection is based on finding the characteristic ova in stool specimens.

Blood and Tissue Nematodes

CUTANEOUS LARVA MIGRANS

ETIOLOGY   Cutaneous larva migrans is caused by larvae of dog hookworms of the genus Ancylostoma.

EPIDEMIOLOGY   The filariform larvae of Ancylostoma caninum or Ancylostoma braziliense will penetrate the skin of humans in much the same manner as Ancylostoma duodenale. However, once the larvae have penetrated the skin, they are unable to complete their migratory pattern in humans. The larvae are trapped in the subcutaneous tissues where they migrate for long periods of time.

PATHOGENESIS   As the larvae migrate in the subcutaneous tissues, they produce erythematous tunnels of up to 2mm in diameter. The larvae evoke an allergic reaction often resulting in an intense itch. When infected people scratch, they often acquire secondary bacterial infections.

DIAGNOSIS   Diagnosis of cutaneous larva migrans (creeping eruption) is made on finding the characteristic larvae in the subcutaneous tissues.

VISCERAL LARVA MIGRANS

ETIOLOGY   Visceral larva migrans is caused by the larvae of dog and cat ascarids, particularly Toxocara canis and Toxocara cati.

EPIDEMIOLOGY   Humans, particularly children, acquire visceral larva migrans through the accidental ingestion of the infective ova of Toxocara canis or Toxocara cati. When humans ingest these infective ova, the ova hatch in the small intestine, releasing larvae. The larvae will penetrate the small intestine, migrate through the viscera, and ultimately encyst as second stage larvae.

PATHOGENESIS   The migration of the larvae of Toxocara produce a variety of symptoms including: fever, cough, hepatomegally, myocarditis, pulmonary infiltrates, and eosinophilia.

DIAGNOSIS   Diagnosis of human infection with Toxocara is made on finding the characteristic larvae in tissue biopsies or surgically removed cysts.

WUCHERERIA BANCROFTI   Wuchereria bancrofti is the causative agent of Bancroftian filariasis.

DISTRIBUTION   The geographical distribution of Wurchereria bancrofti is world-wide particularly in the tropical and subtropical regions.

EPIDEMIOLOGY   Human infection with Wuchereria bancrofti is acquired by way of the bite of mosquitoes of the genera Culex, Anopheles, and Aedes.

LIFE CYCLE   When the mosquito, of the appropriate genus, bites an infected individual, it may ingest microfilariae. Within the mosquito, the microfilariae develop into infective larvae which migrate to the mosquito's proboscis. When the mosquito next bites a human, the infective larvae escape onto the skin of the host. Once on the skin of the host, the larvae enter the puncture hole made by the mosquito's bite. Once the infective larvae are in the host, they migrate through the lymphatic vessels and develop into adult worms in the lymph nodes and larger lymphatic vessels. In the nodes and lymphatic vessels, the adult male and female worms mate and produce microfilariae.

MORPHOLOGY   The adult female of Wuchereria bancrofti measures 60 - 100mm in length by approximately 0.25mm in diameter, while the adult males measure 40mm by 0.1mm. The microfilariae measure approximately 250 - 300 microns in length, contain a large number of nuclei, and are said to be sheathed. The sheath is actually a type of egg shell which protects the microfilariae. The posterior end of the microfilariae is pointed. One of the identifying characteristics is the fact that nuclei are not found in the posterior portion of the sheathed microfilariae.

PATHOGENESIS   Human infection with Wuchereria bancrofti usually results in chills, fever, lymphadenitis and lymphangitis. The presence of large numbers of adult worms rarely produce a painful, disfiguring complication known as elephantiasis. Elephantiasis appears to be the result of an obstruction of the lymphatics by a combination of the actual presence of the worms and the body's allergic reaction to their presence. The blockage of the lymphatics results in enlargement of the affected area. The areas most frequently affected are the limbs, scrota, breasts, and vulva.

DIAGNOSTIC CRITERIA   Diagnosis of human infection is usually made by finding the characteristic microfilariae in blood smears. In those endemic areas where the mosquitoes are night biting mosquitoes, the microfilariae exhibit periodicity and are found in largest numbers between the hours of 10:00 PM and 2:00 AM. Additionally, immunodiagnostic tests may be employed including: complement fixation tests, Bentonite flocculation tests, and indirect hemagglutination tests.

BRUGIA MALAYI   Brugia malayi is the causative agent of Malayan filariasis.

DISTRIBUTION   Brugia malayi is found in Malaysia, India, and Southeast Asia.

EPIDEMIOLOGY   Human infection with Brugia malayi is acquired by way of the bite of several species of mosquitoes, principally by mosquitoes of the genus Mansonia.

LIFE CYCLE   The life cycle of Brugia malayi is similar to that of Wuchereria bancrofti.

MORPHOLOGY   The adult worms of Brugia malayi are similar to those of Wuchereria bancrofti. The microfilariae of Brugia malayi are also similar to those of Wuchereria bancrofti. The microfilariae measure approximately 180 - 220 microns in length, are sheathed, contain many nuclei, and have nuclei that extend to the tip of the tail. The distinguishing characteristic is the presence of two terminal nuclei which are distinctly separated from the other nuclei.

PATHOGENESIS   Humans infected with Brugia malayi have symptoms and complications similar to those who are infected with Wuchereria bancrofti.

DIAGNOSTIC CRITERIA   Diagnosis of human infection with Brugia malayi is made by finding the characteristic microfilariae in blood smears.   Brugia malayi exhibits periodicity with the largest numbers of microfilariae being found at approximately 8:00 PM and again at 4:00 AM.   Immunodiagnostic tests, such as those used for Wuchereria bancrofti may also be employed.

LOA LOA   Loa loa is also known as the African eye worm.

DISTRIBUTION   Loa loa is found in West Africa and Central Africa.

EPIDEMIOLOGY   Human infection with Loa loa is acquired when humans are bitten by infected Chrysops, or mango fly.

LIFE CYCLE   When humans are bitten by the Chrysops, the infective larvae migrate out onto the skin and then into the bite hole.   Development of the infective larvae takes place in the subcutaneous tissues of the infected human.   The adult Loa loa then migrate throughout the subcutaneous and deeper tissues and are particularly noticeable when crossing the conjunctiva.   The microfilariae migrate from the subcutaneous tissues to the blood stream where they may be ingested by the Chrysops.

MORPHOLOGY   The adult worms of Loa loa are threadlike, with the males measuring approximately 3.0 to 3.5 cm in length, while the females measure approximately 5.0 to 7.0 cm in length.   The microfilariae are sheathed, measure 250 - 300 microns in length, and have nuclei which extend to the tip of the tail.   Humans infected with Loa loa commonly complain of localized, temporary, subcutaneous reactions known as Calabar swellings or fugitive swellings.   The Calabar swellings may reach several inches in diameter, and last for several days.   The worms also produce an eosinophilia of 50% or more.

DIAGNOSTIC CRITERIA   Diagnosis of human infection with Loa loa is usually based on a history of Calabar swellings, exposure to an endemic area, observing the worm migrating in the conjunctiva, eosinophilia, or finding the characteristic microfilariae in blood smears.   Most patients are diagnosed long before the appearance of the microfilariae in the blood.

DIPETALONEMA PERSTANS   Dipetalonema perstans is a filarial parasite that is generally considered to be non-pathogenic.

DISTRIBUTION   Dipetalonema perstans is found in many areas of Africa, and South America, as well as in coastal areas of Panama.

EPIDEMIOLOGY   Human infection with Dipetalonema perstans is acquired by way of the bite of midges or gnats of the genus Culicoides.

MORPHOLOGY   The adult worms of Dipetalonema perstans are similar in appearance to other filarial worms.   The microfilariae are characteristically unsheathed, and have nuclei that extend to the tip of the tail.

PATHOGENESIS   Dipetalonema perstans is considered to be non-pathogenic, however, some infected humans have had mild allergic symptoms.

DIAGNOSTIC CRITERIA   Diagnosis of human infection with Dipetalonema perstans is made upon finding the characteristic microfilariae in blood smears.   The microfilariae of Dipetalonema do not exhibit periodicity.

MANSONELLA OZZARDI   Mansonella ozzardi is a filarial parasite that is generally considered to be non-pathogenic.

DISTRIBUTION   Mansonella ozzardi is found in Central America, South America, and parts of the West Indies.

EPIDEMIOLOGY   Human infection with Mansonella ozzardi is acquired from the bite of midges or gnats of the genus Culicoides.

MORPHOLOGY   The adult worms of Mansonella ozzardi are similar in appearance to other filarial worms. The microfilariae are characteristically unsheathed, and have nuclei that do not extend to the tip of the tail.

PATHOGENESIS   Mansonella ozzardi is considered to be non-pathogenic; however, some infected humans have had allergic symptoms.

DIAGNOSTIC CRITERIA   Diagnosis of human infection with Mansonella ozzardi is made upon finding the characteristic microfilariae in blood smears. The microfilariae of Mansonella ozzardi do not exhibit periodicity.

ONCHOCERCA VOLVULUS   Onchocerca volvulus is the causative agent of onchocerciasis or blinding filariasis.

DISTRIBUTION   Onchocerca volvulus is found in Central Africa and parts of Central America and South America.

EPIDEMIOLOGY   Human infection with Onchocerca volvulus is acquired from the bite of black flies or buffalo gnats of the genus Simulium.

MORPHOLOGY   The adult worms of Onchocerca volvulus are thin and wire-like. The male worms measure approximately 2.0 - 4.0 cm in length, while the females measure approximately 35 - 50 cm in length. The microfilariae are unsheathed and measure anywhere from 150 microns in length to as much as 350 microns in length.

PATHOGENESIS   Human infection with Onchocerca volvulus may result in two types of pathologic reactions. Once is caused by the adult worm, and the other is caused by the microfilariae. The pathologic condition associated with the adults of Onchocerca volvulus is nodule or tumor formation. These nodules or tumors are the result of encapsulation of the adult worms in the subcutaneous tissue. Humans who acquire the infection in Africa usually have these nodules or tumors on their thighs and buttocks, while those who acquire the infection in the Americas usually have the nodules or tumors on the head and upper trunk. The second pathologic condition is associated with the microfilariae of Onchocerca volvulus. When the microfilariae are released from the adult female, they migrate through the cutaneous and subcutaneous tissues. The microfilariae often migrate to the eyes where they cause lesions that result in corneal opacities resulting in blindness.

DIAGNOSTIC CRITERIA   Diagnosis of human infection with Onchocerca volvulus is based on finding the characteristic microfilariae in skin snips.

DRACUNCULUS MEDINENSIS   Dracunculus medinensis is also known as the guinea worm. It is one of the oldest known and recognized human parasites. It is believed that Dracunculus medinensis were the "fiery serpents" that plagued the Israelites in the Sinai Peninsula.

DISTRIBUTION   Dracunculus medinensis is found in many parts of Africa, Asia, the Middle East, and in some parts of the U. S. S. R.

EPIDEMIOLOGY   Human infection with Dracunculus medinensis is acquired by ingestion

of larvae bearing copepods of the genus Cyclops. The copepods are contained in contaminated drinking water.

LIFE CYCLE   When humans ingest the larvae bearing copepods, digestion of the copepods releases the larvae which penetrate the intestinal wall. Following penetration,
the larvae develop to maturity in the deeper tissues. In about 8 months to one year,
gravid females migrate to the skin surface. The female worm, when at the skin surface, produces a blister which, when immersed in water, ruptures causing the release
of larvae. The Cyclops ingest the larvae. Development of the larvae, to the infective stage, takes place in the copepod.

MORPHOLOGY   The adult worms of Dracunculus medinensis are elongated and cylindrical.
The adult males are rather inconspicuous, measuring approximately 2.0 - 3.0 cm,
while the adult females measure approximately one meter in length by 1.0 - 1.5mm in
diameter.

PATHOGENESIS   Humans infected with Dracunculus medinensis most frequently suffer
from secondary infection of the ruptured blister. Patients who do have secondary
infections may also develop arthritic symptoms. In addition, patients often have
other symptoms including nausea, vomiting, and diarrhea. These symptoms disappear
after the formation of the ulcer.

DIAGNOSTIC CRITERIA   Diagnosis of human infection is usually made upon examination
of the ulcer to determine the presence of the larvae or the adult female.

TRICHINELLA SPIRALIS   Trichinella spiralis is also known as trichina, and is the
causative agent of trichinosis.

DISTRIBUTION   Trichinella spiralis is cosmopolitan in distribution.

EPIDEMIOLOGY   Human infection with Trichinella spiralis is the result of consuming
raw or improperly cooked animal flesh containing the encysted larvae. Most commonly,
infection occurs from ingestion of improperly cooked pork. However, humans may acquire the infection from other meats, particularly bear meat.

LIFE CYCLE   When humans ingest improperly cooked meat containing the infective larvae, the cysts are digested and the larvae invade the mucosa of the small intestine.
The larvae become sexually mature adults within two days. The fertilized females
burrow futher into the mucosa and the intestinal lymphatics. Once in the intestinal
lymphatics, they release their larvae, which are ultimately carried through the circulatory symtem. Ultimately the larvae penetrate skeletal muscles, coil, and become
encysted. The encysted larvae remain dormant and viable for years. The source of
infection for pigs and other larvae bearing animals is through food scraps containing
infective larvae; ingestion of larvae or adults in fecal material; or ingestion of
meats or animals containing infective larvae.

MORPHOLOGY   The adult males of Trichinella spiralis measure approximately 1.5mm in
length while the females measure 3 - 4mm in length. Freshly deposited larvae measure approximately 100 microns in length, while fully developed larvae measure approximately 1mm in length.

PATHOGENESIS   Depending on the stage of the infection, humans infected with Trichinella spiralis may experience a variety of symptoms. During the intestinal stage,
most patients will be relatively asymptomatic; however, some patients may have gastroenteritis or diarrhea. The next stage of the infection is the muscular invasion
stage. During this stage, patients may experience muscular pain, dyspnea, periorbital
edema, fever, eosinophilia, and lymph node enlargement. The third stage of the in-

fection is the encystation stage. During this stage, patients may experience a wide range of symptoms and disorders including: dehydration, pulmonary hemorrhage, arthralgias, meningitis, myocarditis and death.

DIAGNOSTIC CRITERIA   Diagnosis of infection with Trichinella spiralis is most fre-quently made after a patient presents with a history of having eaten insufficiently cooked pork or bear meat; displays bilateral periorbital edema; eosinophilia; or has a positive muscle biopsy or positive immunodiagnostic test. The immunodiagnostic tests include: the Bachman intradermal reaction, indirect fluorescent-antibody tests, Bentonite flocculation tests, complement fixation tests, and cholesterol flocculation tests.

GNATHOSTOMIASIS

ETIOLOGY   Gnathostomiasis is caused by the larvae of Gnathostoma spinigerum.

EPIDEMIOLOGY   Human infection with Gnathostoma is acquired by way of the ingestion of raw, pickled, or improperly cooked fish containing the larval worms. Infection has also been traced to improperly cooked frog legs and duck imported from Far Eastern countries.

PATHOGENESIS   After humans ingest larvae bearing foods, the larvae are liberated and penetrate the intestinal wall. This penetration and migration may produce a variety of symptoms ranging from fever, anorexia, and vomiting, to edema and blindness.

DIAGNOSTIC CRITERIA   Diagnosis of human infection with Gnathostoma must be distin-guished from sparganosis, cutaneous larva migrans, and visceral larva migrans. The differentiation is best accomplished by recovery and identification of the worm.

ARTHROPODS

SARCOPTES SCABIEI   Sarcoptes scabiei, also known as the itch mite, is the causative agent of scabies.

DISTRIBUTION   Sarcoptes scabiei is cosmopolitan in distribution.

EPIDEMIOLOGY   Human infection with Sarcoptes scabiei is usually acquired by direct contact with other infected individuals, their clothing or linen.

LIFE CYCLE   When humans come in contact with Sarcoptes scabiei, the mites enter the skin and burrow in the upper layers of the skin. As the gravid females burrow, they deposit their ova in the tunnels that they have created. The ova in the tunnels ma-ture in approximately four days and commence burrowing their own tunnels. In approxi-mately two weeks the larvae mature, and the females have been fertilized. The fer-tilized females continue burrowing and depositing ova. The life span of the adult mites is approximately 5 weeks.

MORPHOLOGY   The adults of Sarcoptes scabiei are ovoid, have six legs (2 pair anteri-orly and 1 pair posteriorly). The males measure approximately 0.09 - 0.25 mm in length while the females measure approximately 0.35 - 0.50 mm in length.

PATHOGENESIS   The most prominent symptom of humans infected with Sarcoptes scabiei is an intense itching which is caused by the activity of the mites and their secre-tions. Scratching promotes a secondary infection to other parts of the body.

DIAGNOSTIC CRITERIA   Diagnosis of human infection with Sarcoptes scabiei is usually made upon finding the mature mites in skin scrapings. The most frequently infected areas include the interdigital spaces, axillae, groin and the back of the hands.

Skin scrapings will produce the best results when they are taken toward the terminal end of the tunnels, since this is where the females are usually located.

PEDICULUS HUMANUS   Pediculus humanus are more commonly referred to as head lice or body lice, and are the causative agent of pediculosis.

DISTRIBUTION   Pediculus humanus is cosmopolitan in distribution, and is most frequently seen when personal hygiene is poor. It is most prevalent in institutions and living environments where individual hygiene is not respected or protected. Mental institutions, jails, crammed living quarters and military barracks are examples of such institutions.

EPIDEMIOLOGY   Human infection with Pediculus humanus is most commonly acquired by personal contact or contact with hair or clothing of infected individuals.

MORPHOLOGY   Adult Pediculus humanus are large enough to be seen with the naked eye, measuring approximately 2.5mm, while those of the variety Pediculus humanus capitis are slightly smaller than those of the variety Pediculus humanus. The ova of Pediculus humanus, often called nits, are oval, measure approximately 0.8mm in length, and are found stuck to hairs.

PATHOGENESIS   Humans infected with Pediculus humanus most frequently suffer from intense itching which is due to the biting and sucking of the parasite. The larvae are also vectors of diseases which include: epidemic typhus, trench fever, relapsing fever, impetigo, and cholera.

DIAGNOSTIC CRITERIA   Diagnosis of human infection with Pediculus humanus is made on microscopically confirming the presence of the characteristic organisms in the hair of the head or body.

PHTHIRUS PUBIS   Phthirus pubis is also known as the pubic louse or the crab louse.

DISTRIBUTION   Phthirus pubis is cosmopolitan in distribution and exhibits a prevalence similar to that of Pediculus humanus.

EPIDEMIOLOGY   Humans infected with Phthirus pubis acquire the organisms in much the same way as Pediculus humanus.

MORPHOLOGY   Adult Phthirus pubis are similar to Pediculus humanus and may be distinguished by the size (Phthirus pubis are shorter in length), the size of the legs (Pediculus humanus adults have legs that are all equal in length, while Phthirus pubis adults have an anterior pair, that is significantly shorter than the two posterior pairs), and the size of the abdomen (Pediculus humanus adults have an elongated abdomen while Phthirus pubis adults have a shorter abdomen).

PATHOGENESIS   Human infection with Phthirus pubis results in pathogenesis similar to that of humans infected with Pediculus humanus.

DIAGNOSTIC CRITERIA   Diagnosis of human infection with Phthirus pubis is similar to that of Pediculus humanus.

TUNGA PENETRANS   Tunga penetrans is also known as the chigoe flea.

DISTRIBUTION   Tunga penetrans is found in tropical regions of American and Africa.

EPIDEMIOLOGY   Human infection with Tunga penetrans is usually acquired by walking barefoot in soil containing the fleas.

PATHOGENESIS   Humans infected with Tunga penetrans demonstrate inflammation and ulceration of the skin, particularly the skin beneath the toe nails.   The ulcerations produced are often secondarily infected.

Many other arthropods are of clinical significance as vectors of disease and as stinging or biting organisms.   For more information on these arthropods consult the recommended readings found at the end of this chapter.

TABLE 1

TROPHOZOITES OF INTESTINAL AMEBAS

	SIZE	MOTILITY	NUCLEAR CHROMATIN	NUMBER NUCLEI	CYTOPLASM
E.HISTOLYTICA	10-60 microns	Active and directional	Central karyosomal chromatin mass and evenly distributed peripheral chromatin	1	Generally appears "Clean". May contain red blood cells; usually does not contain bacteria
E.HARTMANI	5-12 microns	Active and directional	Same as E. Histolytica	1	Same as E. Histolytica, but does not contain red blood cells
E.COLI	12-50 microns	Sluggish and non-directional	Large eccentric karyosomal chromatin mass Coarse, unevenly distributed peripheral chromatin	1	Granular, vacuolated, contains bacteria,"dirty" appearance,does not contain red blood cells
E.NANA	6-12 microns	Sluggish	Large karyosomal chromatin mass No peripheral chromatin	1	Granular, vacuolated, may contain bacteria; does not contain red blood cells
I.BUTSCHLII	8-20 microns	Sluggish and progressive	Large karyosomal chromatin mass that is central or eccentric Numerous chromatin granules No peripheral chromatin	1	Vacuolated, contains bacteria Does not contain red blood cells
D.FRAGILIS	5-15 microns	Active and progressive	Karyosomal chromatin is fragmented or clumped No peripheral chromatin	2	Finely granular vacuolated, contains bacteria Does not contain red blood cells

TABLE 2

CYSTS OF INTESTINAL AMEBAS

	SIZE	SHAPE	NUCLEAR CHROMATIN	INCLUSIONS	NUMBER NUCLEI
E.HISTOLYTICA	10-20 microns	Spherical	Central karyosomal Chromatin, Smooth, evenly distributed Peripheral chromatin	Iodine stained: Reddish-brown Diffuse glycogen mass, H & E: Chromatoidal bars that are thick and have round ends	1 - 4
E.HARTMANI	5-9 microns	Spherical	Same as E. Histolytica	Same as E. Histolytica	1 - 4
E.COLI	10-35 microns	Spherical	Eccentric karyosomal Chromatin, Coarse, unevenly distributed Peripheral chromatin	Iodine stained: Dark brown diffuse Glycogen mass, H & E: Chromatoidal bars with square, splintered or pointed ends	1 - 8
E.NANA	6-10 microns	Oval	Blot like karyosomal Chromatin mass, No peripheral chromatin		1 - 4
I.BUTSCHLII	6-20 microns	Irregular	Large karyosomal Chromatin mass with many chromatin granules, No peripheral chromatin	Large prominent glycogen mass, Often vacuolated	Usually only 1

TABLE 3

INTESTINAL FLAGELLATES

	SIZE	SHAPE	NUCLEI	FLAGELLA	CYTOPLASMIC INCLUSIONS	OTHER DIST. CHARACTERIS.
G.LAMBLIA TROPHOZOITE	Average 14 microns	Pear shaped	2 Ovoid or spherical Large karyosomal chromatin mass	4 pair 1 pair anteriorly 2 pair medially 1 pair posteriorly	2 median bodies axonemes sucking disk	Bilaterally symetrical
G.LAMBIA CYST	Average 12 microns	Oval	4 Ovoid or spherical Large karyosomal chromatin mass	8 pair scattered	4 median bodies axonemes fine granulation	Cyst wall: smooth, thin, colorless
C.MESNILI TROPHOZOITE	Average 12 microns	Conical to pear shaped	1 Round Central karyosomal chromatin mass; some peripheral chromatin	3 Located anteriorly	Cytostome Spiral groove fine granulation	Asymetrical
C.MESNILI CYST	Average 6 microns	Lemon shaped	1 Round Central karyosomal chromatin mass	- - -	Cytostome may be visible	Clear zone in the nipple-like protrusion that gives the cyst its characteristic lemon shape
T.HOMINIS TROPHOZOITE	Average 10 microns	Oval	1 Scattered chromatin granules	3-5 anteriorly 1 posteriorly	Axostyle cytostomal cleft	Undulating membrane

TABLE 4   MALARIA

	RED BLOOD CELL PREFERENCE	RED BLOOD CELLS ENLARGED	SCHÜFFNER'S DOTS	MAURER'S DOTS	MULTIPLE INFECTIONS OF A RED BLOOD CELL	NUMBER OF MEROZOITES	DISTINGUISHING CHARACTERISTICS
P.VIVAX	Prefers Reticulocytes	Yes 1.5-2 times normal size	Yes	None	Occasionally	12-24 Average 16	All stages present in peripheral blood; ring occupies 1/3 of the cell; merozoites fill entire red blood cell; schizogony cycle = 48 hrs.
P.OVALE	Prefers Reticulocytes	About 50% of infected cells are enlarged and oval	Yes	None	Occasionally	8-12 Average 8	All stages present in peripheral blood; cells sometimes fimbrinated; ring larger than P. vivax; merozoites sometimes found in rosettes; schizogony cycle = 48 hrs.
P.MALARIAE	Prefers mature red blood cells	No	None	None	Rarely	6-12 Average 8	All stages present in peripheral blood; rings smaller than P. vivax; trophozoites often seen in "band" forms produces an abundance of pigment; merozoites often found in rosettes; schizogony cycle = 72 hrs.
P.FALCIPARUM	Invades all stages of red blood cells equally	No	None	Yes	Commonly	8-24	Ring forms and gametocytes found in peripheral blood; applique forms; are sausage shaped; schizogony cycle = 48 hrs.

TABLE 5

TREMATODE OVA

	SIZE	SHAPE	COLOR	OTHER DISTINGUISHING CHARACTERISTICS
F.BUSKI	130-140 microns by 80-85 microns	Oval	Yellowish Brown	The ova of Fasciolopsis buski are very large, have a small operculum, and cannot be differentiated from the ova of asciola hepatica. Ova are recovered in fecal specimens.
H.HETEROPHYES	28 by 16 microns	Oval	Light Brown	The ova of Opistorchis senensis phyes heterophyes and Metagonimus yokogawai) cannot be easily differentiated from one another. They have an operculum without prominent opercular shoulders. They must be differentiated from the ova of Opisthorchis sinensis.
O.SINENSIS	28 by 16 microns	Ovoid	Yellowish Brown	The ova of Opisthorchis sinensis very closely resemble those of the Heterophyids. They may be differentiated by finding the prominent opercular shoulders, and comma-like process opposite the operculum on the ova of Opisthorchis.
F.HEPATICA	140 by 70 microns	Oval	Yellowish Brown	The ova of Fasciola hepatica are very large, have a small operculum, and cannot be differentiated from the ova of Fasciolopsis buski. Ova may be recovered in fecal specimens and in duodenal aspirates.
S.MANSONI	115-180 microns in length by 45-70 microns in width	Ovoid and elongate	Light Yellow Brown	The ova of Schistosoma mansoni are not operculated, possess a prominent lateral spine that resembles a thorn, and may be found in fecal specimens and rectal tissue biopsies.
S.JAPONICUM	75-105 microns in length by 50-80 microns in width	Round to oval	Pale Yellow	The ova of Schistosoma japonicum are not operculated, possess a minute lateral spine that may not be seen, and may be found in fecal specimens and sometimes in rectal tissue biopsies.

TABLE 5 CONTINUED

S.HAEMATOBIUM	115–180 microns in length by 45–70 microns in width	Oval	Yellowish Brown	The ova of schistosoma haematobium are not operculated, possess a prominent terminal spine, and are found in urine specimens and biopsies of the urinary bladder wall.
P.WESTERMANI	90 by 50 microns	Ovoid	Golden Brown	The ova of Paragonimus westermani possess a distinct flattened operculum with prominent opercular shoulders, must be distinguished from the ova of Diphyllobothrium latum ova, and may be found in fecal specimens and sputum.

TABLE 6

CESTODE OVA

	SIZE	SHAPE	SHELL WALL	OTHER DISTINGUISHING CHARACTERISTICS
D. LATUM	65 X 45 microns	Ovoid	Thick, Yellowish Brown	The ova of diphyllobothrium latum are operculated with opercular shoulders, must be differentiated from the ova of paragonimus westermani, and possess a small knob-like process opposite the operculum which, if seen, is diagnostic. Ova are found in fecal specimens. Diagnosis of human infection with diphyllobothrium latum is based on finding the characteristic ova or proglottids.
T. SOLIUM	35 microns in diameter	Round	Thick, Brown, and radially striated	The ova of the taenias cannot be distinguished from one another, contain a hexacanth larva, and are recovered in fecal specimens. Differential diagnosis of taenia infection is best accomplished by microscopically examining the gravid proglottids which are found in fecal specimens. Differential diagnosis may also be made by examining the scolex when it is recovered.
H. DIMINUTA	35-45 microns	Slightly Ovoid	Moderately thick and may have concentric striations	The ova of hymenolepsis diminuta have a hexacanth embryo enclosed in a rigid membrane. The membrane has polar thickenings, but no filaments projecting. The absence of the filaments serves to differentiate hymenolepsis diminuta from hymenolepsis nana. The ova are found in fecal specimens.
H. NANA	35-45 microns	Ovoid	Thin	The ova of hymenolepsis nana have a hexacanth embryo enclosed in a rigid membrane. The membrane has polar thickenings. Four to eight long, thin filaments project from these polar thickenings. The ova are found in fecal specimens.

TABLE 7

OVA OF INTESTINAL NEMATODES

	SIZE	SHAPE	COLOR	SHELL WALL	OTHER DISTINGUISHING CHARACTERISTICS
A.LUMBRICOIDES	45–70 microns in length by 40–60 microns in width	Oval	Usually bile stained golden brown	Thick and usually covered with a coarsely mammillated albuminoid layer	Occasionally ova will be found that have lost the albuminoid layer. These are referred to as decorticated and may be distinguished from other nematode ova by their thick yellowish shell wall. Infertile ascaris ova are sometimes countered. These are similar to fertilized ova except that they are elongated giving a barrel appearance.
E.VERMICULARIS	55 X 25 microns	Ovoid, with a distinctively flattened side	Colorless	Double, moderately thick, and translucent	Ova are usually fully embryonated when released. Ova are not usually found in fecal specimens since the female migrates out of the anus for egg deposition. Recovery of ova is best accomplished by examining perianal scrapings or scotch tape tests.
A.DUODENA	60 X 45 microns	Oval	Colorless	Thin and colorless	Ova, when passed, are either unsegmented or in early stages of development, usually in the 2–8 cell stage. If fecal samples are left at room temperatures the ova may hatch and will have to be differentiated from the larva of strongyloides stercoralis. Hookworms cannot be speciated on the basis of their ova.
S.STERCORALIS	60 X 45 microns	Oval	Colorless	Thin and colorless	The ova of strongyloides are not usually found in fecal specimens. Diagnosis of human infection with strongyloides stercoralis is based on the proper identification of the rhabditiform larvae which are found in fecal specimens.
T.TRICHIURA	50 X 20 microns	Barrel shaped	Bile stained golden brown	Double and thick	The ova of trichuris trichiura have bipolar refractile plugs giving them the appearance of serving trays. The ova, when passed are unsegmented.

TABLE 7 CONTINUED

TRICHOSTRONGYLUS	75 X 45 microns	Oval elongated	Colorless	Thin and colorless

The ova of trichostrongylus must be differentiated from those of the hookworms. This is most easily done by observing that the ova of trichostrongylus are longer than those of the hookworms, and have ends that are more pointed that those of the hookworm ova.

BIBLIOGRAPHY AND RECOMMENDED READINGS

Beck, J. W. and J. E. Davies, <u>Medical parasitology</u>. 2nd Ed. 1976. The C. V. Mosby Company, Saint Louis.

Cable, R. M., <u>An Illustrated Laboratory Manual of Parasitology</u>. 5th Ed. 1977. Burgess Publishing Company, Minneapolis.

Faust, E. C., Seaver, P. C., and R. C. Jung, <u>Animal Agents and Vectors of Human Disease</u>. 4th Ed. 1975. Lea and Febiger, Philadelphia.

Faust, E. C., Russell, P. F., and R. C. Jung, <u>Craig and Faust's Clinical Parasitology</u>. 8th Ed. 1970. Lea and Febiger, Philadelphia.

Lenette, E. H., Spaulding, E. H., and J. P. Truant, <u>Manual of Clinical Microbiology</u>. 2nd Ed. 1974. American Society for Microbiology, Washington, D. C.

Markell, E. K. and M. Voge, <u>Medical Parasitology</u>. 4th Ed. 1976. W. B. Saunders Company, Philadelphia.

Noble, E. R. and G. A. Noble, <u>Parasitology: The Biology of Animal Parasites</u>. 4th Ed. 1976. Lea and Febiger, Philadelphia.

Chapter 4

Special Topics in Virology

LORRAINE D. DOUCET, CSC, PhD.
Medical Technology Program Director
Professor of Biology
Notre Dame College
Manchester, New Hampshire

OUTLINE

    Hepatitis A Virus
    Hepatitis B Virus
    Parainfluenza Viruses
    Mumps
    Measles (Rubeola)
    German Measles (Rubella)
ONCOGENIC VIRUSES

INTRODUCTION

Most hospital laboratories perform limited diagnostic tests for viruses. To date, most Medical Technologists perform simple and straightforward viral diagnostic test procedures. More complicated test procedures, viral research and viral studies are restricted primarily to either the Center for Disease Control (CDC), a limited number of virology laboratories, or certain research or reference laboratories.

Since this section is geared for the prospective Medical Technologist, the practitioner with a limited background in the area, or the bench-worker preparing for examination, the section will provide the fundamentals of virology. Selected viral diseases and their clinical diagnoses are included.

It is hoped that this section will provide the reader with basic information in virology and impress upon the reader the need to develop a greater knowledge of virology.

A greater knowledge of viruses should be a prime concern to all practicing clinicians. The writer strongly urges all to take clinically oriented programs and seminars conducted by experts in the field.

SPECIAL TOPICS IN VIROLOGY

GENERAL CHARACTERISTICS

Viruses are the smallest infective agents capable of replicating within a living cell system. Viruses average from about 20 nm to 300 nm in size and therefore are filterable, that is, they pass through bacteriological filters. Viruses are obligate intracellular parasites and, to date, have not been cultivated outside of susceptible host cells. Viruses possess only one nucleic acid, (DNA or RNA) but never both nucleic acids together.

Since viruses are devoid of enzymes, they depend upon their host cells for the amino acids, nucleotides and metabolic machinery needed for nucleic acid, protein and lipid synthesis. Once the viral nucleic acid penetrates a host cell, the virus controls the host cell's genetic material and induces it to form new viruses.

VIRION PRODUCTION

Infected host cells may either: (1) burst and release the virions or (2) extrude the virions through their cell membrane. In some instances, a fragment of the host cell's membrane breaks off to form a lipid envelope around the virion's protein coat. In other instances, the lipid envelope is formed independent of the host while other virion's are devoid of the lipid envelope. Virions bearing the lipid envelope are susceptible to treatment with ether while the nonenveloped virions are not susceptible to ether.

The enveloped virions have a lipid bi-layer and glycoproteins which form projections. These projections, extruding from the envelope are called spikes. These spikes contain components which: (1) appear to attach the virion to the host cell, and (2) contain enzymes which destroy the attachment site to give the virion the ability to detach itself from one receptor site and re-attach itself to an intact (or new) host cell's receptor site. Virions (mature infectious virus particles) have a variety of shapes. Some virions are spherical, others are cylindrical or cubical, and still others are polyhedral.

Bacteriophages, which penetrate bacteria, have tail-like structures which are believed to attach these viruses to bacterial receptor sites or to permit the bacteriophages to penetrate bacterial cell walls. The hollow tail structure forms a tube-
like passage for the virus nucleic acid to penetrate the host cell. The attachment
site seems very specific.

Bacteriophage susceptibility testing of different strains within a species is referred to as <u>phage</u> <u>typing</u>. Phage typing facilitates the identification of certain
disease causing bacteria.

VIRUS SHAPES

Capsomeres and capsids determine the shape of viruses. The capsomeres are protein molecules that constitute the virus protein coat (or capsid). When the nucleic
acid is contained within the protein coat of the virus, the protein coat (or capsid)
is then termed the nucleocapsid. The nucleic acid is arranged differently in different viruses. The capsomeres and the nucleic acid are helical in cylindrical viruses while the nucleic acid is coiled randomly in cubical or polyhderal viruses.
Other virus forms display other modes of nucleic acid arrangement.

VIRUS CULTURE

Viruses cannot replicate on artificial media, since they are obligate intracellular parasites. Different viruses need different tissue cell types for in vitro studies. Tissue cultures are essential for diagnostic and vaccine production pruposes.
A variety of tissues, cell types, and embryonated eggs, as well as laboratory animals, have been used for these purposes. The use of laboratory animals has diminished
considerably, but animals are still needed for Togaviruses and many "slow" growing
viruses. Embryonated eggs were used to a great extent before the tissue culture technique was refined. Viruses were propagated in amnionic, allantoic, chorionic or egg
yolk sac membranes. This propagation procedure is used less extensively today.

Many primary cell cultures are obtained directly from tissues. These primary
cultures, grown in vitro, can be subcultured to produce secondary cultures, however,
this cannot be done an unlimited number of times.

VIRAL ASSAY

Viruses can be enumerated by chemical and physical means as well as infectivity.

1. Electron Microscopy

Electron microscopy can be used to enumerate viruses by mixing a viral suspension
with a known number of latex particles. The two particle types can be observed
and counted. However, this technique does not differentiate particle infectivity
or non-infectivity.

2. Hemagglutination

Many viruses have a protein coat that can bind appropriate erythrocytes. These
viruses can be assayed by erythrocyte agglutination. The hemagglutination titer
(HA) refers to the highest dilution which agglutinates appropriate RBC's. The
HA may be derived by using the reciprocal of the last dilution which demonstrated
complete hemagglutination. The HA test can establish the number of hemagglути-
nation viruses in a clinical specimen and aid to serotaxonomically identify the
viruses in the specimen. The latter may be done by adding a specific antibody to

the virus-containing specimen prior to introducing the erythrocytes to the same specimen thereby inhibiting agglutination of the erythrocytes. This is referred to as hemagglutination inhibition (HI or HAI).   HA known viruses are used as antigens to test for the presence of homologous antibodies in serum samples. These tests are performed in diagnostic and research laboratories. The HA test has its limitations since different viruses require different RBC's for agglutination and some viruses fail to cause hemagglutination.

3. Plaque Assay

Bacterial and animal viruses can be enumerated by plaque formation. Phage virions that affect an E. coli strain may be determined as follows:

A. 1.0 ml of a contaminated water sample is filtered and serial dilutions of the filtrate are prepared.

B. 1.0 ml of each of the dilutions is added to active *E. coli* broth cultures, mixed, plated onto appropriate agar preparations, and incubated at 35-37°C for 24 hours.

C. A thick layer of bacterial growth is apparent on the agar plates, but wherever the phages are present, a clear area is formed. This clear area is devoid of bacteria due to the lytic action of the viruses.

D. To determine the number of viruses in the 1.0 ml of the undiluted filtrate, count the number of plaques and multiply by the reciprocal of the dilution factor.

Cytocidal viruses are enumerated by plaque formation.

Non-cytocidal viruses are assayed by hemadsorption.

Tissue cultures may be used to enumerate virions. When this is the case, the tissue cytopathic dose is determined (TCD). The TCD is the smallest viral inoculum needed to induce microscopic or macroscopic damage to susceptible tissue culture cells. The damage or cytopathological effects are usually apparent microscopically, if not macroscopically.

Cell cultures containing confluent monolayered cell growth can be purchased commercially. Most virology or reference laboratories purchase these already prepared.

4.   Interference Test

Certain viruses cannot be determined by either hemagglutination or by cytophathological effects and can only be determined by the interference test. This technique is based on the fact that viruses growing in a tissue culture will limit or stop the growth of a second virus inoculated into the same tissue culture. The rubella virus exhibits this characteristic. CPE producing viruses may be inhibited by rubella and fail to produce cytopathogenic effects if rubella is propagating in the same tissue culture; e.g., herpes simplex virus, which is usually CPE positive by changing infected cells into large multinucleated cells, fails to do so in the presence of a propagating rubella virus.

However, if the herpes simplex virus were inoculated in a cell culture devoid of rubella, the herpes simplex virus would produce its characteristic CPE. These

procedures are not routinely performed in all hospitals, but are done more frequently in reference laboratories, research laboratories, or a limited number of
hospitals.

VIRUS IDENTIFICATION

If a virus is isolated from a clinical specimen by either of the three procedures
listed, i.e., CPE, hemadsorption or interference, the isolated virus can usually be
identified by establishing:

1. The virus' nucleic acid type (DNA or RNA)

2. Whether the virus in question is sensitive to acids, and

3. Whether the isolate is sensitive to ether or chloroform.

It is beyond the scope of this section to describe viral isolate identification
procedures. To date, very few laboratories routinely perform in depth virology testing. Consequently, more detailed texts or manuals along with seminars or workshops
in the area are recommended. One basic laboratory manual containing laboratory procedures in diagnostic virology is that of Christensen's (see Bibliography and Recommended Readings).

MODE OF VIRUS REPLICATION (PROPAGATION)

Since a virus is an obligate intracellular parasite, its propagation is dependent
upon the virus' ability to: (1) penetrate a susceptible host; (2) control the host's
genetic material to thereby produce virus nucleic acid and virus proteins; (3) as-
semble and form new viruses; and (4) cause the release of new viruses from within the
host. The virus does this in five stages or steps which are conventionally listed
as:

1. Attachment or adsorption.

2. Penetration.

3. Uncoating.

4. Eclipse or biosynthesis, and

5. Maturation and release from the host.

The particular biochemical processes that occur within each step seem to vary
somewhat and are dependent upon the virus in question and the specific host cell.

ATTACHMENT OR ADSORPTION

Viral attachment to a host cell surface depends upon the interaction of both the
virus and its host. This is dependent upon electrostatic or chemical bonding between
the sites of attachment on the virus and the receptor sites of the host.

A virus-receptor interaction site is essential for host infection to occur.

PENETRATION

Animal viruses are not injected into the host as are the bacteriophages. There does not seem to be one penetration procedure common to all the viral types. Generally though, viruses enter the host cells via a phagocytic process or directly penetrate the host cell membranes.

UNCOATING

Viral uncoating is initiated by proteolytic enzymes released from the host cells' lysosomes. These enzymes remove the viral capsid and the virus nucleic acid is released. Many studies have been performed to demonstrate the effects of viral penetration and uncoating upon host cells. The details of this process vary somewhat from virus to virus, but ultimately the virus nucleic acid dominates and controls cell activities.

ECLIPSE OR BIOSYNTHESIS

When the uncoating process occurs, the virions cannot be recovered from the infected cell. Once the virions are fully formed, they are infectious. Eclipse can then be defined as that period between loss of infectivity until the formation of progeny. Viral components are believed to be synthesized during the eclipse period. The eclipse period is terminated when virions are fully formed and infectious. The important events during virion replication are: genome replication, RNA transcription, translation and maturation of virus proteins.

MATURATION AND RELEASE

Nucleocapsid formation and envelope formation (when applicable) occur prior to the release of the virions. Viruses that do not bear an envelope are usually released by cellular disruption. These viruses have been reported to be in the host cells even after cytopathologic changes are observed.

In enveloped viruses, the nucleocapsid and surrounding host membrane bulge or push out and a bud pinches off to form the enveloped virion. The envelope proteins are determined by the virus, but the lipids are characteristically similar to the host.

VIRUS REPLICATION EFFECTS UPON THE HOST CELL

Virus replication within the host may:

1. Destroy the host cell.

2. Infect the host, but cause no apparent change within the host-cell, or

3. Transform the host cell.

DESTRUCTION OF HOST CELL

Cytocidal viruses destroy host cells. This is microscopically observed and reported as CPE.

PROLONGED HOST CELL INFECTION

Persistent susceptible tissue culture infections can occur without any observable morphological tissue cell changes. Antiviral antibodies fail to stop the infection in steady state infections in which all of the tissue culture cells are infected. All progeny are infected in this form of culture infection.

In what is termed the carrier state of infection, only a limited number of tissue culture cells are infected. In this type of culture infection, antiviral antibodies are effective.

What viruses do in tissue cultures, they also do within the host. Chronic viral infections or latent viral infections are reported in many viral diseases. For example, after an acute primary infection of herpes simplex or herpes zoster, the patient seems recovered. Later, the disease may reoccur not due to an exogenous re-infection, but due to the reactivation of a latent virus. Although the virus was dormant in a nerve for a while, the virus was resistant to the infected host's immune system and high antiviral antibody titer.

TRANSFORMATION OF HOST CELL

Oncogenic viruses cause permanent changes within susceptible host cells. In vitro virus induced transformation is believed to be similar to tumors in animals, since the tissue culture cells have tumor cell characteristics.

Transformed cells no longer demonstrate contact inhibition; do demonstrate tumor (T) antigens and tumor specific transplant antigens (TSTA); induce tumors when introduced into susceptible hosts and exhibit morphological changes.

LYSOGENY

Bacterial viruses may produce either a lytic or lysogenic reaction, after invading a susceptible bacterial strain. The bacterial viruses are called *temperate bacteriophages*. The lytic reaction results in lysis of the bacterial cell and the ultimate release of viral progeny. However, in the lysogenic reaction, the phage nucleic acid is incorporated into the bacterial chromosome. This change in the procaryotic bacterial cell can be considered analogous to transformation in the eucaryotic cell as induced by oncogenic viruses. The viral nucleic acid is said to be in the prophage state and replicates with the bacterium. UV light can cause the virus to replicate independently. When this occurs lysis follows.

The lysogenic bacterium is not altered morphologically and may not be reinfected by the same bacteriophage or very similar viral types. However, lysogenic bacteria may convert to the lytic phase and lyse.

VIRUS MUTATION

Animal viruses can mutate spontaneously or mutations can be induced. Common mutagens are: nitrous acid, 5-fluorouracil and 5-bromodeoxyuridine. Other viruses are sensitive to temperature change and mutate at an elevated temperature.

ANTIVIRAL AGENTS

Since the virus is an obligate intracellular parasite, inhibition of certain processes which are critical to the virus but not to the host cell can lead to virus inactivation. Several agents are capable of preventing virus replication. Some of these agents are selective in their action others are less specific. Some of the specific inhibitors of virus replication are:

INTERFERON

A glycoprotein of mammalian cell origin which protects cells from viruses. Once susceptible host cells take in (adsorb) interferon, the interferon induces the formation of a protein that inhibits viral transcription. Interferon can be used against different virus types. Interferon is considered to be the least toxic of the antiviral agents. Many fail to observe an immune response in the host after several treatments with interferon.

IODODEOXYURIDINE

This is a halogenated deoxyribonucleoside which inhibits DNA synthesis. Use of this agent is limited, since it may also stop mammalian DNA synthesis. It has been used effectively in the treatment of herpes keratitis.

ADAMANTADINE

This agent is effective against the rubella virus and the influenza A virus. Andamantaderic stops penetration and uncoating of these viruses.

VIAZOLE

Viazole is a nucleoside that prevents nucleic acid production in both DNA and RNA viruses. However, it should be noted that viazole also prevents the formation of nucleic acid in human cells.

VIRAL DISEASES--THE HERPETOVIRUSES

The herpetoviruses include a variety of viruses that cause a diversity of diseases. The herpetoviruses are usually cytocidal for their host and generally these viruses, after a primary infection, tend to remain inactive in the host. However, these viruses can be activated from their latent or inactive state.

HERPESVIRUSES

1. Herpes Simplex Type 1

    Herpes simplex type 1 strains are responsible for (oral infections) cold sores. These viruses form small plaques and CPE in tissue cultures. The CPE produces adherent rounded cells.

2. Herpes simplex Type 2

    Herpes simplex virus type 2 strains are associated with genital infections. In tissue cultures, large plaques and CPE's resulting in clusters of loosely arranged rounded cells with or without syncytial giant cells are evident.

EPIDEMIOLOGY

Herpes simplex type 1 infections are disseminated by the mouth and respiratory tract. Herpes simplex type 2 is considered a veneral disease and is spread by sexual contact. It should be pointed out that clinically type 1 herpes has been recovered from genital lesions and type 2 has been recovered from oral lesions; although this does not occur often, it can occur.

The risk of infection with herpes simplex type 2 (also called herpes genitalis) is greater with sexual activity with a number of different sexual partners (possibility increases as the number of sexual relations increases) but primary infection may not be apparent. In women, versicular lesions may appear in the vulva, vagina, perineum and cervix. In males the lesions are more visible and may occur on the glands of the penis, the prepuce or the shaft.

TABLE 1

VIRAL FAMILIES

VIRAL FAMILIES	SOME FAMILY MEMBERS	NUCLEIC ACID TYPES
Papovaviridae	Human Wart Virus Simian Virus	Double Stranded DNA
Adenoviridae	Adenovirus Type 1 (Human)	Double Stranded DNA
Herpetoviridae	Herpes Zoster Virus Herpes Simplex Virus Epstein-Barr Virus Cytomegalovirus	Double Stranded DNA
Picornaviridae	Poliovirus Rhinovirus ECHO Virus	Single Stranded RNA
Reoviridae	Diarrhea Virus (Newborn)	RNA
Togaviridae	Rubella Virus	RNA
Coronaviridae	Respiratory Viruses	RNA
Paramyxoviridae	Measles Virus Newcastle Disease Virus	RNA
Rhabdoviridae	Rabies Virus	RNA

Newborns may contract neonatal herpes, which may produce no effects at all or cause a systemic infection which could be fatal. Those newborns who contract neonatal herpes may demonstrate central nervous sytem disorders as infants.

Herpes simplex type 1 is contracted very young. Versicular lesions occur in the mouth, and although this infection could spread to the central nervous sytem, it usually remains restricted to the oral cavity, upper respiratory tract and eyes.

LATENT STAGE/RECURRENT INFECTION WITH HERPES SIMPLEX VIRUSES

Recovery from a herpes virus primary infection does not assure destruction of the virus. The latent virus is believed to remain within neurons. Controversy exists as to whether or not the latent virus replicates within the neurons. Latency may be reversed despite the presence of antibodies in the "apparently recovered" person. Fever, emotional stress, hormonal imbalance or another diseases or disorders may cause the reactivation of a latent herpes virus--either type 1 or 2.

Type 2 has been recovered from cervical carcinoma cells in culture and many feel that type 2 could be implicated in cervical cancer.

VARICELLA/HERPES ZOSTER

Varicella or chickenpox is a contagious childhood disease. Chickenpox is a disease characterized by vesicular eruption and the presence of acidophilic intranuclear inclusion bodies in invaded cells. The skin lesions of chickenpox appear as blister-like vesicles that may form pustules before drying and crusting.

Chemotherapeutic agents do not seem to shorten the duration of chickenpox, but antibiotics could be helpful in preventing secondary bacterial infection of the pock lesions.

HERPES ZOSTER

It is believed that the same virus that causes chickenpox in children causes zoster (shingles) in adults, who have recovered from chickenpox. Many believe that shingles is the reaction of the latent virus harbored in sensory ganglia. Shingles is characterized by intensive pain and versicular eruption along the affected nerves. Secondary bacterial infections develop in the pustules. Corneal and conjunctival lesions may occur. Shingles is more painful than chickenpox. The etiologic agent of varicella and zoster is clinically referred to as the V-Z virus.

Since chickenpox is more prevalent than shingles, some host condition or factor is believed to be responsible for shingles in adults. This is supported by the fact that there is a marked increase in the number of shingle cases reported with leukemia patients, and patients receiving immunosuppressive agents.

TRANSMISSION/PREVENTION

Prior to the formation of skin lesions, chickenpox can be transmitted via the respiratory tract.

Isolation of the infected prevents the spread of chickenpox.

The convalescing or high risk patients may receive zoster immune globulin. However, zoster immune globulin is in limited supply and difficult to obtain.

EPSTEIN-BARR VIRUS

E. B. virus is the causative agent of infectious mononucleosis, an acute infectious disease primarily affecting children and young adults. The disease is characterized by the presence of: (1) a high heterophile antibody titer; (2) a large number of monocytes; and (3) abnormal, large lymphocytes. Also, lymphadenitis is apparent in nearly all cases. The clinical symptoms are fever, headache, chills, sore throat, fatigue and sweating.

Virus specific antibodies are produced by those infected. Those antibodies are the basis for serological tests and provide immunity against reinfection of external origin. However, since the E. B. virus is believed to be latent, reactivation of the virus is possible. It is believed that the virus can remain latent in certain body cells without replication. However, some recovered patients disseminate the virus via mouth secretions without demonstrating symptoms of the disease. These people, as well as those in the infectious state, may spread the disease to unsuspecting potential victims.

Infectious mononucleosis is most prevalent among young adults and since kissing is one of the most frequent modes of transmission, it has often been referred to as the "kissing disease".

E. B. VIRUS/BURKITT'S LYMPHOMA

The E. B. virus has been associated with Burkitt's lymphoma (BL), however it is not certain that the E. B. virus is the etiologic agent of BL.

It is theorized that some host factor is present with the E. B. virus to produce BL. Wherever malaria is prevalent, BL seems prevalent. Malaria suppresses the immune system and increases lymphocyte production in patients. Malaria may be the contributing factor which produces tumors in people infected with EB virus. The Epstein-Barr virus has not been observed in BL tumor cells in situ, but tumor cells cultured in vitro do produce the EB virus. This supports the theory that the EB virus genome can be found in a latent state within the tumor cells.

CYTOMEGALOVIRUS INFECTIONS

Most adults have been found to contain circulating CMV antibody against the 3 CMV antigenic types. When adults contract CMV virus, the infection is usually asymptomatic, however, if the unborn fetus contracts CMV, it is less fortunate. Should a pregnant woman contract a primary infection of CMV, the virus can penetrate the placenta and infect the fetus. Fetal infection may either (1) produce no immediate abnormalities in the newborn; (2) cause congenital defects; or (3) be fatal for the fetus.

Fetal infection with CMV is believed to be the most frequent cause of mental retardation caused by a virus. Some DMV congenital defects such as deafness, mental retardation,visual disorders or chronic gastroenteritis are not obvious for some time after birth, and in some cases not apparent until later in life.

CMV, like the other herpesviruses, exists in the latent state and may be reactivated. CMV may be contained in saliva. Anything which impedes the proper functioning of the immune system could reactivate CMV.

CLINICAL DIAGNOSIS

Complement-fixing antibody assays, antibody titer determinations, and fluorescent antibody tests for IgM antibodies are used to diagnose CMV.

Urine and saliva specimens may be grown on human fibroblasts. The fibroblasts are checked for CPE's. Fibroblasts become characteristically enlarged and rounded and contain intranuclear inclusions.

EPIDEMIOLOGY

In adults, infection with CMV is asymptomatic. Consequently, it is difficult to control the spread of CMV. Blood transfusions from asymptomatic adults may contain infected lymphocytes and may also contribute to the dissemination of the infection.

HEPATITIS

The causative agent of viral hepatitis is yet to be propogated in cell cultures. Clinical studies on hepatitis patient specimens (blood, urine, feces) have provided data which indicate that two viruses are the etiologic agents of hepatitis. These two etiologic agents differ in time of incubation and epidemiology. One agent is responsible for viral hepatitis while the second causes serum hepatitis. Viral hepatitis is infectious in nature and is referred to as hepatitis A virus or HAV. The serum hepatitis etiologic agent is designated hepatitis B virus or HBV.

The hepatitis A virus is thought to be made up of a single stranded RNA. Depending upon the stage of the disease, the hepatitis A virus may be recovered from either feces or blood. Urine and nasal secretions have yielded controversial or negative findings.

SYMPTOMS OF HEPATITIS A

Generally, the incubation stage lasts 3 to 5 weeks. Initially, the patient experiences fever, GI tract disorders, headaches, and anorexia and lassitude.

The liver and postcervical lymph nodes are affected and leucopenia may be observed. The patient may jaundice and the liver and spleen are sensitive. Live damage may occur, but this is usually limited and self repair due to cell regeneration is not uncommon. Hepatic dysfunction and bilirubin dysfunction may also occur.

EPIDEMIOLOGY OF HEPATITIS A VIRUS

Viral hepatitis is usually contracted by ingesting the hepatitis A virus contained in contaminated water, milk or food. Contact with infected persons may also contribute to the spread of the disease via the respiratory tract. The disease is more prevalent among the young and the intestinal-oral route is the more common mode of infection. High public health standards and good personal health standards reduce the spread of this disease.

SERUM HEPATITIS (HEPATITIS B)

The hepatitis B virus (or HBV) has not been grown in vitro. In this trait it resembles hepatitis A. Immunological and E/M studies have provided information concerning HBV.

The HBV virus is reported to be spherical with circularly arranged double stranded DNA. The outer surface of the hepatitis B virus contains an antigen. Since this antigen is an outer surface antigen it is referred to as HB_sAG. The HB_sAG surface antigen has four subtypes.

CLINICAL DIAGNOSIS

Since the hepatitis B virus has not been grown in vitro, diagnosis of this disease is dependent primarily upon serological and immunological tests. Gel immunodiffusion, complement-fixation, red blood cell agglutination, radioimmunoassay and counterelec-trophoresis techniques are employed to test for HB_sAG, or anti-HB_s.

The anti HB_s is detectable during the latter phase of the disease. To show the presence of HB_sAG in a serum specimen, specific anti-HB_s serum is needed. This can be obtained from animals immunized with high concentration of HB_sAG. The presence of HB_sAG confirms viral hepatitis. The test antigen is obtained from human serum free of anti-HS antibody (or in minimal amounts). While many workers use the AGD test (Agar Diffusion test), the AGD test is not always sufficient to test for HB_sAG. Counterelectrophoresis is the most widely used procedure for HB_sAG determination. HB_sAG tests are routine in blood banks and diagnostic laboratories.

Also, blood banks check donors for HB_sAG to prevent the spread of hepatitis B. Furthermore, patients with either hepatitis A or B frequently demonstrate liver dis-orders which are clinically observable due to an increase in serum glutamic-pyruvic transaminase and serum glutamic-oxalacetic transaminase (SGPT/SGOT).

HEPATITIS IMMUNITY

Recovery from hepatitis A infection produces a long lasting immunity against the hepatitis A (HAV) virus and recovery from hepatitis B virus provides a solid immunity against that specific virus. THERE IS NO CROSS IMMUNITY. People immune to hepati-tis B could still contract hepatitis A.

Gamma globulin injections yield poor immunological results as a prophylactic against Hepatitis B. Researchers are actively engaged in developing a vaccine against hepatitis B. Immunized experimental animals have demonstrated promising results but more work is needed for this vaccine to be proven safe and to be administered to in-dividuals requiring the vaccine.

TABLE 2

CERTAIN CHARACTERISTICS DIFFERENTIATING HEPATITIS A AND B

CHARACTERISTIC	HEPATITIS A	HEPATITIS B
Incubation Time	2-6 weeks	7-25 weeks
Clinical Diagnosis	Based upon SGOT	Based upon SGOT and the recovery of HB_sAG
Immunity*	Good	Good

---

*No cross immunity for A and B hepatitis.

Passive immunity is dependent upon the effectiveness of anti-HB antibody. Pooled gamma globulin has been used with limited success for high risk cases. Pooled serum provided limited but better results. The HB_sAG is inactivated to prevent infection but permit it to remain immunogenic.

THE PARAMYXOVIRUSES

These viruses are large enveloped RNA viruses. The genome is single stranded.

PARAINFLUENZA VIRUSES

These viruses are etiologic agents of upper respiratory tract infections. Some of the parainfluenza viruses are called hemadsorption or HA viruses because they form hemagglutinin for certain erythrocytes added to tissue cultures containing these viruses.

PARAINFLUENZA VIRUSES - TYPE 1

Two viruses, the Sendai virus and HA 2 virus, are included in this category. Sendai virus causes pneumonitis in the newborn and may be fatal. It is frequently found in Japan and the East. The Sendai virus forms hemagglutinin and is capable of agglutinating red blood cells. Human, monkey, guinea pig and mouse RBC's can be agglutinated by S.V. Since this virus is more frequently prevalent in Japan and since it is a hemagglutinating virus, it is also called hemagglutinating virus of Japan (HVJ). The name influenza virus type D also refers to this virus.

HEMADSORPTION TYPE 2 VIRUS

This virus causes acute respiratory infections in adults and children. This virus has been the causative agent of respiratory infections in the U. S. as well as Japan. In tissue cultures, HA type 2 virus forms hemagglutinin with no apparent CPE.

The pathogenicity of this virus has been exhibited causing acute respiratory infections in inoculated human volunteers.

The third parainfluenzal virus has been recovered from children suffering either from croup or an acute laryngotracheobronchial condition. Respiratory specimens from these children when inoculated into tissue cultures produced the CA (Croup associated) virus or the acute laryngotracheobronchial virus (ALTB). CPEs in the tissue culture demonstrated a syncytial mass, the absence of cell peripheries and the presence of granules in cell cytoplasm. The CA (or ALTB) virus agglutinates RBC's at 4°C, but agglutination is absent at 37°C.

Type 3 parainfluenza virus affects adults and children. Type 3 resembles a sheep virus and serological differentiation of this virus from the sheep virus is difficult.

MUMPS

Mumps is a highly contagious disease spread via saliva. The incubation period is about 18 to 21 days after contraction. The virus replicates in the person's respiratory tract and nearby lymph nodes. The key clinical symptom is the enlargement of the parotid, salivary, sublingual and submaxillary glands. Occasionally, but not generally, the infection could occur in the pancreas, testes, ovaries or meninges. Infection of the testes in males who have reached puberty could result in a condition referred to as orchitis. This may cause sterility and inflammation of the testes and may cause much pain.

CLINICAL DIAGNOSIS

Patient symptoms play a major part in the diagnosis of mumps. Diagnosis of typical and atypical cases can be confirmed by injecting saliva in week old chick embryos or kidney cell cultures. The virus will cause hemagglutination in the chick embryo and will agglutinate guinea pig RBC's added to the tissue culture. Known antisera can be used to prevent hemagglutination.

IMMUNITY

Contraction of and recovery from mumps provides permanent immunity. A vaccine of live attenuated viruses has been used successfully. The inactivated mumps virus has been used (1) for adult males who have never contracted mumps, and (2) as a skin test to determine whether people, who think they never contracted mumps, are susceptible or immune to the virus. Immune persons usually demonstrate a positive skin reaction in 1 or 2 days following inoculation with the inactivated virus.

MEASLES (RUBEOLA)

The measles virus, like the other paramyxoviruses, is an enveloped single stranded RNA virus. The measles virus also demonstrates monkey RBC hemagglutination and produces cytopathic effects (CPE) in cultures. The CPEs reveal giant multinucleated cells and eosinophilic cytoplasmic inclusions. Antisera contain anti-hemagglutination antibodies. The measles virus differs from the other paramyxoviruses in that it lacks neuraminidase.

Measles is most frequently contracted from infected and contaminated respiratory secretions. After contracting the infectious agent, the virus usually replicates in the conjunctiva and upper respiratory tract. When sufficient viruses are produced, they invade the bloodstream (viremia) and are carried to all parts of the body. The patient may demonstrate a relatively high fever, conjunctivitis, a widespread rash, a sore throat, cough and headache. Conjunctival and respiratory secretions contain the infectious virus. Urine specimens may contain the virus during the latter part of the incubation period and for 3 to 4 days after the appearance of the rash.

Generally, measles is not a serious disease, however, one uncommon complication is encephalitis. Encephalitis may be fatal or cause neurological damage.

Furthermore, secondary bacterial infections are common in many measles cases and the patients seem particularly vulnerable to pneumonia.

CLINICAL DIAGNOSIS OF RUBEOLA

Diagnosis 2-3 days before the appearance of the rash is dependent upon the observation of characteristic lesions, called Koplik spots, on the mucosa of the mouth. The spots have bluish-whitish centers and appear in infected throats of at least 95% of all measle cases. During this stage of infection, the virus can be recovered from nasal and throat secretions and may be grown in tissue cultures. Cough and fever may be observed prior to the rash.

The virus can be detected in culture by hemadsorption of the infected cells following the addition of appropriate red blood cells.

The presence of giant cells in nasal secretions is characteristic of measles.

Serologic tests may also be performed for complement-fixing antibodies.

IMMUNITY

There is only one antigenic measles virus type and recovery from measles provides a solid lifelong immunity.

CONTROL/PREVENTION

It is difficult to control the spread of measles (particularly among children), since the patients are infectious six to seven days before the formation and spread of the rash. At this time, the condition is not usually diagnosed.

Pooled gamma globulin may be given to high risk cases after exposure to measles. This may prevent or lessen the effects of the disease. Should this inhibit the disease, the gamma globulin recipient does not have a solid immunity against rubeola and may be vulnerable to a subsequent measles infection.

ACTIVE IMMUNIZATION

Vacines have been developed for the nonimmune. The first vaccine was formed by killing viruses that were grown in cell cultures. These viruses were treated and killed with formalin. The formalin-killed vaccine produced neutralizing antibodies in the recipient but failed to provide a solid immunity. Consequently, a live attenuated measles vaccine was needed to provide greater protection against measles.

The first live attenuated vaccine produced reactions in a great number of recipients. A more recent live attenuated vaccine yielded a high antibody titer in most recipients after a single injection of the vaccine.

GERMAN MEASLES (RUBELLA)

Rubella is not a paramyxovirus, but is a togavirus. Since it is the causative agent of German measles, it will be discussed here. The rubella virus is enveloped and is made up of a single-stranded (+) RNA molecule which functions as mRNA. When grown in cell culture, the rubella virus may or may not cause CPEs. This virus grows in the host cell's cytoplasm and not the nucleus.

PATHOGENICITY

German measles is clinically milder than rubeola measles, however, it has received much medical attention because of its tetratogenic effects upon the fetus should the mother contract the infection within the first 3 to 6 months of pregnancy.

The rubella virus appears to be particularly attracted to fetal tissues and some researchers feel that virus growth in fetal tissues inhibits normal fetal cell proliferation. The tetratogenic effects on the fetus may result in either fetal abortion, stillborns, or cause aberrations resulting in mental retardation, microcephaly or congenital heart defects. The extent of the defects upon the fetus depends upon the stage of fetal development at the time the mother became infected with rubella. Greatest damage seems to occur during the first two months of pregnancy at which time all proliferation and differentiation is greatest.

In children, rubella is a common, infectious, relatively mild disease. Studies performed on human volunteers indicate that neutralizing antibodies inhibit the clinical manifestation of the disease and that the virus may be recovered from serum and urine specimens 6 or 7 days prior to the appearance of the rash. High antibody titers cause the disappearance of the virus in the urine and serum.

Before and after the rash, the rubella virus can be recovered from nasal and pharyngeal secretions.

CLINICAL DIAGNOSIS

Hemagglutinin is formed by this virus and infected tissue culture cells can be detected by hemadsorption. Complement-fixation and antibody neutralization tests may also be used to diagnose rubella. Diagnosis of recent infections can be made by using fluorescent anti-IgM to determine the presence of IgM antibodies in the serum. CPEs are not always present and therefore are not reliable diagnostically.

IMMUNITY

There is only one antigenic type rubella virus. Recovery from rubella seems to provide a life-long immunity. There have been rare reports that second infections with rubella have occurred, but the disease symptoms are very mild or inconspicuous.

IMMUNIZATION

Live attenuated rubella vaccines are used to provide temporary immunity against rubella.

The antibody titer is lower in vaccinated individuals than in individuals who have contracted and recovered from the disease. Also, vaccine recipients have complained of fever and discomfort.

Although no fetal abnormalities have been attributed to the vaccine, it is still strongly suggested that women pregnant within 3-4 months should avoid receiving the rubella vaccine.

Diagnosis of recent infections can also be made by determining the presence of IgM antibodies in the serum. Fluorescently labeled anti-IgM can be used.

CPEs are not always detected in tissue culture cells and cannot be used for reliable diagnosis.

Oncogenic Viruses

DNA VIRUSES

Some viruses may induce a proliferative cellular response which may be limited or result in unlimited disorderly growth thereby causing malignant tumors.

An understanding of the cell-virus relationship is critical to establish the cellular modifications that occur in tumors.

Oncogenic viruses, introduced to cell cultures, changed, transformed and induced uncontrolled proliferation of the cells. The transformed cells grow in clusters rather than in an orderly parallel fashion. Changes have been reported in the cell membrane of the transformed cells. Furthermore, antigens not present in the original cells are present in the transformed cells. These new antigens may be on the cell surface or within the cell itself. Virally transformed cells are malignant and may form tumors in appropriate hosts. Cells from viral tumors, when grown in tissue cultures, exhibit the traits of viral-transformed cells.

DNA viruses which may induce cell transformation may have oncogenic potential.

RNA TUMOR VIRUSES

E/M has differentiated three types of RNA tumor viruses: Types A, B, and C. The type A RNA tumor viruses are intracellular; type B viruses are extracellular, and type C viruses are extracellular and possess a centrally located, electron dense nucleoid.

The murine leukemia viruses and avian viruses are type C RNA tumor viruses. The C type viruses are the most frequently occurring RNA tumor viruses, and like the DNA oncogenic viruses, the C type RNA viruses may be formed as a result of cell transformations.

Replication of RNA tumor viruses does not lead to host cell death, however, the host cell is the site of virus proliferation and cell transformation. Numerous hypotheses exist as to how carcinogenic agents cause RNA viruses to transform or allow viruses to grow.

Many human breast cancers and leukemias are remarkably similar to the RNA tumors induced in experimental animals. This finding has led many to establish a relationship between cancer and RNA viruses.

BIBLIOGRAPHY AND RECOMMENDED READINGS

Acton, J. D., Kucera, L. S., Myrvik, Q. N. and R. S. Weiser. 1974. *FUNDAMENTALS OF MEDICAL VIROLOGY*. Lea and Febiger Publishers. Philadelphia.

Christensen, Mary. *BASIC LABORATORY PROCEDURES IN DIAGNOSTIC VIROLOGY*. 1977. Charles C. Thomas Publishers. Springfield, Illinois.

Dulbecco, R. and H. S. Ginsberg. *VIROLOGY*. 1978. Harper and Row Publishers, Inc. Hagerstown.

Fenner, F. J. and D. O. White. *MEDICAL VIROLOGY*. Second Edition. 1976. Academic Press, Inc. New York.

Freeman, Bob A. *BURROW'S TEXTBOOK OF MICROBIOLOGY*. Twenty-first Edition. 1979. W. B. Saunders Company. Philadelphia.

Grist, N. R., Ross, C. A. and E. J. Bell. *DIAGNOSTIC METHODS IN CLINICAL VIROLOGY*. Second Edition. 1974. J. B. Lippincott Company. Philadelphia.

Horne, Robert W. *STRUCTURE AND FUNCTION OF VIRUSES*. 1978. Edward Arnold Publishers. London.

Luria, S. E., Darnell, J. R., Baltimore, D., and A. Campbell. *GENERAL VIROLOGY*. Third Edition. 1978. John Wiley and Sons. New York.

Volk, W. A. *ESSENTIALS OF MEDICAL MICROBIOLOGY*. 1978. J. B. Lippincott Company. Philadelphia.

Chapter 5

Immunology/Serology

JOYCE M. CUFF, Ph.D.
Assistant Professor of Biology
Notre Dame College
Manchester, New Hampshire

OUTLINE

INTRODUCTION

Most routine serology performed in the clinical laboratory involves identification of antibodies to specific pathogens. The most direct method of determining the causative agent of a disease is to isolate the pathogen from a clinical specimen. Both methods of determining etiology, isolation and serological tests, have limitations. One of the major problems in serology is that conclusive diagnostic evidence depends upon demonstrating a rise in antibody titer during the course of infection or between acute and convalescent stages. Very often, when it is time for the second sample, the patient has been discharged from the hospital or is deceased. In either case the sample is not forthcoming. A second problem with routine serology has been the lack of good antigen preparations resulting either in decreased sensitivity of the test or cross-reactions. Isolation of the pathogen, on the other hand, is specific and usually rapid. Problems with the quality of the specimen as well as culturing problems, offering appropriate media and conditions, have resulted in a fairly low percentage of isolations of a number of pathogens. Consequently, in spite of its limitations, serology is an important diagnostic tool, increasing in importance as the science continues to develop.

This chapter is designed to give the clinical laboratory scientist sufficient theoretical background in immunology to understand the procedures and implications of serological tests. The major serological tests are also briefly reviewed.

IMMUNOLOGY/SEROLOGY

BASIC CONCEPTS

Immunology is the study of the lymphoid specific mechanisms of defense against infectious agents as well as against any substance recognized as foreign by the body. The ability to recognize foreignness resides in, and is a property of lymphoid tissue. Clinical immunology deals primarily with the production and detection of antibodies to infectious disease, but hypersentivities and tissue rejection are also important areas of concern.

In addition to specific lymphoid responses to infectious agents, the body has a number of nonspecific defenses. Externally there are mechanical barriers such as the tough keratin in the skin, the sweeping action of cilia in the respiratory tract, and the flushing action of urine and tears. The chemical external barriers include the acidic pH of sebaceous gland secretions, stomach secretion, and urine, antibiotics produced by natural flora and fauna such as colicins produced in the intestines, and fatty acids and basic proteins present on body surfaces.

Internal defenses are primarily blood related and are both nonspecific and specific. There are five blood cell lines in the body--four of which are involved in fighting infectious disease. Megakaryocytes give rise to the small nonnucleated blood platelets which are involved in clotting. Disruption of platelets begins a sequence of reactions resulting in the formation of a network of fibrin which prevents foreign matter from spreading to other parts of the body. Platelets also release beta lysin, a protein demonstrating Gram + bactericidal action. The granulocytes and the monocytes which give rise to macrophages are involved in three defense activities: phagocytosis, inflammation, and chemotaxis. Phagocytosis is the process in which a particle or cell is engulfed by ameboid movement of a cell forming a vacuole called a phagosome. After the particle is ingested, lysosomes release enzymes into the phagosome, digesting its contents. Phagocytosis is not always followed by intracellular digestion; some microorganisms are capable of resisting lysozyme action and may even multiply within the phagocyte. Inflammation is both a protective and constructive process. Local injury stimulates the release of vasoactive substances and chemotaxins from leukocytes. These substances cause vascular dilation and increased blood flow to the area, increased vascular permeability, and accumulation of phagocytic cells. The increased blood flow and permeability make the area red and swollen, but also serve to dilute the harmful substances causing the inflammation. Platelets are usually disrupted in inflammation, and a clot forms which contains phagocytic cells and foreign particles in the area. Finally, phagocytes ingest microorganisms and other particulate matter, and the source of the inflammation is thereby eliminated. The fourth type of blood cell involved in host protection is the lymphocyte. Lymphocytes are responsible for specific interactions with foreign substances which result in direct lysis, antibody formation, or inactivation through mediators collectively called lymphokines.

Blood is composed of cells and plasma. The latter also has a role in the host response to infection. The basic protein, lysozyme, present in urine and tears, is also present in plasma and exerts a bacteriolytic action by hydrolyzing bacterial cell walls. Lysozyme is more effective against Gram + than Gram - bacteria. Plasma also contains hormones, particularly corticosteroids, which modulate the immune response. There is a group of plasma proteins, complement, which when stimulated by antibody or by another protein, properdin, demonstrates cytolytic, chemotactic, and inflammatory properties. Finally, interferon, an antiviral substance produced by cells in response to viral infection, may be present in plasma, and prevents translation of viral proteins in cells exposed to it.

ANTIGENS

An antigen is any substance capable of inducing antibody formation and reacting specifically with such antibodies. Antigenicity is directly dependent upon the degree of foreignness of the substance. The degrees of foreignness are categorized as follows:

A. Autologous, autogeneic--antigens within the same individual.

B. Isologous, syngeneic, congeneic--antigens of individuals with identical genetic makeup, for example identical twins and inbred animals.

C. Homologous, allogeneic--antigens of individuals of the same species, but not genetically identical.

D. Heterologous, xenogeneic--antigens of individuals of different species.

Antigenicity is also directly proportional to the degree of chemical complexity, diversity, stability, and size of the antigen. Proteins are the most antigenic macromolecules because they are highly diverse, chemically complex, relatively stable molecules, capable of reaching considerable size. Polysaccharides are less antigenic than proteins because polysaccharides are not as diverse nor as stable as proteins. Nucleic acids because of their instability and lack of diversity, and lipids because of their size and simplicity are poor antigens.

Haptens are substances which are capable of reacting with antibodies but do not stimulate antibody production. Haptens are usually small molecules which, when combined with a larger inert carrier molecule become antigenic.

Antigenicity may be increased by increasing the amount of time the antigen is exposed to lymphocytes. Adjuvants are substances which are not readily broken down by the body; when an antigen is combined with an adjuvant it increases the life time of the antigen in the blood and results in an enhanced antibody titer. In addition, adjuvants may increase lymphocyte proliferation, thereby enhancing the immune response. The two most common adjuvants are Freund's adjuvant, an oil-water emulsion which may contain mycobacteria, and BCG, bacille Calmette-Guerin, consisting of an attenuated strain of Mycobacterium bovis, Corynebacterium parvum, and levamisole. BCG is used in tumor therapy to activate the immune response.

Antigenicity is influenced by the route of administration of the antigen. Any antigen administered orally may be modified by digestion. Therefore, the oral route is reserved for local antibody production by stimulation with antigens whose normal route of entry is the digestive system, such as polio virus. For production of high titers of antibody, the intravenous (IV) route is best, but is the least safe. Dosages must be precisely calculated, and toxic and hypersensitivity reactions guarded against if this method is chosen. For these reasons the IV route is usually reserved for production of antibody by laboratory animals. Intraperitoneal administration also gives high titers of antibody. For most immunizations in man, the antigen is given intramuscularly. This results in a lower titer of antibody than the other methods but because some of the antigen is broken down in the muscle and the rest is released slowly into the blood, it is a far safer method and hypersensitivity reactions are far less common. The antibody titer from intradermal administration of antigen is quite low and therefore this route is used primarily for hypersensitivity screening, not immunization.

The primary antigenic activity does not seem to reside in the entire antigen molecule but appears to be restricted to one or more relatively small groups of residues, perhaps 5-10 amino acids in the case of protein antigens, called the antigenic determinants. Antigenicity of a substance is increased as the number of antigenic determinants increases. Similar antigenic determinants in two unrelated organisms results in cross-reactivity. Cross-reactivity refers to the ability of an antibody to one organism to react with a second seemingly unrelated organism. The ability of vaccinia antibodies to react with smallpox is an example of cross-reactivity and is the basis for vaccination.

IMMUNOGLOBULINS

GENERAL PROPERTIES   Immunoglobulins, or antibodies, are globular proteins. As is true of all proteins, the sequence and types of amino acids determine the structure and properties of immunoglobulins. Basically each immunoglobulin contains units made up of two identical heavy chains and two identical light chains of amino acids held together by disulfide bridges and alligned such that free carboxyl groups are at one end and the free amino groups are at the other. The amino end, called the Fab region, reacts with the antigen and therefore the amino acid sequence at this end must differ for every antigen. The carboxyl end, called the Fc region, is the end which reacts with complement, possesses no antigen specificity and is therefore constant or nonvariable. The light chains are always one of two types, lambda (λ) and kappa (κ). There are five types of heavy chains, alpha (α) or A, delta (δ) or D, epsilon (ϵ) or E, gamma (γ) or G, and mu (μ) or M. (Figure 1)

Immunoglobulins are classified into 5 groups on the basis of their heavy chain. Within each class, variations in the heavy chain are grouped as subclasses. Immunoglobulin G (IgG) makes up from about 30-70% of the immunoglobulins in normal serum. It is a monomer, that is, it is made up of one immunoglobulin unit. IgG has a sedimentation coefficient of 7s, and has a half-life of about 24 days. IgG appears late

FIGURE 1

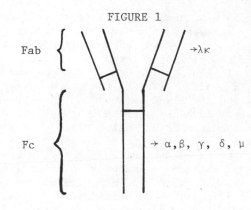

in infection and is responsible for long-term immunity and fetal immunity. There are 4 subclasses of IgG. IgM makes up from 2-10% of circulating antibodies. It is a pentamer, with a sedimentation coefficient of 19s and a half-life of approximately 5 days. IgM appears early in infection and disappears rapidly. There are 2 sub-classes of IgM. IgA constitutes between 5 and 20% of circulating antibodies. Its size ranges from 7 to 17s because it can exist as a monomer, a dimer or a trimer, and it has a half-life of about 5 days. IgA is produced in mucous membranes and other secretory cells. There are 2 subclasses of IgA. IgE is present in trace amounts in normal serum. It is a monomer, with a sedimentation coefficient of 7 or 8s and has a half life of about 2 days. IgE is homocytotropic, causing the release of histamines from mast cells when in combination with appropriate antigen, resulting in an allergic reaction. There are no subclasses of IgE. IgD constitutes about 1-2% of circulating antibodies. It is a 7s monomer with a half life of 2 days. Its physiological function is still undetermined.

IDENTIFICATION   There are three properties of immunoglobulins used as a basis for separation and identification: size, charge and antigen specificity. Filtration is used to separate proteins on the basis of size. Electrophoresis is used to sepa-rate proteins on the basis of charge. Each protein has a pH at which it is neutral, its isoelectric point. At the isoelectric point the proteins will not be attracted to either a negative or a positive charge, and will, therefore, stop migrating in a hydrogen solution in an electric field. When fresh serum proteins are electropho-resed, five peaks are usually distinguishable: albumin, alpha-1, alpha-2, beta, and gamma fractions. Most immunoglobulins migrate with the gamma fraction. The number of peaks corresponds to the number of proteins or protein groups separated. The area under each peak corresponds to the amount of each protein present. Different numbers of peaks can be obtained from the same sample by using different electro-phoretic media. Immunoelectrophoresis is a combination of electrophoresis and immu-nodiffusion. This technique utilizes all three criteria for separation, size, charge, and antigen specificity. Immunoelectrophoresis is usually done on an agar strip and antisera to the various proteins is added in a trough parallel to the line of electrophoretic migration. Diffusion of the various proteins is independent of one another; lines of precipitation will form where antibodies combine with their specific antigens.

Identification of specific antibodies or antigens can be achieved by using an agent that can easily be detected. Radioimmunoassay uses radioactivity to monitor the location of antigen or antibody. Immunofluorescence uses fluorescent dye that can be visualized with a fluorescent microscope to signal the presence of antigen or antibody. Both types of assay can be modified to fit the needs of the test. In the competitive direct binding test a known antibody is affixed to a solid phase such as latex and the complementary antigen in the patient's serum is estimated by allowing a specific amount of serum to compete with a known amount of labelled antigen. The concentration of antigen in the patient's serum is inversely proportional to the amount of radioactivity or fluorescent dye bound. In the noncompetitive direct binding test a known antibody is again affixed to the solid phase. Next the patient's serum is allowed to react with the fixed antibody. Finally labelled antibody to the antigen in the patient's serum is added. The amount of antigen present in the serum is directly proportional to the amount of radioactivity or fluorescent dye bound. In the direct binding assays a variety of labelled antibody is required. These methods tend, therefore, to be expensive and would only be used for screening large amounts (volumes) for a given antigen or antibody. The indirect binding methods require only one type of labelled antibody and are, therefore, preferable for screening large numbers of different antigens or antibodies. In the indirect binding method an antibody from rabbit is fixed to the solid phase. The corresponding antigen from the patient's serum is then allowed to react with the fixed phase. Unlabelled human antibody to the antigen in the patient's serum is then allowed to react with the fixed antigen. Finally, labelled anti-human antibody is allowed to react with the above. The amount of radioactivity or fluorescent dye in the solid phase is directly proportional to the amount of antigen in the patient's serum. All of the binding tests described can be appropriately modified to detect antibody rather than antigen in the test sera.

PATTERNS OF RESPONSE   During the initial exposure of an individual to an infectious agent, IgM specific for that microorganism increases in concentration until a maximum is reached after 7 to 14 days. IgG is not produced at all until IgM reaches its peak; IgG reaches a plateau level between 2 and 3 weeks after the initial exposure. During subsequent exposures to the same infectious agent, the pattern of IgM synthesis remains the same as in the primary exposure, but IgG is produced simultaneously, reaches a higher plateau titer, and consequently lasts longer. This latter response is the amamnestic response.

On the cellular level, when an antigen first reacts with a lymphocyte the cell is stimulated to undergo blast transformation. The blast cells proliferate giving rise to two types of cells, plasma cells and memory cells. Plasma cells produce antibody, initially IgM, subsequently IgG. Memory cells continue to circulate and during the anamnestic response produce additional antibody. In order for blast transformation to occur, a minimum surface area of the lymphocyte must be stimulated by the antigen. This may occur because the antigen contains repetitive determinants, because the antigen naturally forms aggregates, or because helper T cells, another type of lymphocyte, focus or concentrate the antigens.

Immunity may be achieved actively when the individual produces his or her own antibodies in response to a natural infection or to an injection of attenuated or inactivated microorganisms. Immunity is passive when the individual possesses antibodies which he or she did not synthesize, as in the case of infant immunity from mother's antibodies derived from the placenta or colostrum, or immunity from injection of antibodies in the form of antitoxins or antisera.

ANTIGEN-ANTIBODY REACTIONS

DIRECT REACTIONS   Direct interactions of antigen and antibody occur and can be observed without any accessory factors. Direct interactions include precipitation, agglutination and flocculation. These are distinguished on the basis of the antigen involved. Precipitation involves soluble particles, agglutination involves insoluble particles usually cells, and flocculation involves insoluble particles smaller than cells. Agglutination in general is the most sensitive direct test because it involves the largest antigens. Large antigens require fewer reactions with antibody to achieve the critical mass which will fall out of solution.

The simplest direct tests are the tube tests. Dilutions of serum are added to constant amounts of known antigen in suspension. Tubes are shaken, incubated, and observed for precipitation, agglutination, or flocculation. Tubes which contain an excess of antigen exhibit the inhibition or prozone phenomenon. Antigens are present in such high concentration that each antibody is saturated with separate antigens so that the lattice of antigen and antibody necessary for precipitation does not occur. A similar phenomenon, the postzone phenomenon, occurs in the tubes with an excess of antibody. Each antigen is saturated with antibody and the lattice formation fails to occur. To overcome the problem of the prozone and postzone, the ring test has been developed. In the ring test, dilutions of antiserum are placed in the bottom of small tubes and carefully overlaid with antigen. The tubes are incubated at 37°C for periods up to several hours. Diffusion of antigen and antibody results in an equivalence zone and ring of precipitation. The titer is equal to the highest dilution producing a positive ring of precipitation.

Direct tests are also done in agar. There are two basic methods of using diffusion in agar, the Oudin, or quantitative method, and the Ouchterlony, or qualitative method. In the Oudin method, a well in the center of an agar plate containing antigen is filled with the serum to be quantitated. The antibody in the well will diffuse radially forming a ring of precipitation when it reaches the optimal concentration of antibody and antigen. The size of the ring is proportional to the amount of antibody in the well, and the amount of time allowed for diffusion. The Ouchterlony method involves filling a central well with serum to be tested and filling peripheral wells with antigens to be tested. As antigen and antibody diffuse radially from their wells, lines of precipitation will form. The configuration of the lines will depend upon the relationship between antigens in adjacent wells (Figure 2). Reactions of

FIGURE 2

OUCHTERLONY DIFFUSION PLATE

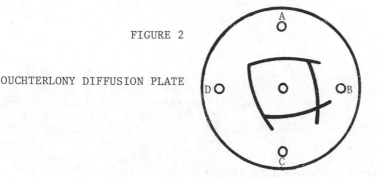

identity are those in which the precipitation lines fuse, as in A and D of Figure 2. Reactions of partial identity, that is, reactions involving some, but not all, of the same determinants are those in which a single spur appears (between D and C, and between A and B of Figure 2). Nonidentity appears as crossed lines of precipitation as between B and C of Figure 2. Antigen B and antigen C have no determinants in common.

INDIRECT REACTIONS   Indirect reactions require accessory factors or indicators in order to be observed. Examples of indirect reactions include immunofluorescence (IF) and radioimmunoassay (RIA), both of which have already been discussed. The other indirect reactions of importance in serology are neutralization, hemagglutination and hemadsorption inhibition, ELISA, and complement fixation.

Damage done to cells by viruses, cytopathic effects (CPE), vary with the type of virus. The neutralization test involves exposing virus to a patient's serum, and then allowing the virus to infect cells in culture. If the patient's serum contains viral antibody, the virus will not produce its CPE. Hemadsorption and hemlagglutination inhibition are also used to detect antibody to certain types of virus. Some viral coat proteins are capable of agglutinating erythrocytes. When these viruses infect a monolayer of cells in culture, the cultured cells adsorb erythrocytes. A patient's serum can be tested for the presence of specific viral antibody by exposing viruses to the serum and seeing if they are still capable of hemagglutination or hemadsorption induction.

ELISA, enzyme-linked immunosorbent assay, is a fairly new technique in which an antigen is attached to a solid matrix, like latex, in a column. The patient's serum is then tested for complementary antibody by exposing the column to the serum. A suspension of antigen to which an enzyme has been attached is passed through the column. The antigen will react with bound patient antibody. Finally, substrate is passed through the column. The substrate will be modified by attached enzyme, and the product observed in the eluent. Usually an enzyme is chosen which will yield a color change or some other easily detected and easily quantitated change in substrate. The amount of product is proportional to the amount of antibody in patient's serum. ELISA is second only to neutralization in sensitivity.

The complement fixation test utilizes the fact that the group of serum proteins, complement, attaches to antibody-antigen complexes. If these complexes are attached to a cell, complement will cause cell lysis. Serum is tested for the presence of antibody by being exposed first to complementary antigen and complement. After the reaction has been allowed to proceed, sensitized sheep red blood cells are added; sensitized cells are coated with antibody. If the patient's serum contains antibody, the antibody-antigen complex formed in the first step will fix the complement, and complement will not be free to lyse the sensitized red blood cells. Therefore, negative hemolysis is positive. Hemolysis occurs when the patient's serum lacks antibody; no antigen-antibody-complement complex forms in the first step, and complement is free to lyse the sensitized red blood cells.

COMPLEMENT

Complement is a group of eleven serum proteins. Complement functions in recognition of the invading substance, enzymatic activation and attack of invader. The C1 protein is responsible for recognition and binds to the Fc portion of the antibody molecule bound to antigen. Enzymatic activation involves C4, C2, and C3 which becomes bound to cell surface receptors. Attack involves components C5-C9. Properdin is a system in the blood which appears to be capable of activating complement when there are insufficient quantities of specific antibody to activate the classical pathway.

Complement component C1a, 4, 2, 3b enhances immune adherence which stimulates phagocytosis. C3 and C5a stimulate the release of histamine from basophils or mast cells and are therefore involved in the inflammatory response. Components C3a, C5a and C567 exhibit chemotactic activity.

CELLULAR IMMUNITY

BIOLOGICAL BASIS   There are two types of lymphocytes responsible for specific immunity, T cells and B cells. The B cells are responsible for antibody production. B cells are processed in areas of the body equivalent to the bursa of Fabricius in chickens, presumably the gut-associated lymphoid tissue. T cells are responsible for cell-mediated immunity and are processed by the thymus gland. T cells like B cells undergo transformation and memory cell formation when stimulated by appropriate antigens.

Cell-mediated immunity is achieved through toxins which lyse the antigen directly or through attraction of phagocytic cells. The mediators of cellular immunity are the lymphokines. Lymphotoxin lyses cells and may be important in routine destruction of cancer cells in the body. Chemotaxin which attracts monocytes, and macrophage inhibitory factor (MIF) and leukocyte inhibitory factor (LIF) which prevent egress of macrophages and polymorphonuclear neutrophils respectively, act to keep phagocytic cells exposed to the antigen. Macrophage activating factor (MAF) enhances the phagocytic and cytolytic activity of macrophages. Blastogenic factor induces multiplication of lymphocytes and thereby increases the immune response.

ASSAYS Cell-mediated toxicity of T cells can be estimated by using vital staining to calculate the percentage of cells killed or by using radioactivity to calculate the percentage of cells capable of incorporating labelled precursor or the percentage of cells leaking prelabelled intracellular constituents. The lymphokines most easily assayed are MIF and LIF. A capillary tube containing macrophages or polymorphonuclear neutrophils is placed in a solution containing T cells. If the T cells have been activated, MIF and LIF will be in solution and the cells will not migrate from the tube. Antigens can be attached to red blood cells; T cells specific for that antigen will form clusters of red cells around them called rosettes.

IMMUNOLOGICAL DISFUNCTIONS

HYPERSENSITIVITY There are two types of hypersensitivity reactions, immediate-type hypersensitivity (ITH) occurring within thirty minutes of exposure and delayed type hypersensitivity (DTH) developing over a 24-48 hour period. In ITH, an allergen stimulates the production of IgE which attaches to mast cells or basophils. During subsequent exposures the allergen combines with IgE on the mast cells causing these cells to release histamine, serotonin, bradykinin, and SRS. These substances cause smooth muscle contraction and vascular dilation and increased vascular permeability. Hay fever, hives, and asthma are examples of ITH. The most severe ITH reaction is systemic anaphylaxis in which smooth muscle contraction can result in death. The mediators of hypersensitivity are inactivated very rapidly by the body. If an individual requires something he or she is hypersensitive to, it may be administered in very small doses at 20 minute intervals so that the mediators do not reach a high level and no serious reaction occurs. Hypersensitive individuals may also be desensitized to an allergen by receiving an initial small dose intramuscularly followed in subsequent weeks by gradually increasing doses. In this way a high titer of IgG is gradually built up which can compete with IgE for allergen and thereby decrease or eliminate the allergic response.

Local anaphylaxis is used diagnostically to test for hypersensitivity. When a sensitized individual's skin is exposed to allergen a typical "wheal and flare" reaction occurs. Mediators cause vascular dilation (flare) and increased vascular permeability (wheal). Agents to be tested are generally scratched on the forearm of the individual and reactions observed. In the Prausnitz-Küstner test serum from an allergic individual is injected intradermally into a non-allergic individual. A period of 1 to 2 days is allowed to elapse while Ig^E attaches locally to mast cells. The allergen is then tested on both arms; the test individual is allergic if the control arm is negative and the test arm demonstrates "wheal and flare".

Sometimes ITH results in immune complexes which are not properly filtered, but are still capable of causing release of lymphokines. Lymphokines cause local vasculitis and may result in local hemorrhage and necrosis. Examples of immune complex diseases are Arthus reaction and serum sickness.

DTH is involved in a number of responses, contact dermatitis, graft and tissue rejection, tissue immunity, chronic responses to microorganisms, and some autoimmune diseases. DTH occurs when the antigen is taken up by receptor T cells; lymphokines are released causing local inflammation and induration.

DTH can be assayed by skin tests such as the patch test in which an adhesive dressing containing the material to be tested is attached to the skin and observed after 1 to 2 days for erythema and the vesticulation. The ability to develop cell mediated immunity can be tested by a patch test using dinitrochlorobenzene. The most common DTH test is the tuberculin or Mantoux test. Five tuberculin units (TU) of purified protein derivative (PPD) of the tubercle bacillus is injected intracutaneously and the diameter of induration produced in 48 to 72 hours is measured. Induration of 10mm or more is considered positive; 0 to 4mm of induration is considered negative.

AUTOIMMUNE DISEASE   Autoimmune disease may occur when a normally sequestered antigen is exposed to lymphocytes, when a body protein is changed by action of drugs or other agents, when an antigenic determinant of a microorganism is similar to a determinant of normal body proteins or when the normal immune mechanisms fail to respond either through a decrease in number or activity of supressor T cells or through production of helper T cells or B cells against self.

A number of autoimmune diseases are known. Autoimmune hemolytic anemias produce symptoms of fever, fatigue, jaundice, and enlarged spleen. Two groups of antibodies based on their optimal reactivity temperatures have been identified in autoimmune hemolytic anemias. Warm agglutinins react optimally at 37°C, are primarily IgG, and appear to be directed against Rh antigen. Cold agglutinins react optimally at 4°C, are primarily IgM, and appear to be directed against red cell antigen I. A class of cold agglutinins cause a rare disease, paroxysmal cold hemoglobinuria, and are distinguished from other cold agglutinins by the fact that they are of the class IgM and are directed against red cell antigen P. Patients demonstrate symptoms of hemolytic anemia after being exposed to the cold, at which time antibody reacts with the red cell. Hemolysis occurs at body temperature, 37°C.

Systemic lupus erythematosis (SLE) is a generalized disorder involving vasculitis in a number of organs. SLE occurs primarily in females between the ages of 10 and 40. In SLE, peripheral leukocytes extrude nuclear material and other cellular components to which the body makes antibody. The antinuclear antibody test is used in diagnosing SLE.

Rheumatoid arthritis is a chronic inflammatory disease producing vasculitis and usually involving the synovial lining of joints. Rheumatoid factor (RF) is an IgM capable of reacting with IgG and is found in the serum of patients with rheumatoid arthritis. RF is used diagnostically, however it should be kept in mind that RF occurs in a number of other diseases, particularly connective tissue disorders.

There are a number of autoimmune diseases that are organ specific, myasthenia gravis in muscle, rheumatic fever in heart tissue, and multiple sclerosis in central nervous tissue.

TRANSPLANTATION AND TUMOR IMMUNOLOGY

HLA ANTIGENS   The antigens which are the most important in transplantation immunology are coded for by the 6th chromosome in a region called the HLA region. Products of these genes combine with mucopolysaccharides on cell surfaces. Histocompatibility depends upon these antigens and is tested for in four steps: first blood typing is done; second, HLA antigens are serotyped; third, recipient's serum is tested for preformed antibody to donor's tissue; finally, if HLA makeup is compatible, the mixed lymphocyte response is tested. If cells are compatible, donor's inactivated cells will not stimulate the recipient's lymphocytes to undergo blastogenesis.

There are four types of rejection reactions with transplanted tissue. In the hyperacute reaction, preformed antibody to donor's antigens results in tissue rejection during the first week. In the acute accelerated reaction, previously sensitized lymphocytes, primarily T cells, stimulate rejection of tissue during the first month. In the chronic reaction, an immune response to weak or minor antigens not screened for in the histocompatibility tests requires months or even years before rejection is complete. The graft versus host reaction occurs in instances where immunologically competent cells are transplanted into immunologically deficient individuals and donor cells stage an immune response to recipient's cells.

TUMOR IMMUNOLOGY   Tumor immunology appears to be primarily a T cell function. There are two types of tumor antigen: tumor specific antigen (TSA), and tumor-associated antigen (TAA). TAA seems to be of viral origin, and is associated with most tumors. TSA varies with the type of tumor, for example alpha fetoprotein is associated with liver cancer. Ordinarily T cells are capable of lysing cells with TAA or TSA. Cancer seems to occur when these cells are not detected by T cells either because TSA or TAA are weak antigens or because the tumor cells secrete excess antigen which competes with the T cells enabling the tumor cells to multiply. The very young and very old, because of their weak immunological status, have the highest incidence of tumors.

IMMUNOREGULATION   Sometimes the body fails to react to a given antigen. Such unresponsiveness may be natural or induced. Total unresponsiveness is called tolerance; partial unresponsiveness is called immunosuppression and is usually induced. Tolerance is usually a natural phenomenon developed during fetal maturation and results in the ability of the body to distinguish between self and non-self or between what is native to the body and what is foreign. Decreasing the immune response is desirable in the case of allergic responses, in transplantation or tissue grafting, and in autoimmune disease. Immunosuppression is achieved through use of chemicals of 5 types:

A. Lympholytic Agents--include alkylating agents and X-rays, both of which kill cells by damaging nucleic acid.

B. Antimetabolites--usually analogues which effect bone marrow stem cells and thereby decrease the number of lymphocytes.

C. Antibiotics--substances which inhibit macromolecular synthesis and are therefore nonspecific.

D. Antibodies to lymphocytes--antilymphocytic serum (ALS) which react with lymphocytes specifically and destroy them.

E. Hormones--corticosteroids, for example, are known to suppress immune responses.

Occasionally it becomes important to increase the immune response, as in the case of tumor therapy. Such potentiation of immunity can be achieved by prolonging the release of antigen or using an antigen that will have a general effect on lymphocyte proliferation like BCG.

SEROLOGICAL TESTS FOR SYPHILIS

Tests for syphilis are based upon the appearance of two types of antibodies during infection: a specific antitreponemal antibody and a nonspecific antibody, reagin, which reacts with lipid antigens.

The serological test for reagin, the Venereal Disease Research Laboratory (VDRL) test, is a modification of the rapid plasma reagin (RPR) test. The antigen used is cardiolipin (usually from beef), lecithin, and cholesterol, and should be stored at room temperature. Control sera should include a weakly reactive and a nonreactive serum for the qualitative test, and a titered reactive serum for the quantitative test. Serum stored at 4°C or -20°C is good for several months. All sera should be heat inactivated at 56°C for 30 minutes, and the test should be performed at room temperature within 4 hours of heating. Serum and antigen are combined, rotated for 4 minutes and read for agglutination. Results are reported as R - reactive, W - weakly reactive, or N - nonreactive. Undiluted serum is used qualitatively to screen for reagin; serial dilutions are performed to quantitate reagin. Positive reactions are obtained in a number of conditions other than syphilis, including malaria, infectious mononucleosis, and upper respiratory tract infections. Some autoimmune diseases also demonstrate elevated reagin levels, particularly rheumatoid arthritis, and systemic lupus erythematosus. Some drugs including heroin and some anti-hypertensive drugs may stimulate the production of reagin.

When the diagnosis of syphilis is difficult on the basis of symptoms and reagin levels, specific antitreponemal antibody tests are performed. Either the Treponema pallidum inhibition test (TPI) or the fluorescent treponemal antibody absorption test (FTA-ABS) is appropriate. The antigen in the TPI test is usually Treponema pallidum from rabbit testicular syphilomas. Antigen and heat-inactivated sera are incubated with guinea pig complement at 37°C overnight in an atmosphere of 95% nitrogen and 5% carbon dioxide. Dark field illumination is used to measure loss of motility. The disadvantages of the TPI test are that the antitreponemal antibody lasts too long for the TPI test to be used to assess therapy, antitreponemal antibody does not distinguish T. pallidum from the treponemas causing pinta and yaws and finally, the antitreponemal antibody titer is not significant in early syphilis.

The FTA-ABS method uses nonviable T. pallidum as antigen on a methanol or acetone fixed slide. Fixed antigen is first exposed to test serum and then treated with anti-human globulin labelled with ferritin isothiocyanate (FITC). Careful standardization of this method is necessary because of the subjectivity of estimating the degree of reactivity.

SEROLOGICAL TESTS - CONDITIONS OTHER THAN SYPHILIS

WIDAL REACTION   The Widal test is used to measure antibodies to O (somatic) and H (flagellar) antigens of the agents of enteric fever. Agglutination is observed in tubes containing twofold dilutions of serum in normal saline and antigen. Tubes are incubated at 50 to 52°C for 2 hours to detect anti-H antibody and for 24 hours to detect anti-O antibodies. At the end of the incubation time tubes are shaken gently. Agglutination of H antigens is seen as a large, flocculur aggregate, which is easily disrupted. Agglutination of O antigen is seen as a small, granular aggregate, less easily disrupted. There are a number of factors affecting antibody titers in enteric fever including (a) the stage of the disease; titers increase during the second week; (b) age, geography, and certain narcotics, as well as vaccination with related organisms may cause false positives; (c) early treatment with antibiotics may prevent a rise in antibody titer; and (d) technical variations cause changes in antibody titer. Because of these difficulties, no minimum titer can be established as diagnostic. A demonstrable rise in titer of at least a factor of four from successive samples frozen and assayed simultaneously may be considered supportive diagnostic evidence.

Tests for Tularemia and Leptospirosis are conducted as Widal-like agglutination tests. Tularemia is endemic in the middle and southern parts of the United States. Agglutination test titers greater than 1:40 or 1:80 are considered diagnostic of infection. Leptospirosis is an acute, febrile septicemic disease caused by Leptospira interrogans. Serological quantitation of antibody is achieved by incubating mixtures of antigen and serum for 2 to 3 hours at room temperature. In sera with high titers, a prozone phenomenon may occur. Therefore, serial dilutions of serum should be tested. Titers greater than 1:100 may be significant, but a rise in titer should be demonstrated in successive samples. Single sample titers greater than 1:1600 may be considered significant.

FEBRILE AGGLUTININS   Febrile agglutinins appear in rickettsial and brucella infections. The Weil-Felix test is based on the fact that antibodies produced in response to some rickettsial infections react with the O antigens of Proteus OX strains. This cross-reactivity is probably due to the fact that the O antigen is a polysaccharide having less diversity and complexity than protein antigens. There are five rickettsial diseases endemic to the United States. The three most common rickettsial diseases, typhus, spotted fever, and scrub fever can be tested using the Weil-Felix reaction (WF). The less common rickettsial diseases, Q fever and rickettsialpox, are negative in the WF test. The WF test has limitations, but its simplicity and the availability of antigens make it the most widely used rickettsial assay. The more specific tests available are usually restricted to rickettsial research labs.

Whole, unflagellated proteus bacilli, viable or killed, are used in the WF test. A rapid slide test may be used, followed by a tube test for confirmation of positives. Tenfold dilutions of serum ranging from 1:10 to 1:2560 are combined with OX-19, OX-2, or OX-K antigens and agitated to mix. The tubes are incubated for 2 hours at 37°C and overnight at 4°C. Results are reported on a 0-4 scale from zero to complete agglutination. Presumptive tests should be forwarded to state labs or to CDC for tests with species specific antigen. Low titers to Proteus antigen are frequent in the general population. Therefore, titers lower than 1:160 are not significant. A fourfold change in antibody titer between acute and convalescent sera tested simultaneously is significant. Convalescent serum showing a dropping antibody titer is a useful tool for retrospective diagnosis.

Brucellosis is determined by detecting antibodies to cell wall antigens A and M(S) of Brucella suis, B. abortus, and B. melitensis. Dilutions of serum from 1:20 to 1:10,240 in 10 tubes are combined with antigen and incubated for 48 hours at 37°C. Usually a titer of 1:320 is considered presumptive; isolation is necessary for confirmation. Antibodies to Brucella cross-react with Vibrio cholera, Francisella tularensis, and Yersinia enterocolitica.

STREPTOCOCCUS   Group A beta-hemolytic streptococcus has a number of antigens which can serve as the basis of serological tests. The most common antibody tested for is that directed against streptolysin O, antistreptolysin O antibody (ASO). Antibodies to hyaluronidase, deoxyribonuclease B, and streptokinase may also be tested for to support a presumptive ASO titer.

The most common ASO test is the neutralization test, based on the finding that reduced streptolysin O lyses erythrocytes. Serum is diluted and incubated with antigen. Erythrocytes are added and hemolysis is observed after the tubes are reincubated. A buffer containing gelatin may be used to inhibit spontaneous lysis and stabilize streptolysin. There are two disadvantages of the ASO neutralization test.

First, other substances can neutralize streptolysin O including beta-lipoprotein of hepatic disease and Bacillus cereus and Pseudomonas infections. Second, oxidized en-zyme is not hemolytic. Streptolysin O fixed to latex particles overcomes both dif-ficulties since only ASO will agglutinate oxidized as well as reduced streptolysin. ASO tests display good reproducibility and use readily available antigen. ASO titers are elevated in 80-85% of rheumatic fever cases and in glomerulonephritis.

Other tests used to diagnose streptococcal infections include the anti-hyaluroni-dase test (AH) and the streptozyme test. AH is often elevated in those individuals with negative ASO titers. In addition, good antibody levels are obtained in skin infections where ASO titers tend to be low. Neither the AH reagents nor the response is as good with respiratory infections as with skin infections. In the streptozyme test, a number of streptococcal antigens fixed to inert particles are reacted with sera and allowed to agglutinate. This test provides an excellent screen for anti-streptococcal antibody. However, because there are a number of antigens and anti-bodies involved, the test cannot be standardized.

C-REACTIVE PROTEIN   C-reactive protein is a 7.5s protein, not an immunoglubulin, appearing in the sera of patients in the acute phase of pneumonia, streptococcus, and staphylococcus infections, in acute rheumatic fever and rheumatoid arthritis, in cirrhosis of the liver, in certain carcinomas and in a number of other disease states. C-reactive protein reacts with a nitrogenous polysaccharide of pneumococcus, C-substance. Liquid or gel precipitation tests are used to determine the presence of C-reactive protein. Antiserum to C-reactive protein is used as a precipitant be-cause it is more specific than C-substance. The presence of C-reactive protein indicates the presence of fever, infection, inflammation, or tissue necrosis.

AUTOIMMUNE ANTIBODIES

NUCLEAR ANTIGENS   Antibodies to nucleic acid (ANA) are screened for most commonly in suspected systemic lupus erythematosus (SLE), but also in chronic active hepatitis with negative hepatitis-associated antibody titers. IF is generally used because it is more sensitive than complement fixation or precipitation tests. Mouse liver cells or leukocytes are first exposed to test sera and subsequently to goat or rabbit FITC-conjugated anti-human antibody. Each laboratory should have control sera of patients with each disease to be tested for in order to compare patterns of fluorescence. Antibodies to double-stranded DNA (as in SLE) produce a peripheral or diffuse pat-tern. Since 10% of normal individuals have ANA titers as high as 1:16, titers higher than this and hemagglutination titers to DNA antibody are important in confirming SLE diagnosis.

RHEUMATOID FACTORS   A group of immunoglobulins reactive with the F_c portion of IgG is associated with rheumatoid arthritis. All tests for rheumatoid factors use an indicator system with IgG bound to a carrier such as bentonite or erythrocytes and detect agglutination, flocculation, and precipitation, primarily due to IgM. Human IgG bound to carrier is incubated with the heat inactivated test serum for 30 minutes at 4°C and for 90 minutes at 56°C. Tubes are then observed for agglutination. False positives may occur if the test serum is not completely inactivated or in the pre-sence of excess lipid in the serum. In addition, rheumatoid factors may be elevated in other chronic inflammatory diseases such as tuberculosis, leprosy, and bacterial endocarditis, or in infectious mononucleosis.

TISSUE-SPECIFIC ANTIGENS   Indirect immunofluorescence tests have been developed to detect antibodies to a number of tissue specific antigens appearing during certain autoimmune diseases: (a) anti-thyroglobulin appears in chronic thyroiditis, goiter and thyroid tumors as well as in some instances of diabetes melitis and pernicious anemia; (b) anti-mitochondrial antibodies appear primarily in biliary cirrhosis and (c) anti-smooth muscle antibody is associated with chronic active hepatitis.

ANTI-SPERM ANTIBODY   Production of antibody to human spermatozoa may have a role in unexplained infertility.   In addition, anti-sperm antibody production has been found to be a possible sequella to vasectomy.   Immobilization of spermatozoa in the presence of complement is measured after incubating antigen and serum for 1 hour at 37°C.   In one experimental group, 15% of the cases of unexplained infertility displayed anti-spermatozoan antibody.

INFECTIOUS MONONUCLEOSIS   Two types of antigens are associated with infectious mononucleosis, heterophile antigens and Epstein-Barr antigens.   Heterophile antigens are serologically related substances in cells from different species.   Forsmann first discovered the phenomenon, and often the name Forsmann is improperly used as synonymous with heterophile antigen.   The heterophile antigen associated with infectious mononucleosis is the Paul-Bunnel antigen (PB) which reacts with both sheep and beef erythrocytes.   The Monospot test differentiates anti-heterophile antibodies on the basis of absorption.   Normal and test sera are first reacted with guinea pig cells which absorb Forsmann antibodies but not PB antibodies, and separately with beef cells which absorb PB antibodies.   Fresh horse cells which agglutinate all available heterophile antibodies are added to all test solutions.   Sera exposed to guinea pig cells will show no agglutination with normal serum but strong agglutination with serum from individuals with infectious mononucleosis.

EB virus is widespread throughout the world.   Economically deprived areas have a greater EB seropositive population than economically advanced countries.   In seronegative adolescents, primary exposure to EB virus often appears as infectious mononucleosis.   EB virus is also associated with Burkitt's lymphoma and nasopharyngeal carcinoma in some populations.   Immunofluorescence is used to detect antibodies to a number of EB antigens.   These tests are used primarily to screen for susceptibility to infectious mononucleosis, to discover the etiology of heterophile-negative mononucleosis, and to determine the etiology of a number of other diseases.

PREGNANCY   The simplest test for pregnancy is the agglutination test for human chorionic gonadotrophin (HCG) in urine.   HCG is a glycoprotein similar in structure to human luteinizing hormone (HLH), and less closely related to human follicle-stimulating hormone (HFSH) and human thyroid stimulating hormone.   The test is performed using urine; first voided morning specimen provides the best titer.   The urine sample may be kept at room temperature if used within 12 hours, otherwise the specimen should be frozen until tested.   HCG fixed to erythrocytes or latex particles is mixed with serum containing anti-HCG antibody and the urine sample, and the mixture is incubated at 37°C for 90 minutes.   High levels of HCG in the serum will compete with the fixed HCG for antibody, thereby inhibiting erythrocyte or latex agglutination.   The test reagents are available in kits, and the test is 75-95% reliable for detection of pregnancy at 6 weeks.   False positives may result from low levels of HLH in the urine or from nonspecific interference from high levels of protein.   Lower than normal values of HCG during pregnancy may reflect ectopic pregnancy or threatened abortion.   In these instances human placental lactogen (HPL) levels should be checked.   Ectopic pregnancies will show no HPL; threatened abortion will show decreased HPL.   Increases in HCG late in pregnancy may reflect toxemia or diabetes melitis.   In the former condition HPL will be decreased; in the latter, HPL will be increased.   HCG in the urine of nonpregnant, non-aborted females who have not been recently pregnant is a sign of trophoblasic or neoplastic disease.

PARASITIC DISEASES   Serology is useful in the diagnosis of parasitic infections when identification of parasites in blood or stool specimens is difficult. Serological tests are most commonly performed in the detection of trichinosis, amebiasis, toxoplasmosis and hydatid disease caused by Echinococcus. Antibody titers in these infections are often quite high. Serology is also useful in parasitic epidemiology.

AMEBIASIS   A number of tests are available to detect antibodies in invasive amebiasis. The sensitivity of these tests increases with the invasiveness of the parasite; serological methods do not detect cyst carriers. The indirect hemagglutination (IHA) test is the most widely used; titers greater than 1:128 are considered positive.

TOXOPLASMOSIS   The methylene blue dye test (MBD) once popular, has been replaced by immunofluorescence (IF) and IHA tests which are safer, simpler, and more economical. Low persistent antibody titers to toxoplasma are found in a large percentage of the population. Therefore, IHA titers of 1:256 are of questionable significance. IF titers tend to be lower than IHA titers; titers exceeding 1:64 may be clinically significant. Since the IF and IHA tests use separate toxoplasma antigens, some labs choose to run both tests.

ECHINOCOCCUS   High IHA titers (greater than 1:256) are usually CF positive and indicate echinococcal infection. Elevated IHA titers have also been observed in collagen disease, cirrhosis, and other parasitic infections. CF and IF titers drop during the first year after removal of hydatid cysts, whereas IHA antibodies persist. Therefore IHA titers alone are diagnostically insufficient.

TRICHINOSIS   Bentonite flocculation (BF) is a sensitive (approximately 97%) reproducible test. Antibodies to trichina may be detected 3 weeks after onset of primary infection. The antibody titer rises for several weeks, gradually reaches a peak, and declines over a two-year period. A titer of 1:5 is significant; a rise in titer during infection is an important corollary for diagnosis.

FUNGAL DISEASES   As is true of parasitic infections, serology in mycotic infections is important when direct isolation and diagnosis is difficult. In general, a positive high titer may be significant, even in the absence of subsequent samples. Low titers, however, may result from a previous infection, an early primary infection, or cross-reactivity, since a number of fungal antigens are widespread. Low titers should be accompanied by successive sampling and titering, trying a variety of antigen preparations, and studying hypersensitivity (skin) reactions. Negative titers do not necessarily mean the absence of infection by the given agent; some mycoses render the individual immunologically unresponsive. In addition, antibodies do not usually appear from 1-4 weeks after the onset of infection.

Hypersensitivity often accompanies histoplasmosis and coccidioidomycosis. An intradermal injection of 0.1 ml of dilute antigen is read after 48-72 hours in the case of histoplasmosis, and after 24-36 hours for coccidioidomycosis. A diameter of induration of 5mm or more is positive. The skin test is used as a screen for endemic disease and not diagnostically unless a negative titer is obtained from an infant with a presumptive mycotic infection. A negative skin reaction demonstrates a definite absence of the disease except in very early stages of infection, in terminal infections, or in cases of anergy. A skin test is useful in prognosis; a positive skin test followed by negative tests indicates a poor prognosis.

Blood samples for fungal serology are collected aseptically, and the serum diluted 1:10,000 with merthiolate. Samples stored in this way do not have to be refrigerated. Samples to be used for culturing specimens should not be diluted with preservative, but should be stored and shipped frozen or refrigerated.

ASPERGILLOSIS   The most commonly used tests for aspergillosis are complement fixation (CF) and immunodiffusion (ID). Aspergillus fumigatus, A. flavus, and A. niger
antigens are used in the ID test. Lines of identity with known reference sera are
highly specific. Nonspecific bands may result from precipitation of C-reactive protein by C-substance of Aspergillus ssp. Sera from patients with invasive disease
may have to be concentrated; all other sera need not be concentrated.

BLASTOMYCOSIS   CF and ID tests are commonly used to identify blastomycoses. Positive lines of identity with B. dermatitidis indicate recent or current infection. In
established cases, a decrease in titer indicates a positive prognosis. CF, although
less sensitive and less specific than ID, is more widely used. At least 50% of
positive CF sera reacts with other antigens, and sera from patients with other mycotic
infections also react positively in the CF test for B. dermatitidis. In general,
titers greater than 1:8 are considered positive; a rise in titer in sequential samples is more significant.

CANDIDIASIS   Latex agglutination (LA) and ID tests show a sensitivity of 80-90%,
and are often used to test the significance of Candida ssp. in clinical specimens.
ID is the more specific of the two tests; the only cross-reactivity occurs with
Torulopsis glabrata antisera. LA titers of 1:8 are considered presumptive.

COCCIDIOIDOMYCOSIS   The CF and tube precipitin (TP) tests use separate antigens and
are therefore often used together. TP precipitins appear early in primary infections,
and decline within 6 months. Three dilutions of serum are used for the TP test to
obviate the zonal inhibition problem. CF antibody titers parallel the course of infection, appearing later than precipitins and persisting as long as candidiasis is
active. A CF titer of 1:16 indicates disseminating disease.

HISTOPLASMOSIS   CF and ID tests are widely used to detect histoplasmosis antibodies. A CF titer greater than 1:16 or a rising titer is strong evidence of histoplasma infection. ID bands, h and m, are significant indicators of histoplasmosis.
The m band may appear after skin tests in histoplasmosis-negative individuals.

BIBLIOGRAPHY AND RECOMMENDED READINGS

Barrett, J. T. *TEXTBOOK OF IMMUNOLOGY.* Third Edition. 1978. W. B. Saunders, Co., Philadelphia.

Bellanti, J. B. *IMMUNOLOGY II.* 1978. W. B. Saunders, Co., Philadelphia.

Carpenter, P. C. *IMMUNOLOGY AND SEROLOGY.* Third Edition. 1975. W. B. Saunders, Co. Philadelphia.

Daniels, J. C. "Immunoglobuline Disorders". Directions in Immunology. Monograph. 1976.

Hyde, R. M. and R. A. Patnode. *IMMUNOLOGY.* 1978. Prentice-Hall. Reston, VA.

Neter, E. "Bacterial Hemagglutination and Hemolysis". Bact. Rev. 20:166, 1956.

Pike, R. M. "Antibody Heterogeneity and Serological Reactions. Bact. Rev. 31:157, 1967.

Roitt, I. *ESSENTIAL IMMUNOLOGY.* Third Edition. 1977. Blackwell Scientific Publishers. London.

Rowley, D. "Phagocytosis". Adv. Immunol. 2:24, 1962.

Uhr, J. W. "Delayed Hypersensitivity". Physiol. Rev. 46:360, 1966.

Yalow, R. S. "Radioimmunoassay: A Probe for the Fine Structure of Biological Systems" Science. 200:1236, 1978.

Chapter 6

Immunohematology

MARGARET MUELLER-SHORE
MT (ASCP), CLS (NCA), MS
Medical Technology Program Director
Central Maine Medical Center
Lewiston, Maine

INTRODUCTION
THEORY REVIEW
    A Review of Immunology
    Genetic Concepts
BLOOD GROUP SYSTEMS
    The ABO System
        Introduction
        Inheritance
        Chemical Characteristics of A, B, H Antigens
        Bombay Phenotype
        Anti-H
        Se Gene
        Subgroups of A
        Notes on ABO Testing
        Other tests
    Rh
        Nomenclatures
        Du
    Lewis
    MNSs
    Li System
    P System
    Lutheran
    Kell, Duffy, and Kidd
    Study Guide for Blood Group Systems
IMMUNOHEMATOLOGICAL DISORDERS
    Auto Immune Hemolytic Anemia (A.I.H.A.)
        "Warm" Type
        "Cold" Type
        Paroxysmal Cold Hemoglobinuria
        Drug-induced Hemolytic Anemia
    Hemolytic Disease of the Newborn
        Sensitization of Mother
        Prognosis of HDN Infant
        Prevention of HDN

INTRODUCTION

This chapter is a comprehensive review of important topics in Immunohematology. It is designed to help the student preparing for a general certification examination, the practitioner rotating through Blood Bank, and the student currently studying Immunohematology.

The chapter contains applicable academic material with clinical applications, when possible. The chapter is not designed to replace a technical text, but rather to provide a broad foundation upon which technical details may later be assimilated. The reader will find headings for each topic.

The chapter is dedicated to all my students whose constant questions give me new perspective.

IMMUNOHEMATOLOGY

THEORY REVIEW

REVIEW OF IMMUNOLOGY

An antigen is a foreign particle that stimulates the formation of antibodies, and once formed, the antibody can react with that antigen. An antibody is a serum protein (immunoglobulin) which reacts with the antigen that stimulated its formation. There are 5 kinds of antibodies: IgG which is acquired, IgM which occurs naturally, IgA which is found in secretions such as tears, saliva, etc., IgD which is found in high amounts in patients with Multiple Myeloma, and IgE which occurs with allergies. An excess of antibody will prevent visible agglutination, and is known as the prozone phenomenon. Likewise an excess of antigen also prevents visible agglutination, and is called the postzone phenomenon.

An IgG antibody consists of 2 light chains and 2 heavy chains interconnected by disulfide linkages. The area where the 2 heavy chains meet is called the Fragment Constant (Fc). This area is composed of an invariable sequence of amino acids, terminated by a carboxyl group. This is the portion of the antibody molecule which fixes complement, macrophages, and skin. The opposite terminal ends of the light and heavy chain are called the fragment variable or fragment antigen binding site (Fab). The amino acid sequence in this region varies among different antibodies, and is responsible for the specificity of the particular antibody (Figure 1).

FIGURE 1

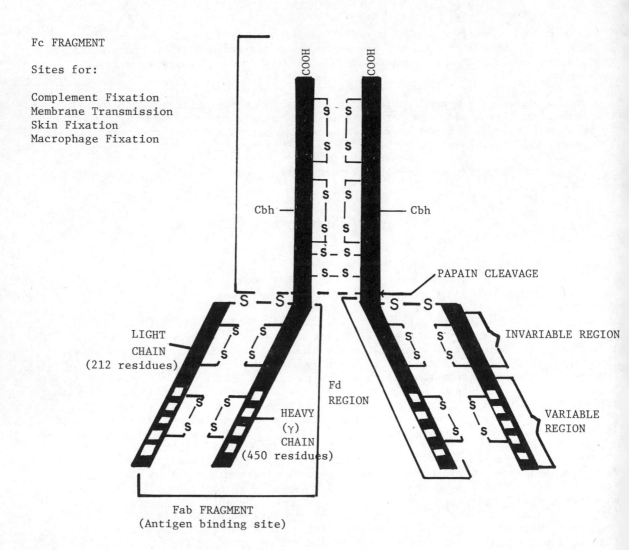

Fc FRAGMENT

Sites for:

Complement Fixation
Membrane Transmission
Skin Fixation
Macrophage Fixation

Cbh

Cbh

PAPAIN CLEAVAGE

LIGHT
CHAIN
(212 residues)

INVARIABLE REGION

Fd
REGION

HEAVY
(γ)
CHAIN
(450 residues)

VARIABLE
REGION

Fab FRAGMENT
(Antigen binding site)

COOH   COOH

TABLE 1

PROPERTIES OF SERUM IMMUNOGLOBULINS

Characteristic	IgG	IgA	IgM
Concentration in serum mg/100 ml	800–1,680	140–420	50–190
Usual temperature of reaction	$37^{\circ}C$	$37^{\circ}C$	$20^{\circ}C$
Usual Ag. stimulus	Transfusion or pregnancy		Often occurring naturally
Reactivity Best in:	albumin or AHG		Saline
Molecular weight	160,000	170,000	900,000
Molecular formula	(Monomer)	(Monomer/Dimer)	(Pentamer)
External Secretions	No	Yes	No
Complement fixation	Yes	No	Yes
Placental Transfer	Yes	No	No
Half-life (days)	25	6	5

Agglutination and/or hemolysis are the two most common reactions observed in blood banking. Hemolysis is dependent on the presence of complement, therefore, it can only be seen if fresh serum is used. Agglutination is a two step process. In the first place, sensitization occurs. Here, the agglutinin (antibody) combines with the agglutinogen (antigen) which is usually located on the cell. Agglutination, the second and visible phase, usually follows quickly.

GENETIC CONCEPTS

Each human cell has 23 pairs of chromosomes; 22 pairs are autosomes, the 23rd pair is a set of sex chromosomes. Females possess XX, while males have XY sex chromosomes.

The gene is the basic unit of inheritance. Imagine a chromosome as a string of beads. Each bead is a gene. Since you inherit a set of chromosomes, 2 genes that are located at the same place (locus) on the pair of bead strings, these are called alleles. If these beads (alleles) are both blue (identical), the individual is homozygous for that trait. If one bead is blue, and the other black, the individual is heterozygous. If the black bead is always expressed whether it is matched with black (BB) or with blue (Bb), it is a dominant gene. In this case (Bb), blue is recessive, and will only be expressed when found in the homozygous state (bb). One other possibility remains: the genes may be codominant or egalitarian, in which case products of both alleles will be detectable. An example of codominance is the ABO system, in which A is codominant with B, and if both are inherited, the individual is AB.

Other genetic terms of importance in immunohematology are:

PHENOTYPE	An observable trait (ex. blue eyes)
GENOTYPE	A list of genes for a particular trait (ex. bb for blue eyes). Phenotype can be observed or tested, however, the genotype must be deduced by patient and family history.
PENETRANCE	The amount of which a gene will be expressed in a certain population (ex. if 25% of the offspring from a Bb X Bb mating is expected to have blue eyes (bb), we state that the trait is 25% penetrant).
EXPRESSIVITY	The degree of expression of a gene in an individual; a graded response which is different in each individual.
EPISTATIC GENE INTERACTION	The interaction of genes located at different loci (ex. although the se gene is located away from the AB genes, a combination of sese will inhibit secretion of ABH substance, thus acting as an epistatic recessive supressor).
ALLELIC GENE INTERACTION	The interaction of genes occurs at the same loci (ex. A activity is reduced in the presence of B in AB individuals).
WILD ALLELE	A "normal" gene, often indicated by +.

There are 4 modes of inheritance which are of importance to blood bankers. The first is autosomal dominant or condominant inheritance. With this type of inheritance, the trait never skips a generation. An example is the crossing of two heterozygous individuals (Cc x Cc) in which 3 out of 4 children will have the trait C. Most blood group antigens fit into this category.

Autosomal recessive inheritance is demonstrated in thalessemia. The disease is a product of 2 heterozyous recessive parents (th/+) who produce a homozygous recessive (th/th) child. Both parents will not show signs of thalassemia, because of the presence of the wild allele. Therefore, carriers are often undetected in a population. Also, the problem of "normal" carriers producing affected children increases with consanguinity. Autosomal recessive traits are expressed equally in males and females, and the trait may skip a generation, then reappear.

Sex-linked dominant or codominant occurs when a normal woman marries an affected man. The trait is transmitted to the daughters but not to the sons. Few diseases are inherited this way, among them are hereditary hematuria and vitamin D resistant rickets. In the blood groups, Xg^a and Xm systems are inherited this way.

Sex-linked recessive inheritance occurs with the transmission of a trait from a carrier mother to her sons. An example is Classic hemophilia. As is seen in Figure 2 a carrier female mates with a normal male. One of her X genes carries the trait. When this gene is inherited by the son, he will be a hemophiliac. Fifty percent of the daughters will be carriers, and 50% of the sons will be hemophiliacs.

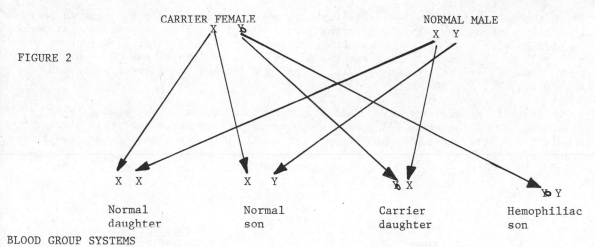

FIGURE 2

BLOOD GROUP SYSTEMS

The Abo System

Introduction

    In 1900, Landsteiner discovered the A and B Antigen on red blood cells. His conclusions are summarized in 3 basic rules:

1. The antigen on the red blood cell determines the blood groups.
2. The corresponding antibody is never found in the individual's serum.
3. The opposite antibody is always present in the individual's serum.

The antibodies of the ABO system are usually IgM.

    Table 2 demonstrates these rules. For example, an individual who is Group A has the A Antigen on his red blood cells, has no Anti-A in his serum, but always has Anti-B in his serum.

TABLE 2

Antigen on Surface of RBC	Naturally Occurring Antibody in Serum	Group	Possible Genotypes	% in U. S. White	Black	Amer* Ind.	Oriental
A	Anti-B	A	AA, AO	40	27	16	28
B	Anti-A	B	BB, BO	11	20	4	27
AB	none	AB	AB	4	4	4	5
O	Anti-A Anti-B	O	OO	45	49	79	40

INHERITANCE

    In 1930, Thomson suggested that 4 alleles were involved. They are A, A_2, B, and O (an amorph which produces no antigen product). Each person inherits two genes, one from each parent.

---

*American Indian

In the ABO system, the A gene is found on one chromosome and the B gene is found on another chromosome. Each is codominant. If a person's phenotype is A, that person may possess either AA or AO as his/her genotype. Likewise, a B person may be either BB or BO. An AB person has the genotype AB, and an O individual has OO as his genotype. Thus, there are 4 phenotypes (A, B, AB, and O), but there are 6 genotypes (AA, AO, BB, BO, AB, OO).

In order to determine the possible offspring from parents whose phenotype is known, one must first write all possible genotypes of each parent and then proceed to select 1 of the genes of each. From your resulting combinations, determine the phenotypes.

FIGURE 3

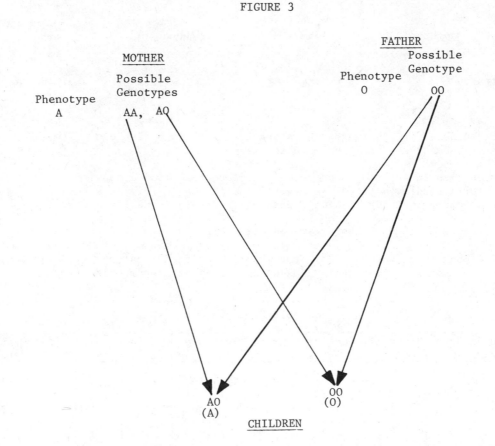

Although newborns inherit the A, B, and O genes, the antigens are not expressed in full strength until the child is 3 years of age or older. Newborns have <u>no</u> anti-A or anti-B in their serum. Any anti-A or anti-B detected in a newborn is of maternal origin.

The expression of the A and B genes depends on the action of the H gene. Most people are homozygous HH. The genotype hh is extremely rare, and is referred to as the "Bombay phenotype."

In the ABO system, the H gene works in the following manner:

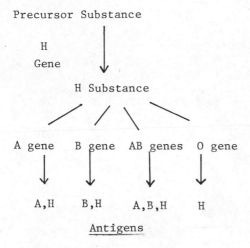

1. A precursor substance (mucopoly-saccharide) is converted by the H gene to H substance

2. The A or B genes convert part of the H substance to A or B antigen.

3. Since O is amorphic, no conversion takes place; therefore, the H antigen is found in highest concentration in O individuals.

4. The order of greatest to least RBC reactivity with anti-H is:
$O > A_2 > A_2B > B > A_1$

CHEMICAL CHARACTERISTICS OF A, B, H ANTIGENS

There are unvarying chemical traits concerning the A, B, and H Antigens. The precursor substance discussed earlier consists of 4 sugars: 2 molecules of D-galactose, one molecule of N-acetylgalactosamine, and one molecule of N-acetylglucosamine. The terminal sugar which attaches to the D-galactose determines the antigen. See Figure 4.

Protein or + Precursor + Fucose → H Antigen
lipid base   substance
on RBC   (4 sugars)

Protein or + Precursor + N-acetylgalactosamine → A Antigen
lipid base   substance
on RBC   (4 sugars)

Protein or + Precursor + Fucose + Galactose → B Antigen
lipid base   substance
on RBC   (4 sugars)

The A, B, and H antigens are present in almost all human tissues, therefore, the ABO system is important in histocompatibility.

BOMBAY PHENOTYPE

A "Bombay" individual has inherited an hh genotype, and cannot make H substance. Although he/she may have inherited A or B genes, the lack of H substance will prevent their expression. Thus, a "Bombay" individual has notated in superscript the antigen which is suppressed. ($O_h{}^{A_1}$, $O_h{}^{A_2}$, $O_h{}^{B}$, etc.) When the suppressed gene is not known, the individual is classed as O_h. Bombay individuals are compatible only with other Bombay individuals. Some Bombay individuals will produce Anti-H.

FIGURE 4

H ANTIGEN

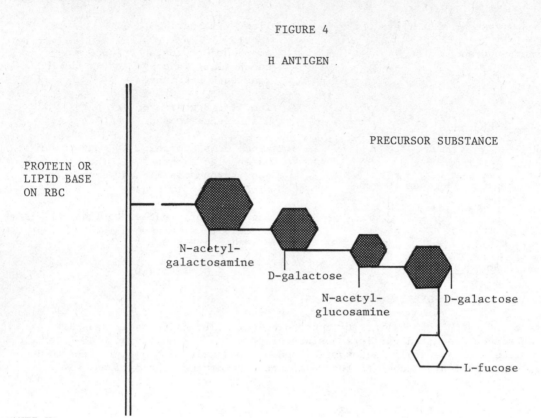

PRECURSOR SUBSTANCE

PROTEIN OR
LIPID BASE
ON RBC

N-acetyl-
galactosamine

D-galactose

N-acetyl-
glucosamine

D-galactose

L-fucose

ANTI-H

There are 2 forms of Anti-H. The first is an antibody formed in Bombay indivi-duals. The second is a cold agglutinin which may be produced by A_1 and A_1B indivi-duals. Because they have converted much of their H substance to make A_1 or A_1B_1 antigens, they may produce an antibody to the H antigen.

Lectin anti-H comes from seeds of <u>Ulex</u> <u>europaeus</u>.

Se GENE

The Se gene controls the presence of A, B, and H Antigens in saliva, sweat, tears, breast milk, urine, and semen. There are 3 genotypes: SeSe, Sese, sese. Se is dominant, therefore SeSe and Sese are secretors, i.e., these individuals will se-crete A, B, and H Antigens. In the Caucasian population, 80% are secretors. Non-secretors are sese.

TABLE 3

SECRETORS

BLOOD GROUP	ANTIGEN IN SALIVA AND BODY FLUIDS
A	A, H
B	B, H
AB	A, B, H
O	H

The most common subgroup is A_2, comprising 20% of A and AB individuals. 1-2% of A_2 individuals and 26% of A_2B persons produce Anti-A_1. These individuals will have confusing results in the forward and reverse ABO testing. For example, an A_2B cell will agglutinate in Anti-A, Anti-B, and Anti-AB sera since Anti-A usually reacts equally with A_1 or A_2 cells. The serum (which contains Anti-A_1) will agglutinate A_1 cells, but not B cells. Therefore, the person will forward group as an AB but reverse group as a B.

   <u>Dilochos biflorus</u> is a lectin which simulates Anti-A_1. It reads strongly with A_1 cells but weakly or not at all with A_2 cells, and is used to test for subgroups of A. See subgroup testing below.

NOTES ON ABO TESTING

   ABO testing consists of a forward grouping (patient cells with known Anti-A, Anti-B, and Anti-AB and a reverse grouping (patients serum with known reagent A and B cells). The tubes are checked for hemolysis and agglutination. A slide test is also available.

   Hemolysin testing may be employed to determine High-Titer Anti-A and Anti-B in Group O blood if it must be given as unmatched blood in an emergency situation. Fresh serum is incubated at 37°C with A and B cells for 1 1/2 hours, and then checked for hemolysis.

   An error in technique will cause discrepancies between the forward and reverse grouping. False positives will be seen with dirty glassware, too strong a concentration of cells, and over centrifuging. False negatives are seen with weak cell suspensions, careless reading, and warming of the cell-serum mixture.

   The presence of Wharton's jelly from cord blood, a high protein serum content, multiple myeloma, Anti-I, or injected materials such as dextran, dyes or drugs will all cause false agglutination in ABO testing.

   Remember that infants have no ABO antibodies. Elderly people can also have low antibody levels.

OTHER TESTS

   Saliva testing, to determine secretor status, utilizes <u>Ulex</u> <u>europaeus</u> lectin. This is an inhibition test.

   Subgrouping of A individuals used to be done by using absorbed Group B serum. Group B serum contains Anti-A (which reacts with A_1 or A_2 cells) and Anti-A_1 (which reacts with A_1 cells <u>only</u>). Group B serum is added to questionable A_2 cells. If the cells are A_2, they will combine with Anti-A. The absorbed serum (containing Anti-A_1) is now placed in 2 tubes, one containing known A_1 cells, the other containing known A_2 cells. If a reaction is seen with only the A_1 cells, the original cells in question are A_2.

   The more common method for subgrouping of A employs <u>Dilochus</u> <u>biflorus</u>, which reacts strongly with A_1 cells, but weakly or not at all with A_2 cells.

Rh

Eighty-five percent of the U. S. population is Rh positive. The "positive" means that these people possess the D antigen on their red blood cells. This antigen was discovered in 1939 by Levine and Stetson. By the mid-1940's, CcEe antigens were discovered. We now know that the Rh system is comprised of more than 30 antigens, however, in clinical practice, 99% of the work deals with DCcEe antigens.

Nomenclatures

There are 3 nomenclatures involved in the Rh system: Fisher-Race (DCcEe), Weiner (Rh, rh) and Rosenfield (Rh:1).

The Fisher-Race system describes 8 different Rh complexes: Dce, DCe, DcE, dce, dCe, dcE, DCE, and dCE. To convert them to the Weiner nomenclature, follow these rules:

1. If a capital D is present the Weiner system will use a capital R. Likewise, if a small d is present, a small r is used.

2. If the following letters (ce) are not capitalized, it is designated in the Weiner system as an o or blank, example Dce - Rh_o; dce = rh.

3. If the C is capitalized, the Weiner system will use a' or 1, example dCe = rh' or DCe = Rh_1.

4. If the E is capitalized, it is designated as" or 2; example dcE = rh" or DcE = Rh_2.

5. If both are capitalized, they are ascribed an alphabetical letter; example DCE = Rh_z and dCE = rh^y.

The agglutinogens are written for each of the D, C, and E's. If the C is not a capital, it is written in reverse (hr'). When dealing with agglutinogens, each antigen must be described. For example, the agglutinogens describing Dce are (Rh_o, hr', hr").

FISHER-RACE	WEINER	GENE SYMBOL	AGGLUTINOGENS
Dce	Rh_o	R	(Rh_o, hr', hr")
DCe	Rh_1	R_1	(Rh_o, rh', hr")
DcE	Rh_2	R_2	(Rh_o, hr', rh")
dce	rh	r	(-, hr', hr")*
dCe	rh'	r'	(-, rh', hr")*
dcE	rh"	r"	(r, rh', hr")*
DCE	Rh_z	R_z	(Rho, rh', rh")
dCE	rh^y	r^y	(-, rh', rh")

*Left blank, since d is an amorph, and not an antigen.

The Rosenfield system assigns a number to each of the antigens:

D = Rh:1
C = Rh:2

E = Rh:3
c = Rh:4
e = Rh:5

   The system indicates whether cells reacted with specific numbered antisera.   For
example, DCE is written as Rh:1, 2, 3.   The system is very awkward when dealing with
a large number of antiseras.   DCe/dce is written as Rh:1, 2,-3, 4, 5, 6, 7,-8,-9,-11,
12 and possibly more, depending on the number of antisera used.

   If a mate possesses DCE/Dce, either DCE or Dce will be <u>inherited</u> by the offspring.
Mixtures are not possible because the antigens are closely linked on the chromosome,
and no crossing-over takes place.   Therefore, the whole gene combination is inherited.

   In counseling cases of HDN (Hemolytic Disease of the Newborn) caused by maternal
Anti-D, it is important to determine whether the father is homozygous for D or
heterozygous (DD vs Dd).   If the father is DD, all his offspring will be Rh positive.
If the father is heterozygous Dd, there is a 50% chance that the offspring will <u>not</u>
inherit D, and be Rh negative.   That means that 50% of the children will be unaffected.

   To determine the risk, the father's blood is phenotyped.   (The term "phenotype"
is used because the cells are only tested for the presence of DCcEe, and not the 25
other Rh antigens).   Rh phenotype testing uses the individual's cells against known
anti-seras (anti-D, -C, -c, -E, -e).   Because d is an amorph and cannot be tested
for, this test does not prove the father to be DD or Dd.   To best determine this,
familial studies must be done, along with the use of phenotype frequency statistics.
The rates of occurrence are as follows:

1st order   R1   R2   r   = > 15% of the population

2nd order   r'   r" R_o =   .1 - 2%

3rd order r^y Rz   = < .1%

   As an example, the red blood cells of father X are tested with known antiseras.
The results are:

Antisera -D	-C	-E	-c	-e
Plus Father's RBC				
Agglutination Results +	0	0	+	+

+ = agglutination
- = no agglutination

   Therefore, the father possesses D, c, e, antigens.   But there are several possible
combinations.   The D may be homozygous or heterozygous.

D/D
D/d

Since c and e are present, here are their possible combinations:

Dce/Dce
Dce/dce

   The most likely combination can be determined by assigning each the percentage
of occurrence, and tallying.

Dce/Dce
(R_o) + (R_o)
2% + 2% = 4% at maximum

$$\begin{array}{lll} \text{Dce} & /\text{dce} \\ (R_o) & (r) \\ 2\% \quad + & > 15\% \quad = \quad > 17\% \end{array}$$

Therefore, the father is most likely heterozygous for D (Dd). And if heterozygous, only 50% of the offspring will inherit D. The other 50% will not be affected by maternal Anti-D, and will not have HDN.

<u>Rh antibodies</u> are usually IgG and react best at 37^oC. The agglutination is greatly enhanced by a high protein medium, such as albumin. Rh antibodies are usually stimulated by pregnancy or transfusion. The most severe forms of HDN involve Anti-D, -CD, and -DE. Less severe forms involve Anti-c, -E, or -k. For prevention of Rh_o (D) immunization, refer to the section on HDN.

D^u is a variant of the Rh system which is of practical importance. A possible explanation for D^u is that it represents a portion of D.

FIGURE 5

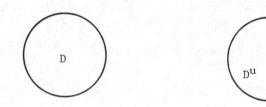

Rh D cells will usually react with anti-D after an immediate spin. To check for the presence of D^u, the cells are incubated and Anti-Human Globulin is added. This indirect Coomb's test will be positive if D^u is present.

Since a D^u individual has part of the D antigen, it is safest to treat him as Rh positive when a donor, and as Rh negative as a recipient. As a donor, he donates part of the antigen to a patient who already has the entire antigen. As a recipient, he will receive cells containing no antigen. If he were to receive Rh positive blood, he might produce an antibody to the part of the antigen which he does not possess.

LEWIS

The Lewis antigen differs from all other blood groups in that it is <u>soluble</u> and found in saliva and plasma. This antigen is <u>adsorbed</u> onto the red blood cell membrane as Le^a or Le^b. Since it is not indigenous to red blood cells and must be adsorbed, most infants type as Le(a-b-). The antigen is fully developed by the age of six.

There are two allelic genes in the Lewis system: Le and le. Both are inherited independently of the ABH and secretor genes, but the expression of the Lewis antigens is <u>influenced</u> by the presence of Hh and Sese genes. As can be seen in the table below, there are 3 Lewis phenotypes: Le(a-b+), Le(a+b-), and Le(a-b-). Here are some rules regarding Le antigen expression:

1. An lele individual will not produce any antigen, i.e., is Le(a-b-).

2. A person who inherits at least 1 Le gene and at least 1 Se gene will be Le^b positive i.e., Le(a-b+).

3. A person with at least 1 Le gene and sese genes will be Le(a+b-).

Genes Inherited	Phenotype	Adult Levels Reaction with Anti-Le^a, -Le^b		Secretes
Le H Se	Le(a-b+) 70%	0	+	ABH substance Le^a and Le^b substance
Le H se	Le(a+b-) 20%	+	0	only Le^a substance*
le H Se	Le(a-b-) 10%	0	0	80% of Le(a-b-)
le H se	Le(a-b-)	0	0	are secretors

*Se controls ABH secretion, but has no control over Le secretion.

One theory concerning the expression of the Lewis antigens is that the H and Le genes compete for a common precursor substance to make H and Le antigens present in body fluids. If you are a secretor, Le and H must compete for this common substance, and there is not enough Le^a produced to make the red cells Le^a positive. Le^b, a hybrid of these interactions, is produced.

Likewise, if a nonsecretor, the H substance precursor is not in the body fluids, but in the blood. Therefore, the Le gene can convert large amounts of this substance into Le^a for the red cells.

Two Le^a positive individuals can have an Le^a negative child, if both are heterozygous Lele.

FIGURE 6

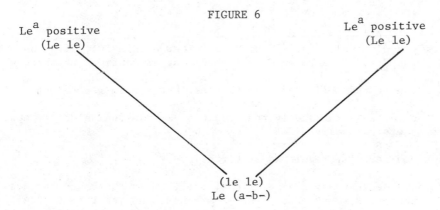

Le^a positive
(Le le)

Le^a positive
(Le le)

(le le)
Le (a-b-)

Also, two Le(a-b+) individuals can produce an Le(a+b-) child, if they are heterozygous for Sese. (See Figure 7).

Lewis <u>antibodies</u> are IgM and therefore not usually found in HDN, since they cannot cross the placenta.

Anti-Le^a is a relatively common antibody and occurs only in Le(a-b-) individuals. It binds complement, and will be incompatible with 20% of the adult caucasion population.

There are 2 forms of Anti-Le^b: Anti Le^{bL} and Anti Le^{bH}. Anti-Le^{bL} reacts with Le^b positive individuals. Anti-Le^{bH} doesn't react with Le^b positive cells of a

FIGURE 7

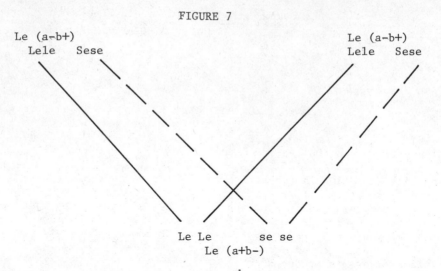

Le (a-b+)   Le (a-b+)
Lele   Sese   Lele   Sese

Le Le   se se
Le (a+b-)

Group A or B individual, but does react with Le^b antigen from O cells.

Anti-Le^x is a specific agglutinin which will bind to a cell only if Le^a is present.

People with Lewis antibodies should be given Le(a-b-) blood. Lewis antibodies are common in pregnant women who may type as Le(a-b-) when pregnant. To detect the presence of Le substance, saliva tests are better than blood tests.

MNSs

This system was discovered in 1927 by Landsteiner and Levine. Everyone is either MM, MN, or NN. The M and N antigen differs from the ABO antigen in three ways:

1. It is found on red cells and some tissues, but not in secretions.

2. Anti-M and Anti-N are usually the result of a transfusion or pregnancy, and
3. rarely occurs naturally.

The antigen is fully developed at birth.

The system does demonstrate dosage effect, i.e., MM or NN reacts stronger than MN with Anti-M and Anti-N. Anti-M and Anti-M are IgM, and react best at 4°C.

S, s are allelic genes located close to the Mn loci. s^u is a 3rd allele and when present in a homozygous state (s^{u}s^u), can produce Anti-U, which reacts with both S and s antigens. Anti-S, -s, -U are infrequent antibodies, but can cause HDN and transfusion reactions.

Ii SYSTEM

I is a public antigen, i.e., most adults possess the I antigen.i is found on cord blood cells. By the time the child is 1½-2 years old, he/she will have mostly I. It is transitional between I and i (See Table 5).

TABLE 5
AMOUNTS OF I ANTIGEN

	I	i	I^1
I adult	Much	Trace	Moderate
i cord	Little	Much	Much
i adult	Trace	Much	Trace

As can be seen in the above table, no cell completely lacks i or I antigen.

Anti-I is a cold agglutinin which is present in low titers in healthy adults. High titers are seen during and following infections with <u>Hycoplasma</u> <u>pneumoniae</u>, in less than .01% of those adults who have no I, in elderly individuals with autoimmune hemolytic anemia, and in some patients who have cancer of the reticuloendothelial system. Anti-I is an IgM and has never caused HDN.

Anti-I may cause problems in the laboratory, since it will agglutinate all adult cells, including the patient's own cells at room temperature. Such problems can be resolved by autoabsorption prior to compatibility tests, and by performing a prewarmed crossmatch. Blood should be warmed when given to a recipient who has Anti-I.

Identification of Anti-I is usually based on its decreased reactivity with cord cells and high reactivity with adult cells.

P SYSTEM

Most individuals are either P_1 or P_2. P_2 individuals often have Anti-P_1, a cold agglutinin. There are rare individuals with a "p" phenotype' their serum contains anti-PP_1p^k (anti-Tj^a).

Anti-P_1 is found in 67% of P_2 individuals. It is an IgM and has never caused HDN, but has occasionally caused a transfusion reaction. In transfusing recipients with Anti-P_1, it is best to use P_1 negative units.

Anti-PP_1p^k (Anti-Tj^a) is mostly IgM, and present in persons with "p" phenotype. It can cause HDN and transfusion reactions.

Anti-P is present in all known p^k individuals, and reacts with both P_1 and P_2 cells.

LUTHERAN (Lu)

There are many antibodies associated with this system; however, only 3 will be discussed. Anti-Lu^a (Anti-Lu^1) is a rare IgM antibody which does not cause HDN and is unlikely to cause a transfusion reaction. It will be incompatible with 7% of the population.

Anti-Lu^b (Anti-Lu^2) is an IgA (though some are IgM) which can cause HDN and transfusion reactions. It will be incompatible with 99.8% of the population.

Anti-Lu^aLu^b (Anti-Lu^3) is IgM or IgA, and is active at 37^oC in anti-human globulin or enzymes. It will be incompatible with 100% of the population.

KELL, DUFFY, AND KIDD

All three produce antibodies which cause HDN and transfusion reactions. The antibodies are IgG, and react best at 37^oC with antihuman globulin. Of the three, Kell is most antigenic and Kidd is least antigenic. However, anti-Kell is not commonly found because only 7% of the population have the Kell antigen.

TABLE 6

STUDY GUIDE FOR BLOOD GROUP SYSTEMS

ANTIBODY	IgG or IgM		BINDS COMPLEMENT	CAUSES HTR or HDN	
Anti-A		X	X	X	
Anti-B		X	X	X	
Anti-AB		X	X	X	
Anti-A		X	X	X(rare)	
Anti-H (Non-Bombay)		X	X	X	
Anti-Le^a		X	X	X	
Anti-Le^b		X	X	X	
Anti-Le^x		X	X	X	
Anti-M		X	X	X	
Anti-N		X	X(rare)		
Anti-S	X	X	X(rare)	X	X
Anti-s	X		X	X	X
Anti-I		X	I(some)		
Anti-P$_1$		X	P(some)	P$_1$(rare)	
Anti-Lu^a		X			
Anti-C	X			X	X
Anti-D	X			X	X
Anti-E	X			X	X
Anti-c	X			X	X
Anti-e	X			X	X
Anti-f	X			X	X
Anti-G	X			X	X

TABLE 6 (continued)

STUDY GUIDE FOR BLOOD GROUP SYSTEMS

APPROXIMATE FREQUENCY IN PROBLEM CROSSMATCH	ANTIGEN INCIDENCE IN CAUCASIONS	COMMENTS
Universal	44%	IgG form possible. May be hemolytic.
Universal	14%	IgG form possible. May be hemolytic
	58%	
E. R.	37%	Occurs in A_2 and A_2B ind.
R.	100%	Sometimes encountered when crossmatching A or AB bloods
R. C.	20–25%	Occurs only in Le(a-b-) ind.
E. R.	70–75%	2 forms: Le^{bL} AND Le^{bH}; Le^a and Le^b show hemolysis, increase rx with enzymes.
	90–95%	Binds only if Le^a is present
R.	78%	Not in secretions, fully developed at birth.
	72%	Not in secretions, fully developed at birth
R.	55%	
E. R	89%	
R.	100%	Public Ag_1 cold agglutinin use cord cells to I. D.
R. C.	78–80%	Found in 67% P_2 ind.
E. R.	7%	= (Anti-Lu1)
	70%	Anti-C alone is rare, combinations are more frequent.
R. C.	85%	Most common immune Ab
R. C.	30%	Enzyme method best
R. C.	80%	Most common immunization of Rh pos. inds.
E. R.	98%	Warm AIHA resembles-c
	64%	= Anti-ce
R. C.	84%	= Anti-CD, very common

TABLE 6 (continued)

STUDY GUIDE FOR BLOOD GROUP SYSTEMS

ANTIBODY	IgG or IgM	BINDS COMPLEMENT	CAUSES HTR or HDN	
Anti-K (K:1)X		K(some)	X	X
Anti-K (K:2)X			X	X
Anti-Fy^a	X	Fy^a(some)	X	X
Anti-Fy^b	X	Fy^b(some)	X	
Anti-JK^a	X	X	X	X
Anti-JK^b	X	X	X	X

HTR = Hemolytic Transfusion Reactions
HDN = Hemolytic Disease of the Newborn

TABLE 6 (continued)

STUDY GUIDE FOR BLOOD GROUP SYSTEMS

APPROXIMATE FREQUENCY IN PROBLEM CROSSMATCH	ANTIGEN INCIDENCE IN CAUCASIONS	COMMENTS
R. C.	9%	Potent antibody
E. R.	99%	Easily acquired by rare KK individual
R. C.	65%	Acquired by transfusion or pregnancy
	80%	Both – NOT reactive with enzymes

Frequency:

R.C. = Relatively common (1 in 200 to 1 in 5,000)
R.   = Rare (1 in 5,000 to 1 in 10,000)
E.R. = Extremely Rare (<1 in 10,000)

There are 18 known kell antigens, but only Anti-k:1 and k:2 will be discussed. Anti-K (k:1) is usually an IgG which can cause death in hemolytic disease of newborn. It is best detected at $37^{o}C$, and is enhanced by enzyme techniques. It is usually present as a result of pregnancy or a previous transfusion. Compatible blood is usually not a problem, since 93% of the population is K negative. Anti-k (k:2) (Cellano) is a rare antibody and is usually IgG. It can be detected in anti-human globulin and its production is usually stimulated by pregnancy or transfusion.

Duffy consists of 2 antigens: Fy^{a} and Fy^{b}. 66% of the Caucasion population possess Fy^{a}, and 80% have Fy^{b}. Anti-Fy^{a} and anti-Fy^{b} are both IgG and are detected in anti-human globulin. Both cause transfusion reactions. Only Fy^{a} has been implicated in hemolytic disease of the newborn.

The Kidd system was discovered in 1951 by Allen. Two antigens are involved: Jk^{a} and Jk^{b}. 70% of Caucasions have the Jk^{a} antigen, and it is most commonly found as $Jk(a+b+)$. Homozygous $Jk(a-b-)$ is extremely rare. When both antigens are present ($Jk^{a}Jk^{b}$), they are found on neutrophilic leukocytes and red blood cells. When found alone (Jk^{a} or Jk^{b}), it will be present on the red blood cells only. Both Anti-Jk^{a} and Anti-Jk^{b} are IgG, bind complement, react best in AHG or enzymes, and can produce transfusion reactions. Anti-Jk^{a} has not been implicated in HDN, but Anti-Jk^{b} has.

For additional information, please use the following study guide.

STUDY GUIDE FOR BLOOD GROUP SYSTEMS

1. IgM antibodies are "naturally" occurring, and react best in saline at room temperatures. Systems with IgM antibodies include: ABO, Lewis, MNSs, Ii, P, and Lutheran.

2. IgG antibodies are "immune" antibodies, and are usually produced as a result of pregnancy or a transfusion of a foreign antigen. These react best at $37^{o}C$ in anti-human globulin and in albumin. Because IgG antibodies cross the placenta, they can cause HDN.

3. Only Rh antibodies do not bind complement. ABO, Lewis, and Kidd antibodies do bind complement. The others sometime bind complement.

4. All antibodies listed are clinically significant except anti-N and most cases of Anti-I.

IMMUNOHEMATOLOGIC DISORDERS

Autoimmune Hemolytic Anemia (AIHA)

Some individuals fail to recognize 'self', and as a result, form autoantibodies. Some autoantibodies cause a shortened red blood cell survival, and can cause a hemolytic anemia. There are four types of AIHA which will be discussed:

1. "warm" type
2. "cold" type

3. paroxysmal cold hemoglobinuria
4. drug-induced hemolytic anemia

Most autoimmune hemolytic anemias (66%) are caused by "warm" antibodies of the IgG variety. Most "warm" autoantibodies have no specificity; however, if specificity is shown, it usually resembles an Rh antibody (Core). If there is no apparent cause for the development of the autoantibody, the disease is called primary or idiopathic AIHA. AIHA can be secondary if it appears after an infection, or in a lymphoma or cancer patient. The direct antihuman globulin test is positive in the "warm" type.

The DAT is less positive in AIHA of the "cold" type. The "cold" auto antibody reacts best at room temperature or colder, and is usually an IgM. The specificity of the "cold" autoantibody is usually an anti-I or anti-i. Cold AIHA can be idiopathic or can be secondary to an infection of Mycoplasma pneumoniae, or lymphoma or infectious mononucleosis. The "cold" variety is the most commonly encountered type, though it usually does not produce an anemia. Most patients with the "cold agglutinin syndrome" are elderly.

Paroxysmal Cold Hemoglobinuria is characterized by the presence of hemoglobin or methemoglobin in the urine after exposure to cold. This can occur in 'cold agglutinin syndrome' or secondary to a syphilis infection. The autoantibody reacts like anti-$P + P_1$ and sensitizes the cell in the cold, hemolyzing them at $37^{\circ}C$. The Donath-Landsteiner test is diagnostic for PCH.

Drug-induced AIHA is like a 'warm' autoantibody in that it is usually of Rh specificity. The DAT will also be positive; however, the eluate of a drug-induced AIHA will show no agglutination with normal cells. The most common causative agent is alpha-methyldopa (Aldomet) which is used as an anti-hypertensive. Other drugs which cause drug-induced AIHA are: phenacetin (an analgesic), quinine (anti-malarial), quinidine (a cardiac medication), penicillin, and keflin (antibiotics).

Tests done to determine if the hemolytic anemia has an immune basis are:

1. Direct antihuman globulin test (DAT).

2. If the DAT is positive, the antibody should be eluted from an EDTA specimen and identified.

3. Antibody screening should be done on both eluate and the serum.

4. When performing the ABO grouping, wash RBC in $37^{\circ}C$ saline to remove the auto antibodies. Always be suspicious of AB positive results, and check your controls carefully.

Transfusion should be avoided unless absolutely necessary, and in this case, give the least incompatible unit. If due to a "cold" autoantibody, prewarm the blood before administering.

Hemolytic Disease of the Newborn

Hemolytic Disease of the Newborn, also called Erythroblastosis fetalis, is a disease which results from the destruction of fetal RBCs by maternal IgG antibodies. The child must possess an antigen that is foreign to the mother. When this child is delivered, the placenta separates from the uterus, and causes a small fetomaternal hemorrhage. The child's cells enter the mother's circulation, and are removed by the spleen. Because they contain a foreign antigen, antibodies form. This process is called sensitization.

When the mother becomes pregnant for a second child who possesses the same antigen, the antibodies formed in the previous pregnancy pass through the placenta. They attach to the antigen on the fetal cells, causing a shortened RBC survival which will lead to anemia. The destruction of the cell releases hemoglobin which is converted to bilirubin. While the child is in utero, the mother's serum albumin transports the fetal bilirubin to her liver. Once in the liver, her enzyme glucoronyl transferase will convert the unconjugated bilirubin to the excretable (direct) conjugated bilirubin. Bilirubin becomes a problem once the child is delivered, since the infant's liver does not produce this enzyme. Hence, the unconjugated bilirubin accumulates and collects in the infant's tissues causing jaundice and brain damage (kernicterus).

The prognosis of HDN varies considerably. A severe anemia can cause edema (hydrops fetalis) which may result in heart failure, causing either intrauterine death or neonatal death. If the HDN baby lives, the primary danger is the accumulation of unconjugated (indirect) bilirubin which may result in kernicturus. A useful index for prognosis is based on the cord hemoglobin:

Normal infant	13.6-19.6	gm/dl hemoglobin
Mild HDN	13	gm/dl hemoglobin
Moderate HDN	8-13	gm/dl hemoglobin
Severe HDN	<8	gm/dl hemoglobin

(If a heelstick is used, the hemoglobin will be slightly higher).

The most severe form of HDN is seen with anti-D, anti-CD, and anti-DE. Moderate forms are associated with anti-c, anti-E, and anti-kell. ABO incompatibility causes the least severe form. The reason for the decreased severity is that the mother has Anti-A, Anti-B, and/or Anti-A, B in her serum naturally. When the incompatible cells enter her system, the already-made antibodies quickly attack and destroy the fetal cells, preventing sensitization. Therefore, an ABO and Rh incompatibility is likely to be less severe than a plain Rh incompatibility.

It was this observation which led to the discovery of Rh_o Immune Globulin as a means of preventing HDN. By injecting the mother with Rh_o Immune Globulin within 72 hours of the delivery, sensitization is prevented. The fetal Rh positive cells are destroyed by the injected antibody (anti-Rh_o) before the mother can produce her own antibodies. This form of passive immunity prevents active immunization. Passive immunity is short-lived, and will not be detected beyond 5 months of the injection. If anti-D is found in the serum after 6 months, it is assumed to be the result of active immunization. The failure of the Rh_o Immune Globulin may be due to a massive fetomaternal hemorrhage (greater than 30 ml of whole blood) or greater then 72 hours elapsing between the delivery and the injection. One injection of 300 Mg is sufficient for 30 ml of whole fetal blood entering the mother. If more than 30 ml is suspected a Kleinhauer test should be performed on a postdelivery sample of material blood, and an increased dose given. A smaller portion is available for pregnancies which are interrupted at or before 12 weeks gestation, and protects the mother against 5 ml of whole fetal blood. In order to be qualified as a candidate for the injection, the mother must be Rh negative and have no detectable Anti-D in her serum. Her child must be Rh positive and the direct Coombs on the cord blood must be negative. The minor crossmatch performed on the mother's cells with the material to be injected must be compatible.   In a miscarriage or abortion, the fetus is assumed to have been Rh positive. A smaller dose is available for such cases.

Prediction of HDN uses prenatal and postnatal studies. An ABO grouping and Rh typing is performed on the mother's first prenatal specimen, usually obtained on or before the 13th week of gestation. This specimen is also screened for unexpected antibodies. If an antibody is discovered, it should be identified. All significant antibodies should be titered at least monthly. The titer does not always correlate with the severity of the disease; however, a 1:32 titer or greater of an unexpected antibody capable of producing HDN and a history of a previously affected baby indicate amniocentesis should be performed on the 26th week of gestation.

The amniotic fluid should be centrifuged, and the sedimented red blood cells should be grouped and typed. There are special procedures (Kleinhauer test) which can determine whether the cells belong to the mother or the fetus. The fluid is also examined for a bilirubin-like substance which indicates the degree of hemolysis occurring in the infant.

If the mother tested is D-positive or D^u-positive, another specimen should be requested at 28-32 weeks of gestation. An Rh negative mother with a negative antibody screening should be phenotyped. The father should also be phenotyped. If he is also D-negative, a 28-32 week of gestation specimen from the mother is all that is required. If the father is positive, the pregnancy should be closely monitored from the 28th week for the appearance of antibodies.

In the postnatal investigation, the cord cells are ABO grouped, Rh typed, and a direct Coomb's is performed. The cord cells should first be washed 6 times to remove Wharton's jelly which, when present, may cause false agglutination. Only a front ABO grouping is possible, since the infant's anti-A and anti-B are not fully developed at birth. Use of the cord serum is misleading, since any antibodies found there are probably the mother's. The eluate from the cord cells, however, can be tested against adult A and B cells, and is of value in the diagnosis of an ABO HDN.

As mentioned earlier, the mother is again tested postnatally for her group and type, and screened for unexpected antibodies to determine if she is an Rh_o Immune Globulin candidate.

The treatment goal in HDN is to repair the anemia and get rid of the excess bilirubin. There are 3 ways to accomplish this goal:

1. Give an exchange transfusion in the first hours of life.

2. Induce labor early, especially if amnioscentesis indicates that the fetus won't live until the normal delivery.

3. If the fetus will die before it is mature enough for early delivery, intrauterine transfusion is indicated. However, there is a high risk of fetal mortality.

Blood chosen for an exchange transfusion should be less than 5 days old, and should be compatible with the infant's cells and the mother's serum. If possible, use blood that is of the infant's ABO group. If an ABO incompatibility exists, use group O blood. The blood should be of the same Rh phenotype as the infant, and be compatible with the mother's ABO antibody.

BLOOD SELECTION FOR EXCHANGE TRANSFUSION

Mother	Baby	Blood for Exchange
O	O, A, or B	O
A	O or B	O
	A or AB	A or O
B	O or A	O
	B or AB	B or D
AB	A	A or O
	B	B or O
	AB	A or B or AB or O

*If an exchange is repeated, subsequent units must be of the same group and type as the previous unit.

The mother's serum and the donor's cells should be used for pretransfusion compatibility testing, since the mother's serum contains the greatest concentration of antibody and is more likely to demonstrate an incompatibility. If the mother's serum is not available, the eluate from the cord cells may be used. Lastly, the baby's serum can be used if time is very critical.

BLOOD DONATION

Blood Donors: Selection

The following requirements must be met by the donor:

1. Age: the donor must be between 17 and 66 years old.

2. Medical history:

   a. must not have <u>donated</u> within 8 weeks
   b. must not be <u>pregnant</u>. The donor must be deferred for 6 weeks after termination of the pregnancy
   c. must have no long term <u>illness</u>, nor can they be ill at the time of donation
   d. must have no <u>drug addiction</u>. Therapy with the following drugs should be evaluated by a physician: antibiotics, corticosteroids, digitalis, insulin, quinidine, dilantin, diuretics, nitroglycerin, anticoagulants, or other potent drugs
   e. must not have been <u>vaccinated</u> with anti-tetanus (horse) for 3 months, or received a vaccine of killed bacteria, virus, or rickettsia in the last 24 hours, or received therapeutic rabies vaccine in the last year
   f. must not have had bronchial asthma or a hyposensitization injection in the last 3 days. If other <u>allergic</u> symptoms are present, the Medical Director should evaluate them.
   g. must have no history of <u>convulsions</u> or abnormal <u>bleeding</u> tendencies
   h. if the donor ever had <u>malaria</u>, they must have been symptom-free for the last 3 years, or have been off treatment for 3 years
   i. must be free of HB Ag or anti-HB A_g. Any donor with a history of viral <u>hepatitis</u> or drug addiction is excluded permanently.
   j. must not have received blood or a blood component <u>transfusion</u> in the last 6 months
   k. must be seronegative for <u>syphilis</u>

3. Physical Exam

   a. weight: must be equal to or greater than 110 pounds
   b. Temperature: $\leq$ 99.6°F or $\leq$ 37.5°C
   c. Pulse: 50-100 beats per minute
   d. Blood Pressure: Systolic 90-180 mm Hg; Diastolic< 100
   e. Skin: should be free of infection and boils
   f. Hemoglobin: Female $\geq$ 12.5 gm/dl; Male $\geq$ 13.5 gm/dl
         or
      Hematocrit: Female $\geq$ 38%; Male $\geq$ 41%

Blood Donors: Collection

1. Gather all materials necessary, check containers for sterility and amount of anticoagulant, and use a numerical system to identify the donor record, pilot tubes, and container.

2. To prepare for the venipuncture, select the best vein. A tourniquet or blood pressure cuff can be used. (If a sphygmomanometer is used, the pressure should be 20-40 mm Hg to find the vein, 100 mm Hg to insert the needle, and then 40 mm H$_g$ when collecting the blood). Prepare a 1 1/2 inch area around the proposed site. Beginning at the intended venipuncture site, scrub with a surgical soap for thirty seconds in a circular motion moving outward. Remove the soap with 10% acetone in 70% alcohol, and allow to dry. Apply 3% iodine in 70% alcohol and let dry. Remove the iodine with acetone alcohol and let dry. Cover with a sterile gauze. (A second method is to scrub the area with a .75% aqueous iodophor compound for 2 minutes, and let stand for 1 minute).

   Do <u>not</u> repalpate the vein once cleaned!

3. Perform the venipuncture, cover with sterile gauze, and tape the needle into position.

4. Mix the collecting blood gently and often.

5. Stop collection when bag is at appropriate weight.

6. Remove the tourniquet and then remove the needle, and apply pressure to the phlebotomy site.

Testing of Blood Donation

All donations should be tested as follows:

Donor's Cells

    a. forward group for ABO
    b. test for D and D^u

Donor's Serum

    a. reverse grouping for ABO
    b. antibody screening test using antiglobulin and enzyme testing
    c. V. D. R. L. test
    d. HBAg and anti-HBAg tests

Autologous Blood Donation

In an autologous blood transfusion, the recipient receives his own blood. This blood can be obtained by predeposit, or by intraoperative salvage. The advantages of an autologous transfusion are:

1. It avoids many of the hazards of homologous transfusion, i.e., hepatitis, malaria, and allergic reactions.

2. It is a way of supplying blood to patients with rare blood types, or those who, due to religious beliefs, refuse donated blood.

   Predeposit autologous transfusion requires a physician's written request, and the Medical Director of the facility collecting the blood must determine whether the patient can donate. The patient must sign a written consent form. If the blood is not used by the donor, the donor must sign for the release of the blood before it can be given to another patient.

   The criteria for predeposit donation is that the patient be in good health. There is no age or weight limit. If, however, the donor is less than 110 pounds, the volume of anticoagulant must be reduced according to this formula:

$$V_1 = V_o \ \frac{V_B}{450}$$

V_1 = amount of anticoagulant to be left in the container
V^1 = amount of anticoagulant usually used for 450 ml blood
V^o_B = ml blood to be collected based on the weight of the donor. V_B is calculated as follows:

$$V_B = \frac{Donor's \ weight \ X \ 450}{110}$$

   As an example, let us say that the donor weighs 88 pounds. How much CPD should be used?

(1) $V_B = \dfrac{88 \ lbs \ X \ 450 \ ml}{110 \ lbs}$ (2) $V_B = 360 \ ml$

(3) $V_1 = V_o \ \dfrac{V_B}{450}$ (4) $V_1 = 63 \ ml \ X \ \dfrac{360 \ ml}{450 \ ml}$

(5) = 50.4 ml of CPD should be used.

The donor's hemoglobin must be ≥ 11 grams/dl, the hematocrit must be $\geq 34\%$. A pregnant woman can donate, as long as the pregnancy has no complications. Donors may be drawn every 4 days up to 4 units. With iron supplements, 8 units may be drawn in 20 days. The unit should be labelled "For Autologous Use Only" and should be serologically tested as if a homologous unit. A cross-match is optional.

   Intraoperative autologous transfusion uses equipment which collects blood during surgery, filters the blood, and returns it to circulation. This method is still in the developmental stage, and is contraindicated if the patient has cancer, a perforated viscera, gross infection, a hepatic or renal dysfunction, or has received high amounts of anticoagulant. This technique causes significant hemolysis. A coagulation profile consisting of a P. T., P. T. T., fibrinogen assay, and platelet count should be performed prior to the surgery.

Common Anticoagulants

   CPD (Citrate Phosphate Dextrose) Outdate = 21 days. 63 ml CPD prevents 450 ml of whole blood from clotting. This anticoagulant is widely used, causes less hemolysis and higher levels of 2, 3 DPG than ACD, and a prolonged survival of red cells.

   CPD-adenine is a new product currently being used which gives added RBC survival. Blood in CPD-adenine outdates in 28 days.

   ACD (Acid Citrate Dextrose) Outdate = 21 days. Although the outdate is the same as CPD, the RBC survival is less.

Heparin Outdate = 48 hours after collection. 15 ml heparin prevents 500 ml of blood from clotting. It is a safe anticoagulant, since it has a low toxicity, but blood collected in heparin cannot be stored.

Whole Blood and Blood Component Therapy

WHOLE BLOOD

Whole blood should not be used if a specific component is available. Infusion of large amounts of whole blood can increase bleeding, because the infused blood does not contain the labile coagulation factors, and can also cause circulatory overload.

Whole blood is indicated to restore blood volume, and in the event of an exchange transfusion.

RED BLOOD CELLS (HUMAN)

Packed cells have a hemotocrit of 80% and should be used in patients with cardiac disease, chronic anemias, or patients with restricted sodium, potassium, or citrate intake. If the unit is opened during the packing process, it outdates in 24 hours. If done in a closed system, the outdate is the same as whole blood, 21 days.

RBC (Human) Frozen are stored in glycerol-lactate at $-85^{\circ}C$, and can be used for 2 years. Once thawed and deglycerolized, they outdate in 24 hours. They are indicated in organ transplants, since Histocompatible Leukocyte Antigens (HLA) are destroyed and removed by the freezing and washing. It is also for patients with long term transfusion therapy or those patients with post-transfusion febrile reactions.

LEUKOCYTE POOR RBC

These reconstituted frozen cells are filtered, collected in heparin, centrifuged, and the plasma is expressed. 25% of the white cells are adsorbed to the nylon. This component is used in patients who suffer from repeated febrile nonhemolytic transfusion reactions.

WBC CONCENTRATE

This component is used to treat septicemia or a life threatening infection in a patient with granulocytopenia.

30-50 units of whole blood are used to make 1 unit of WBC concentrate.

FRESH FROZEN PLASMA

A unit of whole blood collected in CPD or ACD is separated and froze within 4 hours of collection. The resultant plasma is rich in clotting factors, including factor VIII. Fresh frozen plasma is used to control bleeding in hemophiliacs, expand blood volume, and prevent shock, especially in burn patients. When stored at $-30^{\circ}C$ or lower, it outdates in 1 year.

CRYOPRECIPITATED ANTIHEMOPHILIC FACTOR (HUMAN)

Cryoprecipitate is made by freezing plasma at $-60^{\circ}C$, then thawing at $4^{\circ}C$ for 24 hours. This forms 3 ml of white precipitate rich in AFH. The component is used to correct Factor VIII deficiencies and control bleeding in Hemophilia A patients. At $-30^{\circ}C$, the product outdates in 1 year. Once the product is thawed at $37^{\circ}C$, it must be used in 6 hours.

PLATELET CONCENTRATE (HUMAN)

Platelet concentrate can be prepared from a unit of whole blood. The product will
be 15 ml in volume, and contain 5 X 10^{10} platelets. It can also be obtained by
plateletpheresis, whereby whole blood is removed from the donor, separated, a portion retained, and the rest returned to the donor. It outdates 72 hours after collection when stored at 20-24°C. The outdate is longer if frozen.

Platelet concentrate is used to correct thrombocytopenia due to aplastic anemia,
leukemia, cancer, chemotherapy, or radiation.

Standard Colors of Blood Group Tags

            Blood Group O   - blue
                       A   - yellow
                       B   - pink
                       AB   - white

METHODOLOGY

Antibody Screening and Identification

The purpose of antibody screening and identification is to detect alloantibodies,
which are unexpected antibodies resulting from exposure to a foreign antigen by
pregnancy, previous transfusion, or injections. Both tests employ anti-human globulin sera, which henceforth will be referred to as AHG. The principle of AHG is to
cause sensitized cells to agglutinate. IgG antibodies, because of their short bridging span, can sometimes sensitize the cell, but are not able to tie cells together.
Anti-human globulin is antibody, made from goats or rabbits, to human globulin. When
sensitized cells (which are coated with globulin) are incubated with AHG, the AHG
attacks the globulin, and bridges the gap between cells. The end result is visible
agglutination.

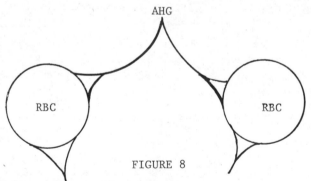

FIGURE 8

There are 2 ways of using AHG: directly (also known as the Direct Coombs) or indirectly (Indirect Coombs). In the direct antiglobulin test (DAT), the patient's
washed red blood cells are directly mixed with AHG. If agglutination results, it
indicates in vivo sensitization of the red cells has occurred. This test is useful
in the diagnosis of H. D. N., A. I. H. A., and in the investigation of RBC sensitization by drugs, and transfusion reactions.

The Indirect antiglobulin test (IAT) detects in vitro sensitization of red blood
cells. It does so by incubating pooled O + red blood cells that contain a high number of antigens with patient serum which is suspected of containing an antibody. If

the antibody is present it will attach to the antigen on the RBC. When AHG is added, the antibodies will be bridged, and visible agglutination will form. This is known as "antibody screening." Antibody identification expands the same.principle. Here, 10 or more sets of cells with known antigens are used. Patient serum containing an unknown antibody is incubated in 10 different tubes, each containing cells of known antigens. By observing which tubes show agglutination, one may deduce which antibody is present.

The IAT is used not only in antibody screening and antibody identification, but also in the crossmatch and in some special tests.

The IAT is performed at 2 temperatures (25°C, 37°C) and in several mediums (saline, high protein or albumin, and AHG).

IgM antibodies are 300 $\overset{\circ}{A}$ in diameter and react strongly at 25°C but less strongly at 37°C. IgM antibodies also react better in saline, and may not show a reaction in AHG. The <u>IgG antibodies</u> are 140 $\overset{\circ}{A}$ in diameter, prefer 37°C, and react more strongly in a high protein medium (such as 22% bovine albumin) or in AHG. Again, because of the short bridging span of IgG, anything which brings cells closer together will enhance agglutination of sensitized cells. Red blood cells are negatively charged, and attract positively charged cations, such as sodium (Na+). These ions form a cloud around the RBC which will repel other RBCs, causing them to "slip" by. The edge of this cationic cloud is called the "slipping plane", or plane of shear. The voltage or potential at the slipping plane is known as the zeta potential. The lower the zeta potential, the less repulsion there is between cells, and the greater the chances of agglutination by IgG antibodies.

FIGURE 9

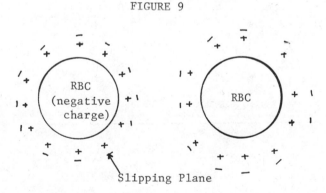

Slipping Plane

<u>Lowering the zeta potential</u> is made possible by increasing the dielectric constant, as occurs with the addition of a high protein medium such as 22% bovine albumin. This lessens the repulsion between cells, and allows cells coated with IgG to interact and show agglutination.

The addition of enzymes to red blood cells cleaves sialic acid (OH-) from the red cell surface, which lowers the negative charge of the cell, and subsequently reduces the zeta potential.

Another method is to replace the saline which contains sodium cations with a glucose solution which contains few cations. The net result will be a decrease in the zeta potential.

Another factor important in the IAT is the incubation time. If the time is too short, it will not allow sufficient association between antibodies and antigens, and interaction between red cells. If the time is too long, antibodies may elute off the cell.

To identify an antibody, a panel of cells is used. This panel may contain 10 to 15 different vials of cells. The antigens present on each cell population is indicated by a (+) on an enclosed form, with space to write in results as they occur at each phase of testing. Here is an example of a single antibody which was identified using a 10 cell panel.

A SINGLE ANTIBODY IDENTIFIED USING A SIMPLIFIED 10 CELL PANEL

Panel Cell Number	D	C	E	c	e	K	k	Fy^a	Fy^b	Saline	Albumin	AHG	Enzyme
1	+	0	0	+	+	0	+	0	0	0	+	3+	3+
2	0	0	0	+	+	+	+	0	+	0	0	0	0
3	0	+	0	+	+	0	+	+	0	0	0	0	0
4	+	+	0	0	+	0	+	+	+	0	0	3+	3+
5	+	0	+	+	0	0	+	+	0	+/-	2+	4+	4+
6	0	0	+	+	+	0	+	0	+	0	0	0	0
7	+	0	0	0	+	0	+	0	0	0	+	3+	3+
8	0	+	0	+	+	0	+	0	+	0	0	0	0
9	+	+	0	0	+	0	+	0	0	0	0	3+	4+
10	0	+	0	0	0	0	+	0	+	0	0	0	0
Autocontrol										0	0	0	0

To analyze which is the problem antibody:

1. Cross out all antigenic determinants present in the first cell sample which did not react with the serum, i.e., go to your first set of results which produced all zeros, then cross out any plusses in that row.

2. Repeat this with each set of negative results, crossing out any plusses which were not crossed out previously.

3. Look for any antigenic determinant which has not any (+) crossed out. In this example, anti-D is identified.

4. Do the reactions agree with this result? Again, in this case, the results are consistent with anti-D. The reactions were usually not present in saline, and increased in albumin, AHG, and Enzyme.

Here are some rules which should be used to be sure that results are consistent with the characteristics of the antibody:

A. IgM reacts best at 25°C. Examples are: Anti-Le^a, Le^b, I, M, N, P$_1$.

B. IgG reacts best at 37°C. Anti-Rh, K, S, and s react best in saline or albumin.

C. Anti K, Fy^a, Fy^b, Jk^a, and Jk^b will react strongly in AHG.

D. Anti-Le^a and Jk^a or Jk^b will often form hemolysis.

E. Enzymes will enhance Anti-Rh, and anti-Kidd and consequently they will <u>PREVENT</u> detection of Duffy and MNS antibodies.

Lastly, here are some <u>interpretations of common panel problems</u>:

1. If all the panel cells agglutinate, but the autocontrol is negative, there is either an antibody present against a high frequency antigen, or there is a mixture of antibodies.

2. If all panel cells <u>and</u> autocontrol are positive at room temperature, weakly positive at 37°C, and weakly positive in AHG, there are 3 possible explanations:

    a. a cold antibody, usually anti-I, is present
    b. rouleaux is present and can be caused by an abnormal protein or the presence of Wharton's <u>jelly</u>
    c. an antibody specific for the stabilizer substance in the reagent is present

3. If the cells and the autocontrol are positive only in the AHG, a warm autoimmune antibody is the problem.

4. If the panel cells are negative or variable positive, and the autocontrol is positive in AHG, it is probably a case of AIHA, where most of the antibody is attached to the patient's cell, and not in the serum.

5. If the panel is negative, the autocontrol negative, yet there are many incompatible crossmatches, either the panel was not done properly, or the pre-panel work is incorrect. For example, an A$_2$ individual may have anti-A$_1$ in his serum, which will cause him to be incompatible with A$_1$ units. The panel won't identify the antibody, since all panel cells are Group O. This anti-A$_1$ should have been noticed in the reverse grouping.

Once an antibody has been identified, donor cells should be screened for that antibody, and only those units which don't contain the antigen should be transfused.

There are lectin preparations which are useful in screening donor units for the presence of an antigen. Lectins are extracts from plants which react like a specific antibody. Here are a few lectins:

```
Dilochos biflorus    =  Anti-A₁
Ulex europaeus       =  Anti-H
Vicia graminae       =  Anti-N
Iberis amara         =  Anti-M
Arachis hypogaea     =  Anti-T
```

Compatibility Testing

Since correct <u>identification of the recipient</u> is crucial in blood transfusion, requests should be written and include the patient's name, identification number, sex, age, and the amount and type of blood to be transfused. The specimen drawn from the recipient should be labelled with the patient's name, identification number, the time, date, and location. If the specimen was obtained from an I. V. line, the tubing must be fresh or flushed prior to drawing. If the patient has no identification band, it is safest to provide the patient with a band, and use that same means of identification when transfusing blood to the patient.

The purpose of a crossmatch is to provide the patient with relatively compatible blood. ('Relative' is used because there is only a 1:30,000 chance of finding perfectly compatible blood for any given recipient.) The <u>major crossmatch</u> mixes 1 part donor cells to 2 parts recipient serum. This will insure that the blood given does not contain antigens to which the recipient has antibodies. It will <u>not</u> guarantee RBC survival, nor will it prevent the recipient from forming antibodies to the transfused cells.

The minor crossmatch uses 1 part recipient's cells and 2 parts donor serum. It determines whether the donor contains an antibody which will attach the recipient's red cells. However, if donor units are screened in advance for unexpected antibodies, the minor crossmatch is not necessary. Minor crossmatches are in order if the component to be used is plasma in nature, e.g., fresh frozen plasma, or Rh gamma globulin. Both major and minor crossmatches use 2 temperatures (25°C, 37°C), 2 mediums (saline, high protein), and are further tested with AHG and check cells.

Pretransfusion testing should include ABO group, Rh type, and an antibody screening. The serum should be fresh to assure the presence of complement, and should not be hemolyzed. If the patient already received a transfusion 2 days ago (48°) or more, a new specimen should be drawn to check if antibodies are detectable.

Select a unit that is the same as the ABO and Rh group of the recipient. If the same ABO group is not available, give cells that are compatible and give only as packed cells. A change from nongroup specific units to group specific units requires a change of infusion line. Rh positive blood may be given in an emergency to an Rh negative patient, provided the patient has no anti-D. If a patient does possess an unexpected antibody, the donors should be screened for that antigen. Only those units free of the corresponding antigen should be transfused.

If the <u>crossmatch is incompatible</u>, recheck the work. If the autocontrol is negative, and the crossmatch is incompatible at 25°C, but only weakly incompatible at 37°C, the problem antibody is most likely an IgM. If the reverse occurs, the alloantibody is probably an IgG. If the patient's serum is incompatible with only 1 unit of several being tested, do a DAT on that unit, to check if perhaps the donor's cells themselves have the troublesome antibody. If the autocontrol is positive, the incompatibility may be due to cold autoantibodies, a protein abnormality, or warm autoantibodies.

When giving the compatible unit, records of compatibility must be complete, the blood must be labelled, and identification of the unit and the patient should be checked by 2 people. The blood samples of recipient and donor should be stored at 1-6°C for 7 days. If uncrossmatched blood is given in an emergencysituation, the blood bank physician should be notified, a release form signed by the attending physician, and O negative or group specific blood should be given. Compatibility tests should be done, and if they prove to be incompatible, the physician should be notified immediately.

If a prolonged clotting time prevents testing, one drop of thrombin per ml sera or dry thrombin on the tip of an applicator stick may be added. Caution: excessive thrombin will cause nonspecific agglutination!

Transfusion Reaction

A transfusion reaction encompasses any unfavorable event which occurs in the patient either during or following the transfusion, that is related to that transfusion. Most problems are caused by leukocytes, platelets, and plasma proteins of the infused component. All reactions should be reported to the Medical Director. When a reaction is observed, the transfusion should be discontinued immediately, and the intravenous line should be kept open. (If hives is the only symptom, the transfusion may be continued.) The remaining blood, a new sample of blood from the recipient, and a reaction report should be sent to the Blood Bank.

There are 2 types of transfusion reactions: immediate and delayed reactions. Among the immediate reactions are: circulatory overload, febrile nonhemolytic reactions, allergic reactions, hemolytic transfusion reactions, reactions caused by bacterial contamination, hypothermia, bleeding diathesis, hyperkalemia, and microemboli. Circulatory overload is caused by the sudden expansion of blood volumes, which is not well tolerated by infants, cardiac patients, or persons with chronic anemias. The symptoms include coughing, cyanosis and dypsnea. It may be prevented by using packed RBC, and transfusing it slowly (1 ml/kg body weight/hour). The most common type of reaction is the febrile nonhemolytic reaction, which is often preceded by chills. It is caused by antibodies against antigens found on the leukocytes or platelet membranes, or can be caused by contaminating pyrogenic bacteria. If the recipient repeatedly demonstrates a febrile reaction, he should be given Leukocyte Poor RBC or deglycerolized RBC. Allergic reactions occur when the patient is exposed to an antigen to which he is hypersensitive. The symptoms are usually mild, and include hives and itching. An antihistamine such as Benadryl is usually sufficient treatment; however, if the patient shows signs of anaphylaxis, he must be treated with epinephrine. Hemolytic transfusion reactions occurs infrequently; they may cause a severe reaction, since transfused cells will be hemolyzed. Lab findings include: hemoglobinuria. hypohaptoglobinemia, uremia, and an elevated indirect bilirubin. This can occur as a result of an ABO or Rh incompatibility. Bacterial contamination reactions occur rarely, and are most severe if the organism is gram negative and capable of growing at refrigeration temperatures. Bleeding diathesis will occur if the patient has either factor V or VIII deficiency. It can be corrected by administering fresh frozen plasma or platelet concentrate. Hyperkalemia may be prevented by using blood less than 5 days old. If a massive transfusion is planned, filtering the blood will prevent microemboli from occurring.

Hemolytic reactions can occur days to weeks after the transfusion, and will show a positive DAT, but a negative indirect antiglobulin test (IAT). The IAT will become positive once the body has had time to remove the antigen from circulation and produce antibodies. Viral hepatitis is always a risk in transfusion. Other delayed reactions are: cytomegalovirus infection (which mimics infectious mononucleosis), malaria, and syphilis (although the syphilis spirochete cannot survive regrigeration temperatures for more than 72 hours.)

INVESTIGATION OF A SUSPECTED TRANSFUSION REACTION

First and foremost, check for clerical errors. Four specimens are needed:

A. The pretransfusion recipient blood.

B. The posttransfusion recipient blood (a clot tube and an EDTA tube).

C. Blood from the unit given.

D. A posttransfusion urine specimen.

Check all specimens for gross hemolysis. Repeat the ABO and Rh tests on a, b, and c. Perform a DAT on a and b. Repeat the cross-match (both major and minor) and screen for antibodies on all three blood specimens. Corroborative tests include: the identification of an unexpected antibody, incompatible crossmatch findings, or the presence of bacteria in the direct smear from the unit.

Tests for haptoglobin (a, b), methemalbumin (a, b), bilirubin (b), creatinine, and direct antiglobulin (c) are optional.

Special Techniques

Since this is a comprehensive review of Immunohematology, this section will be brief, and include only the more commonly used techniques.

When a cold agglutinin causes crossmatching difficulty, a prewarmed crossmatch may solve the problem. Its purpose is to prevent the cold antibody from attaching to the red cell. The prewarmed major crossmatch is set up exactly as the routine crossmatch except that cells and serum and saline are prewarmed to 37°. After incubation, the cells are hand washed with warm saline prior to the addition of AHG.

Rouleaux formation will also cause difficulties, because it appears as agglutination. When observed microscopically, it will appear as "stacked coins." Rouleaux is dispersed in saline, whereas true agglutination will not. One solution is to respin the serum-cell mixture, remove all the serum and replace it with 2 drops of saline. Mix, spin, and check for agglutination. If Rouleaux was present, it will no longer show agglutination.

Enzyme testing enhances the reactivity of certain antibodies, namely Kidd, Lewis, Rh, and P. Note, however, that it prevents the detection of Duffy and MNS. It functions by cleaning sialic acid from the red blood cell membrane, thereby allowing the antibody to come closer to the antigen. Four types of commonly used enzymes are: papain, bromelin, trypsin, and ficin. Papain is obtained from pawpaw, bromelin from pineapple, trypsin from hog stomach, and ficin from figs. The enzyme is usually added directly to the test cell/serum mixture. Enzymes are often used in cross-matches, antibody screening, and antibody identification.

Elution reverses the antigen-antibody complex, and releases the antibody from the cell. The eluate contains antibodies which were attached to the cell's antigens. Two common methods employ heat or ether to reverse the complex. Eluates may be used to:

1. Identify an antibody from a positive direct antiglobulin test in an individual possessing acquired hemolytic anemia.

2. Single out an antibody if 2 or more exist in a serum specimen. (The mixture is first separated by adsorption, then an eluate from the cells used in adsorption will identify one of the antibodies.)

3. Identify the implicating antibody attacking the infant's cells in HDN, especially if the mother's serum is unavailable.

Absorption removes the antibodies from the serum by reacting the antibody with a specific antigen. When cells are used to take up the antibody, the process is called adsorption. Absorption is used to separate a mixture of antibodies, or to remove anti-A or anti-B when making antisera (e.g., to make Kell antisera from a Group A person). Absorption is also helpful in removing cold or warm autoantibodies, or to prove that a cell has a certain antigen because it can remove the corresponding antibody from serum.

Records

Both AABB standards and FDA regulations state that patient's records (ABO and Rh type, antibody screening and identification, and pretransfusion test results and transfusion reaction workups) must be kept for 5 years. All records should be legible, indelible, and contain the identification of the person who performed the test.

FDA mandates that records must include the date, results, interpretation, lot number of reagents, and expiration dates of the reagents.

The record system should allow a person to trace any unit or component from its source to its deposition.

Quality Control

In general, 2 people should check the identification, recording of results, and administration of blood. For specifics concerning transfusion requests, donor units, pretransfusion testing, administration of blood, and personnel I refer the reader to the AABB Technical Manual, Chapter 22, 7th edition. The following equipment should be monitored: centrifuge (speed and time), Rh viewbox if using a slide technique, water baths and other incubators (should have temperatures recorded daily). Reagents should also be tested daily to ensure their reactivity.

BIBLIOGRAPHY AND RECOMMENDED READINGS

American Association of Blood Banks. <u>Technical Manual</u>. Seventh Edition. 1977.
   American Association of Blood Banks. Washington, D. C.

Bryant, N. J. <u>An Introduction to Immunohematology</u>. 1976. First Edition. W. B.
   Saunders Company. Philadelphia.

Crispens C. G., Jr. <u>Essentials of Medical Genetics</u>. 1971. Harper and Row Publishers. New York.

Levine, L. <u>Biology of the Gene</u>. 1973. Second Edition. The C. V. Mosby Company.
   St. Louis.

Mollison, P. L. <u>Blood Transfusion in Clinical Medicine</u>. 1979. Sixth Edition.
   Blackwell Scientific Publications. Oxford.

Chapter 7

Hematology

PAULA M. MILLER, MST, CLS
MLT Program Director
Assistant Professor of Medical Technology
Department of Biological Science
Anna Maria College
Paxton, Massachusetts

OUTLINE

THE THROMBOCYTE
     Morphology
     Function
     Structure
     Production
     Survival
     Diseases
COAGULATION
     Hemostasis
         Blood vessels
         Platelets
         Coagulation factors
     Pathways
     Fibrinolysis and Anticoagulants
     Diseases (other than platelets
BIBLIOGRAPHY AND RECOMMENDED READINGS

INTRODUCTION

This chapter is intended to serve as a basic review in hematology. Normal states and common diseases are emphasized throughout the chapter. Clinicopathologic correlations are emphasized in an attempt to bridge academic and clinical situations. Typical laboratory profiles are used to illustrate cases which may be commonly encountered in the clinical laboratory. However, no procedures have been delineated for laboratory tests. A procedure manual is recommended for this information

HEMATOLOGY

The Erythrocyte
Morphology

The normal mature red blood cell is a hemoglobin filled anucleated biconcave disc which measures 6-8 microns in diameter and is approximately 2.0 microns in thickness. The red blood cell is the predominant cell found in the peripheral blood. There are on the average 5.4 million red blood cells per cubic millimeter of blood in the male, and 4.8 million per cubic millimeter of blood in the female. Unstained, the red blood cell appears as seen in Figure 1. Stained with Wright's stain or Giemsa stain, as in a differential count, a red cell has a pink color with a central light staining area called the area of central pallor.

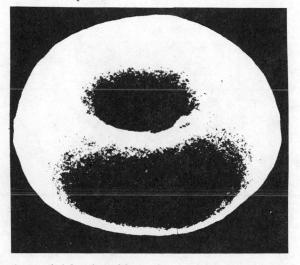

FIGURE 1

The morphology of the red blood cell is best quantitated by laboratory tests known as indices. Indices are a set of tests which include the Mean Corpuscular Volume (MCV), the Mean Corpuscular Hemoglobin (MCH), and the Mean Corpuscular Hemoglobin Concentration (MCHC). Automated hematology instruments may generate these results, but in order to understand them, one should be able to calculate these indices. The indices may be calculated as follows:

$$\text{Mean Corpuscular Volume} = \frac{\text{Hematocrit x 10}}{\text{Red Blood Cell count}}$$

The normal MVC range is 80-99 cubic microns (μ^3) or femtoliters (fl).

The Mean Corpuscular Hemoglobin (MCH) index is derived in the following manner:

$$\text{MCH} = \frac{\text{Hemoglobin x 10}}{\text{Red Blood Cell Count}}$$

The normal MCH value range is 28-33 micro-micro grams per cell.

The Mean Corpuscular Hemoglobin Concentration (MCHC) index is determined as follows:

$$MCHC = \frac{Hemoglobin}{Hematocrit} \times 100$$

The normal MCHC value range is 31-35 g/dl RBC's.

The MCV is an indicator of size. Cells having a low MCV are said to be microcytic. Cells within the normal range are said to be normocytic, and cells above the normal range are said to be macrocytic.

The MCH is an indicator of color. Cells having a low MCH are termed hypochromic. Cells within the normal color range are normochromic, and cells above the normal color range are hyperchromic.

The MCHC is an indicator of color independent of cell size. Cells having a low MCH usually have a low MCHC and are hypochromic, but microcytic cells may have a normal MCHC and a low MCH in some cases. Only sphereocytes give a high MCHC.

Variation in red cell shape is called poikilocytosis. Red cells are extremely pliable and may have a little normal variation. However, the degree of poikiliocytosis in a differential smear may be recorded as slight, moderate or marked. Normal poikiliocytosis is illustrated in Figure 2.

FIGURE 2

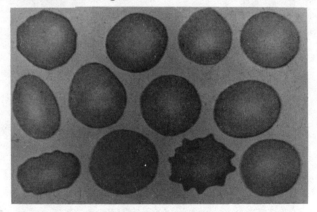

Variation in RBC size is called anisocytosis. This is usually noted as slight, moderate or marked, with additional comments as to the presence of microcytes or macrocytes.

FUNCTION

Simply stated, the function of the red blood cell is gas exchange. This is essential to bring oxygen to the tissues of the body (to be used in cellular respiration), and to remove carbon dioxide.

Several factors influence this process. The most important factors are: the partial pressure of O_2 (pO_2), pH and temperature. The partial pressure of CO_2 (pCO_2) also has to be considered, but this is mainly believed to be an influence on pH. The gas transporting molecule, hemoglobin, will be discussed in detail later. When hemoglobin is combined with O_2, it is called oxyhemoglobin, and when hemoglobin is combined with CO_2, it is called carbamino-hemoglobin.

More oxyhemoglobin is formed at high pO_2 levels (in the lungs). Conversely, at the tissue site, where there is less pO_2, the hemoglobin molecule gives up O_2 and accepts CO_2.

As the pH increases, the percent oxygen saturation increases. However, an increase in temperature causes a lowering of the percent oxygen saturation.

For the hemoglobin molecule to accept a molecule of O_2, the iron atoms must be in the reduced or ferrous (+2) state. It should also be noted that different hemoglobins have different affinities for oxygen.

STRUCTURE

Cell membranes are the subject of active research. Many models have been proposed but it is generally agreed upon that the red blood cell membrane is composed of proteins, lipids, and carbohydrates.

The lipids are predominantly phospholipids, cholesterol and glycolipids.

All of the proteins are not identified, but two appear to be important. These are spectrin and an erythrocyte glycophorin, believed to be a glycoprotein. Although the glycoprotein of the membrane has many functions, one major function is to carry the blood group antigens.

The cell membrane is generally considered to be responsible for the shape of the erythrocyte.

Hemoglobin is classified as a conjugated protein. The globin or protein protion is composed of four polypeptide chains occurring in pairs. These are named using Greek letters. The most common are alpha and beta chains which have between 141 and 146 amino acids respectively.

In the normal adult, there are three types of hemoglobin. Hbg A has two alpha and two beta chains, usually written $\alpha_2\beta_2$. Hgb A_2 has two alpha and two delta chains and Hgb F, fetal hemoglobin, has two alpha and two gamma chains. Another normal hemoglobin found only in the embryo (Gower II) has two alpha and two epsilon chains. As with all proteins in the body, the amino acid sequence, rate of production, and shape are genetically controlled.

The heme moiety is composed of a protoporphyrin ring with an iron atom in the center. There are four heme groups per molecule of hemoglobin. Oxygen is carried bound to the iron atom or atoms but ONLY when the iron is in the ferrous (2+) state. CO_2 is carried on the amino acid chains.

Other substances of clinical importance can combine with hemoglobin. The basis of the laboratory quantitation of hemoglobin relies on the production of cyanmethemoglobin, a laboratory compound ONLY. This should not be confused with methemoglobin which is a hemoglobin with trivalent (ferric 3+) iron which cannot carry oxygen. Carboxyhemoglobin, HgbCO, is hemoglobin with carbon monoxide. The toxic gas, CO, has an affinity for hemoglobin which is 218 times greater than its affinity for oxygen.

PRODUCTION

Heme biosythesis is a long and complicated biochemical process, some steps of which require mitochondria. Since the mature red cell is devoid of all organelles, the process is necessarily restricted to developing cells.

Glycine and succinyl CoA form delta-aminolevulinic acid. Two of these combine to form porphobilinogen. Four porphobilinogens, in turn, are needed to form uroporphyrinogen. Uroporphyrinogen is eventually converted to protoporphyrin. Heme is formed when the enzyme, ferrochetalase, places an iron atom in the center of the protoporpyrin ring (Figure 3).

FIGURE 3

HEME NUCLEUS

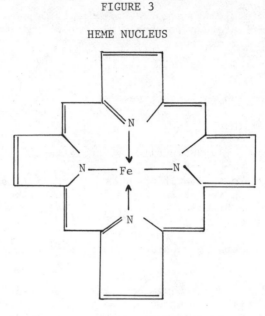

The iron for the production of heme is made available to the normablasts via the iron cycle of the body. Transferrin, a plasma transport protein, is a key factor in the cycle. Polypeptide chain synthesis is associated with the polyribisomes of the normoblast cell. The hemoglobin polypeptide chain follows the normal pattern of all protein production. However, special note should be made of the amino acid sequence, rate of production, tertiary and quaternary structure in the polypeptide chains in question. The primary structure, amino acid sequence, and composition are governed by DNA which uses a template of three bases called triplets or codons. The rate of production of the chain is genetically controlled. The tertiary structure of the polypeptide chains refers to the 3-dimensional shape which is helical and conventionally labelled A through H. The quaternary structure of the hemoglobin molecule is the shape formed by fitting four polypeptide chains together.

In blood formation, the most primitive stem cell is called a hemocytoblast or a pluripotential stem cell. However, the first identifiable member of the erythroid series is the next cell, the pronormoblast, which is followed by the basophilic normoblast, polychromatophilic normoblast, acidophilic normoblast, reticulocyte, and finally the mature erythrocyte. This sequence is listed as follows:

pluripotential stem cell
↓
polychromatophilic normoblast
↓
acidophilic normoblast
↓
reticulocyte
↓
erythrocyte

Pronormoblasts through erythrocyte may be seen in Figure 4. In general, as the cell matures, the nucleus contracts and is extruded at the late acidophilic normoblast stage. At this time, the cytoplasm turns from blue (basophilic) to pink (acidophilic), the RNA content decreases, and the hemoglobin content increases. The last red cell capable of dividing is the polychromatophilic normoblast.

FIGURE 4

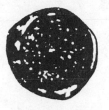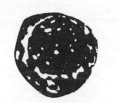

Erythropoietin is a hormone which regulates the differentiation of stem cells into pronormoblasts. Erythropoietin is believed to have an accelerating effect on red cell maturation in general. Plasma globulin precursor from the liver, and renal factor from the kidney, make up erythropoietin.

The blood forming organs are mesenchymal in origin. Blood islands in the yolk sac can be detected at approximately 19 days of gestation. At 5-6 weeks of gestation, the liver begins to produce blood and peaks at 6 months. At 13 weeks, the bone marrow begins production, and at term, erythropoiesis takes place only in this compartment.

Figure 5 illustrates blood formation in the embryo.

SURVIVAL

The life span of the normal red cell is approximately 120 days. In aging red cells, enzymes eventually lose their activity and the cell loses its ability to do work and maintain its integrity.

About 85% of normal red cell destruction takes place within the macrophages of the reticuloendothelial (RE) system. This is termed extravascular hemolysis.

The RE system consists of the reticulum cells of the spleen and lymph nodes, the cells lining the sinusoids of the liver, bone marrow and lymph sinuses, and similar cells in the adrenal and pituitary glands plus free histiocytes.

The remainder of red cell destruction takes place intravascularly or within the blood vessels causing some hemoglobinemia. Most of the hemoglobin is picked up immediately by haptoglobin, a serum protein.

The iron and globin portions are recycled by the body, while the protoporphyrin undergoes a series of reactions to eventually become bilirubin.

FIGURE 5

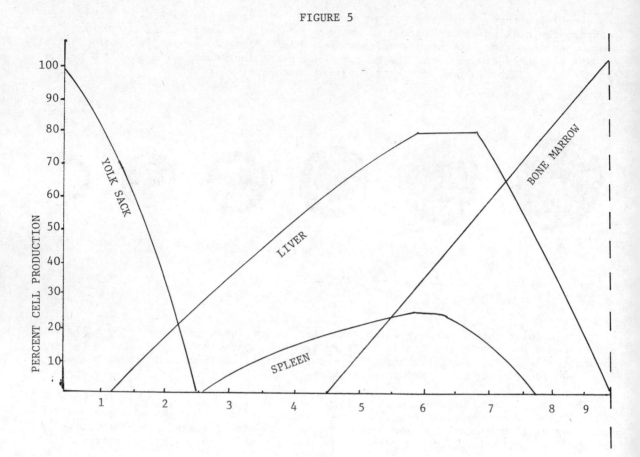

DYSCRASIAS

In this text, the term dyscrasias is used in the broadest possible sense so as to include all abnormalities. Table 1 lists the inclusion bodies which are found in peripheral blood smears stained with Wright's stain and Vital stain.

TABLE 1

RBC INCLUSION BODIES	INCLUSION BODY COMPOSITION
Basophilic Stippling	Precipitated ribosomal material
Siderocytes	Bunched Ferritin Granules
Howell-Jolly Bodies	Nuclear Pieces
Polychromatophilic Macrocytes	Residual RNA

RETICULOCYTE COUNT (VITAL STAIN)	INCLUSION BODY COMPOSITION
Reticulocytes	Residual RNA
Heinz Bodies	Clumps Of Oxidized Hemoglobin

Anomalies are irregular states which generally do not cause signs or symptoms. Hereditary Elliptocytosis is sometimes called an anomaly because the majority of the patients show no clinical manifestations of this state.

Classification of Anemias

The most meaningful classification for the laboratorian is morphologic. The following outline lists only the common anemias. However, note that more overlap occurs than has been listed.

I. Microcytic, hypochromic

    A.   Iron Deficiency Anemia
    B.   Thalassemia

II. Normocytic, normochromic

    A.   Acute Blood Loss
    B.   Hemolytic Anemias
    C.   Aplastic Anemias
    D.   Hemoglobinopathies

III. Macrocytic, normochromic

    A.   Megaloblastic Anemias
    B.   Hemolytic Anemias
    C.   Sideroblastic Anemias

Iron deficiency anemia is the most common microcytic hypochromic anemia. There are many reasons for a deficiency, but the most frequently encountered in the U. S. are blood losses due to: (1) gastrointestinal bleeding; (2) excessive menstrual bleeding; (3) multiple pregnancies; and (4) infants who only have been fed milk.

The typical case of severe iron deficiency anemia will have an MCV of less than 83 cubic microns, an MCH of less than 28 micro-micrograms and an MCHC of less than 31%. The patient will also demonstrate a reticulocyte count less than 1%, and a low serum iron with an increased TIBC (total iron binding capacity). If a bone marrow test is performed, an iron stain (prussian blue reaction) will reveal little to no iron in the reticuloendothelial cells.

Thalassemia is the second most common microcytic hypochromic anemia encountered in the U. S. and it should be considered as a group of syndromes because of the variety of inherited defects.

In general, the disease is due to an impaired rate of synthesis of a polypeptide chain of the globin portion of the hemoglobin molecule.

A mild or severe thalassemia may be inherited. Heterozygous or homozygous genes for either the alpha or beta chains are involved. If the defect is in the alpha chain production, the disease is called alpha thalassemia. If the defect is in the beta chain production, the disease is called beta thalassemia. Cooley's anemia is a homozygous beta thalassemia.

The typical Cooley's anemia patient would show low indices, a marked anemia, and numerous nucleated red blood cells. The reticulocyte count would be increased. Hemoglobin electrophoresis would show approximately 40% hemoglobin F. In some cases,

Hgb A$_2$ would also be increased. In the heterozygous disease, Hgb A$_2$ is expected to be increased.

Acute blood loss will not appear as an anemia until the body has begun to compensate the blood compartment with other body fluids. This may take a few days, and until then, the patient may have an increased hemoglobin, hematocrit and red count due to vasoconstriction.

When the anemia develops, the red blood cell will be normocytic and normochromic with slight anisocytosis and poikilocytosis. The reticulocyte count will be increased, and following severe bleeding, nucleated red cells may be seen.

Many anemias may have a hemolytic component. However, true hemolytic anemias are disorders in which the rate of red cell destruction is accelerated while red cell production is normal. Two broad areas are recognized: intrinsic and extrinsic. In intrinsic hemolytic anemia the red cell survival is shortened due to a defect of the cell, i.e., paroxysmal nocturnal hemoglobinuria (PNH). In extrinsic hemolytic anemia, the red cells are normal, but their survival time is shortened by an outside factor, i.e., malaria or antibody formation.

A typical case will be normocytic and normochromic with an increased reticulocyte count. Heinz bodies may be seen in the reticulocyte count. The indirect bilirubin will be increased along with the urinary urobilinogen. In acute states, hemoglobinemia and hemoglobinuria will occur. Chromium 51 (Cr^{51}) red cell survival studies will show a decreased % survival.

Specific special testing may be in order. Such special testing may include the "sugar water" test, and acid hemolysis test (Ham test) which will both be positive in PNH or a Coombs' test which will be positive in hemolytic diseases of the newborn (HDN).

Aplastic anemia may occur as a congenital, idiopathic or secondary anemia. It is characterized by pancytopenia, a reduction in all three formed elements of the blood.

The typical case will have a marked leukopenia and thrombocytopenia with a severe anemia. The anemia is normocytic, normochromic with a severely decreased to negative reticulocyte count. The bone marrow, in severe cases, will show almost total replacement of cells by fat.

Hemoglobinopathies are inherited abnormal globin structural variants. The majority of the cases are due to a single amino acid substitution. The best known is hemoglobin S (Hgb S). In this case, valine replaces a glutamic acid at the sixth position of the beta chain. There are over 100 abnormal hemoglobins which may be inherited as traits in the heterozygous state or as diseases in the homozygous state.

The typical disease case will have a severe anemia with an elevated white blood count. The reticulocyte count will be increased. The total bilirubin is elevated reflecting the hemolytic component. Hemoglobin electrophoresis is recommended as a test procedure.

Megaloblastic anemias are a group of disorders in which DNA synthesis is defective. The resultant cell, the megaloblast, suffers from asynchrony of the nucleus and cytoplasm, and has been said to be an old cytoplasm with a young nucleus. Folic acid and vitamin B_{12} are necessary for normal DNA synthesis so that anything that interferes, with or deprives the body of them, will cause a megaloblastic anemia.

Pernicious anemia is a syndrome made up of a megaloblastic anemia which is secondary to marked gastric atrophy. The gastric atrophy results in the failure of the cells of the gastric mucosa to secrete intrinsic factor. Intrinsic factor is necessary for the proper absorption of dietary B_{12}. The test of choice is the Schilling test which will be abnormal for Part I and normal for Part II.

The typical megaloblastic anemia case will have macrocytosis with an MCV greater than $100\mu^3$. However, the cells will be normochromic. The white cell count and platelet count are usually decreased but hypersegmented PMN's are seen. The reticulocyte count is less than 1% before treatment. Additional special tests such as the folic acid level, vitamin B_{12} level, gastric analysis and the Schilling test would be essential to determine the cause.

Hemolytic anemias with accelerated erythropoiesis are macrocytic, as are the anemias that occur in response to a prior hemorrhage.

Sideroblastic anemias are a group of disorders characterized by the presence of excessive iron deposits in the mitochondria of the normoblasts. These anemias vary from moderate to severe with idiopathic refractory sideroblastic anemia (IRSA) being macrocytic and normochromic. The reticulyocyte is normal to slightly increased.

Erythrocytosis is an increase in the concentration of red blood cells. Erythremia is an increase in all the formed elements; this is more commonly called polycythemia vera.

The typical case of polycythemia vera will have a red cell count of 9 million/m^3, making the blood so thick that it is difficult to pipette. As the disease progresses, the MCV, MCH and MCHC drop and the bone marrow struggles to keep up with the increased production. Nevertheless, the reticulocyte count is not significantly increased. However, a marked leukocytosis and thrombocytosis may be noted.

Di Guglielmo's syndrome is considered to be an erythroleukemia. The peripheral blood of patients with this syndrome contains erythroblasts in all states of maturation. There is also a slight leukopenia, but the reticulocyte count is normal.

The Leukocyte

MORPHOLOGY

Granulocytes are the predominant white cells found in the peripheral blood of healthy adults. The granulocytes account for approximately 70% of the cells in a differential stain. Mature granulocytes are about twice the size of the average red blood cells.

The mature granulocyte cells are round with a lobate nucleus. The majority of these cells have two to three lobes, but as many as five lobes may occur. If six or more lobes are formed, the cells are said to be hypersegmented.

As the name indicates, these cells have a granular cytoplasm. If the granules take up the blue or basic dye, the cells are said to be basophils. If the cells have granules which do not stain intensely with either the basic or acidic dyes, they are called neutrophils or polymorphonuclear neutrophils.

FUNCTION AND STRUCTURE

Neutrophils phagocytize bacteria. To this end, two types of granules are found: fine and course. The fine granules contain strong acid hydrolases which are said to be responsible for the "toxic granulation" phenomenon. The coarse granules are believed to contain heparin and are not directly involved in the phagocytic process.

PRODUCTION

Granulocytes develop in the bone marrow from a cell line most frequently referred to as the myelocytic series. "Myelo" comes from the Greek word myelos meaning marrow. However, the terms granulocytic and myelocytic are used interchangeably.

The first identifiable member of the series is called a myeloblast followed by a promyelocyte, myelocyte, metamyelocyte, band or non-segmented polymorphonuclear neutrophil (nsp) and PMN. This series is listed below:

```
          Pluripotential Stem Cell
                     ↓
             Myeloblast
                  ↓
               Promyelocyte
                    ↓
                 Myelocyte
                    ↓
                  Metamyelocyte
                      ↓
                    Band
                     ↓
          Polymorphonuclear Neutrophil
```

As the cells mature, they decrease in size and increase in granulation. Also, the nucleus of each decreases in size while gradually becoming lobate.

Among the white cells, blast cells are extremely hard to differentiate between series. To do so, special stains are required.

It is presently believed that the myelocyte is the last cell in the series capable of division.

The bone marrow has approximately a 9-10 day supply of granulocytes in reserve. These granulocytes can be released into the peripheral blood in response to a sudden need, i.e., infection or other stress conditions.

During stress conditions, a "shift to the left" may occur. This results in the increased formation of immature granulocytes (usually bands and occasionally metamyelocytes). Patients with infections or leukemia may have this "shift".

SURVIVAL

The intravascular life of the granulocytes lasts but a few hours. Their half-life has been calculated at seven (7) hours. The granulocytes travel into the tissues and do not re-enter the peripheral blood.

DISEASES

A decrease in granulocytes is referred to as neutropenia. Neutropenia may have many causes. An absolute decrease or absense of granulocytes is called agranulocytosis.

The majority of patients will have an increased or marked over production of granulocytes. If this over production is malignant (an uncontrolled or wild proliferation with abnormal cells) the disease is referred to as a leukemia. If this over production is benign or regular with normal cells, the disease is called a leukemoid reaction.

A typical case of acute granulocytic (myelogenous) leukemia will have approximately 60% or more myeloblast forms in the peripheral blood. These cells may show Auer rods. The white blood count may be increased, decreased or normal, but an anemia and thrombocytopenia are usually present due to bone marrow crowding.

Specific, special stains are used in order to classify the myeloblast cells which are practically indistinguishable from one cell line to another. However, the presence of Auer rods will rule out lymphoblasts. The peroxidase stain and sudan black B stain will be positive in acute granulocytic leukemia (AGL).

The typical case of chronic granulocytic (myelogenous) leukemia will have less than 10% myeloblasts in the peripheral blood. The white blood count is usually markedly increased and an increase in thrombocytes (platelets) is generally present.

The Philadelphia chromosome, a deletion of one arm in chromosomal pair number 22, is found in 85% of the cases of CGL.

In order to distinguish CGL from a leukemoid reaction, a leukocyte alkaline phosphatase stain is performed. In CGL, the granulocytes do not pick up the stain and consequently a low test value is obtained. In myelomonocytic leukemia, Naegeli Type, the acute form usually occurs. Many blast forms, myeloblasts and monoblasts, are present in the peripheral blood.

Monocytic leukemia (Schilling Type) is very rare, but usually occurs in the acute form, with many monoblasts in the peripheral blood.

The Lymphocyte

MORPHOLOGY

In the healthy child, lymphocytes constitute approximately 70% of the white cells found in the peripheral blood. In the adult, the lymphocytes account for approximately 25% of the white cell population.

The mature lymphocytes vary from 8-16 microns in diameter. The larger the cells, the more the cytoplasm will be visible. The smaller cells are more perfectly round with scant cytoplasm, while the larger cells have a tendency to have slightly oval nuclei with cytoplasm that may become indented by surrounding red cells.

With Wright's stain, the Lymphocyte nucleus stains dark blue-purple and the cytoplasm stains a clear pale blue. Some cells may also contain a few nonspecific azurophilic granules.

FUNCTION

Lymphocytes are immunocytes and as such are responsible for cell-mediated immunity and antibody production.

PRODUCTION

Lymphocytes develop in the lymph nodes, spleen, thymus and bone marrow.

Embryonically, it is believed that a lymphoid stem cell, from the bone marrow, seeds the thymus and bursal equivalent (gut associated) tissue. The thymus is considered to populate and maintain the para-cortical area of the lymph nodes and the white pulp of the spleen. The bursal equivalent tissue is considered to be responsible for the lymphatic follicles and splenic cords.

Consequently, lymphocytes in the peripheral blood are either T cells (thymus dependent cells) or B cells (bursa dependent cells). The following diagram illustrates lymphocyte maturation.

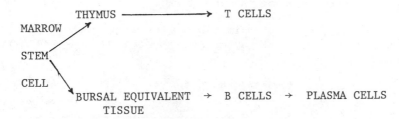

T cells function in cell-mediated immunity. The most common example is a positive tuberculin skin test which is a delayed hypersensitivity reaction. T cells are also capable of reverting to their primative form and thus regain the ability to divide.

T cells may live for as long as ten years, and are therefore frequently referred to as memory cells.

B cells account for approximately 20% of the lymphocytes and function in humoral immunity (antibody production). Upon stimulation, it is generally believed that these cells can transform into plasma cells which synthesize immunoglobulins.

IMMUNOGLOBULINS

TABLE 2

CLASSIFICATION OF IMMUNOGLOBULINS

	Heavy Chains	Molecular Weight
IgG	α	150,000
IgA	γ	180,000 or
		390,000
IgM	μ	900,000
IgD	δ	150,000
IgE	ϵ	200,000

DISEASES

Swiss-type agamma globulinemia is a hereditary, total, immunologic deficiency state due to a failure in the marrow stem cell. No humoral or cellular immunity is present.

In *Di George's syndrome* the thymus fails to form. The result is impaired cellular immunity with normal antibody production.

In *Bruton agamma globulinemia*, there is normal cellular immunity with no antibody production.

Infectious mononucleosis is a syndrome which may be caused by one or more viruses. The Epstein-Barr virus and the cytomegalovirus have been implicated. The typical case will have large numbers, sometimes as much as 60% of atypical lymphocytes in the peripheral blood. The white count may be increased, decreased or normal. Anemia and thrombocytopenia are rare. The heterophile antibody test will be positive.

Acute lymphocytic leukemia is said to be the childhood leukemia because of the increased frequency of the disease in children.

The typical case will have approximately 60% or more lymphoblast forms in the peripheral blood. The white count may be increased, decreased or normal, with anemia and thrombocytopenia.

The peroxidase stain negative and the leukocyte alkaline phosphatase stain is normal.

Chronic lymphocytic leukemia is most frequently found in people who are over 60 years of age.

The typical case will have approximately 80% mature lymphocytes in the peripheral blood, with an increased white count and a normal number of platelets. The diagnosis can be confirmed by the finding of more than 10% mature lymphocytes in a bone marrow biopsy.

Lymphomas are neoplasms (tumors) which arise from lymphoid tissue. The diagnosis is made histologically from biopsy material. If the malignant cells spread to the peripheral blood, the disease is called a leukemia.

The classification of lymphomas differs from author to author; however, two general divisions are generally agreed upon: Hodgkin's disease which constitutes about 40% of the cases and Non-Hodgkin's Lymphoma which makes up about 60% of the cases.

The diagnosis of *Hodgkin's disease* is made upon seeing the characteristic malignant histocyte, the Reed-Sternberg cell, in the biopsied lymphoid tissue. The disease is subclassified into four categories according to histology. Staging--the extent of spread--is done for treatment and prognosis.

In general, most cases have a normocytic anemia with advanced disease showing a lymphopenia. Also, impaired hypersensitivity reactions sometimes occur.

The Thrombocyte

Thrombocytes (platelets) are megakaryocyte cytoplasm fragments. The megakaryocytes are normally found in the bone marrow. Platelets enter the peripheral blood. Platelet are approximately three (3) microns in diameter and appear pale blue when stained with Wright's stain. Purple granules are also apparent in the Wright stain preparation.

At the site of injury, platelets participate in: (1) the formation of a hemostatic plug and, (2) the clotting process.

Platelet production takes about ten (10) days. The production process is as follows:

$$\begin{array}{c}
\text{Committed Stem Cell (?) (Presence uncertain)} \\
\downarrow \\
\text{Megakaryoblast (cannot divide)} \\
\downarrow \\
\text{Promegakaryocyte} \\
\downarrow \\
\text{Megakaryocyte} \\
\downarrow \\
\text{Platelets}
\end{array}$$

Platelets are not kept in reserve in the bone marrow. However, the techniques employed to determine platelet survival time produce different survival time results. In brief, reported platelet survival varies with the method used. Nevertheless, a three (3) to ten (10) day survival time is usually reported. Old platelets are removed by the reticuloendothelial (R.E.) cells of the spleen and liver. Damaged platelets are removed by the spleen, primarily.

Thrombocytopenia is a reduction in the number of platelets in the peripheral blood. Thrombocytopenia may be caused by many conditions, i.e., hemorrhage or toxins. If the origin of the reduction of platelets is unknown, the condition is called idiopathic thrombocytopenia.

Thrombocythemia is an increase in the number of platelets in the peripheral blood.

Thrombocytopathies are diseases attributed to platelet functional defects.

Coagulation

The balance between clot formation and dissolution (hemostasis) should be viewed as a three-part system, the three parts being: the platelets, the blood vessels, and the coagulation factors.

Platelets (thrombocytes) are measured quantitatively by observing them on a stained smear or by performing a platelet count. The latter is reported to be more accurate. Qualitatively, platelets are evaluated by performing a bleeding time (for the formation of the primary plug) and by performing a clot retraction test (for participation in the clotting process). Further, special tests are available which test for the platelets' adhesion and aggregation functions.

The blood vessels must not allow leakage into the surrounding tissue. This factor is referred to as *vascular integrity*. Blood vessels must also construct at the site of injury. To assess vascular function, two tests are performed: (1) the tourniquet test (for vascular integrity), and (2) the bleeding time (for construction. If the blood vessels are constricting normally, there should be a 5-second pre-bleeding time, i.e., there should be a 5-second delay before bleeding time is recorded.

The coagulation factors are:

   I.   Fibrinogen
  II.   Prothrombin
 III.   Tissue Thromboplastin
  IV.   Calcium
   V.   Labile Factor (proaccelerin)
 VII.   Stable Factor (proconvertin)
VIII.   Antihemophilic Factor (AHF)
  IX.   Christmas Factor (Plasma Thromboplastin Component)
   X.   Stuart-Prower
  XI.   Plasma Thromboplastin Antecedent (PTA)
 XII.   Hageman Factor
XIII.   Fibrin Stabilizing Factor (FSF)

The coagulation factors work, by activating each other in a two-part system, to form a stable fibrin clot. The two parts of the system, which are sometimes called pathways, are the extrinsic part and the intrinsic part.

The sequential action of the coagulation factors in fibrin formation is listed below:

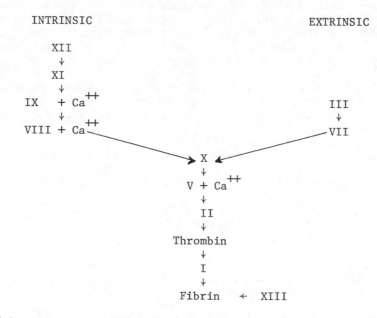

The two laboratory tests which measure the intrinsic and extrinsic system are: (1) the prothrombin time (PT) test; and (2) the activated partial thromboplastin time (APTT). The PT test evaluates the factors of the extrinsic part of the system. The APTT test evaluates the intrinsic part of the system. These two system components must function properly for normal hemostasis to occur.

Fibrinolysis and Anticoagulants

Every time a clot is formed it must be dissolved in order to bring back normal or near normal function of the blood vessel in which it was formed. This process is called fibrinolysis. Fibrinolysis is a function of the enzyme plasmin. Normal blood contains only trace amounts of plasmin.

As a preventative or therapeutic measure, it may be desirable to stop or reduce the natural clotting process with an anticoagulant. Two anticoagulants are in common use: (1) Heparin is an anticoagulant which is an antagonist of thrombin and is sometimes referred to as an anti-thrombin; (2) sodium warfarin (coumarin) is an anticoagulant which blocks the action of vitamin K in the production of factors II, VII, IX and X. With the exception of heparin, the routine anticoagulants used to collect plasma for laboratory testing are binders of calcium.

DISEASES

In the absence of a circulating fibrinolysin or anticoagulant, the most common diseases are Hemophilia, in the hereditary group, and Disseminated Intravascular Coagulation (DIC), in the acquired group.

Hemophilia or Factor VIII deficiency results from an inadequate amount of circulating Factor VIII. Genetically it is transmitted as an X-linked recessive trait. Therefore, it affects males while the females are the carriers.

The typical hemophiliac case will have a normal PT with an elevated APTT, with a normal bleeding time, platelet count and tournique test. Frequently the Lee and White clotting time is prolonged.

Disseminated Intravascular Coagulation (DIC) results from a spontaneous clotting process triggered throughout the body. There are many compounds which will trigger the clotting process. Endotoxin produced by Gram negative bacteria frequently triggers the clotting process. Therefore, DIC may often follow a Gram negative septicemia.

The typical case will have a prolonged bleeding time and a very low platelet count. Both PT and APTT will be prolonged. The thrombin time will be elevated, and the fibrinogen level will be low.

BIBLIOGRAPHY AND RECOMMENDED READINGS

Brown, B. A. *WHITE CELL MANUAL.* Third Edition 1975. F. A. Davis. Philadelphia.

Davidsohn, I. and J. B. Henry (Editors). *TODD-SANFORD CLINICAL DIAGNOSIS BY LABORA-TORY METHODS.* Fifteenth Edition 1974. W. B. Saunders Company. Philadelphia.

Harris, J. W. and R. W. Kellermeyer. *THE RED CELL.* Revised Edition 1974. Harvard University Press. Cambridge.

Miale, J. B. *LABORATORY MEDICINE: HEMATOLOGY.* 1972. C. V. Mosby. St. Louis.

Rapaport, S. S. (Senior Author). Lynch's Medical *LABORATORY TECHNOLOGY.* Volume II. Third Edition 1976. W. B. Saunders Company. Philadelphia.

Williams, W. J., Beutler, E., Erslev, A. J., and R. W. Rundles. *HEMATOLOGY.* 1972. McGraw Hill Company. New York.

Wintrobe, M. W., Lee, G. R., Boggs, D. R., Bithell, T. C., Athens, J. W., and J. Foerster. *CLINICAL HEMATOLOGY.* Seventh Edition 1974. Lea and Febiger. Philadelphia.

Chapter 8

Special Topics in Clinical Chemistry

JAMES J. VAILLANCOURT, MT (ASCP)
Supervisor Clinical Chemistry
Concord Hospital
Concord, New Hampshire

OUTLINE

INTRODUCTION
INORGANIC IONS AND WATER BALANCE
    Water Balance
        Fluid Movement and Properties
        Osmolality
ELECTROLYTES
    Sodium
    Physiology of the Kidney
    Potassium
    Calcium
    Ionized Calcium
    Magnesium
    Other Essential Elements
    Chloride
    Phosphate
    Carbon Dioxide
    Acid/Base Disturbances
    Organic Acid Anions

BLOOD UREA NITROGEN
    Creatinine
    Uric Acid
CARBOHYDRATES
    Glucose
    Methods of Analysis
    Glucose Tolerance Test
    Glycosylated Hemoglobin
PROTEINS
    Chemistry
METHODS OF ANALYSIS
    Clinical Significance

LIPIDS
    Chemistry
    Metabolism of Lipids
    Methods of Analysis
    Clinical Significance
ENZYMES
    Introductions
    Definition of Terms
    Mode of Action
    Specific Enzymes
        Creatine Kinase
        Lactate Dehydrogenase
        Aminotransferase
        Phosphatases
        5' Nucleotidase
        Lipase
        Amylase
        Aldolase
        Cholinesterase
    Diagnostic Applications
BILIRUBIN
BIBLIOGRAPHY AND RECOMMENDED READINGS

SELECTED TOPICS IN CLINICAL CHEMISTRY

To write fully and completely in the field of clinical chemistry would certainly fill a room rather than a book. To condense for the sake of condensation and distillation too often leads one to confusion rather than knowledge. I chose what I believe to be important areas in the field of practicing clinical chemistry at the hospital level and presented them in this chapter.

Electrolytes and water balance are presented in a different manner, hopefully filling a void that appears in recent clinical chemistry textbooks. With the rise in enzyme linked assays (EIA, ELISA) which are replacing some RIA procedure, I chose to stress the enzymes and their applications. The other sections represent the presenting of basic information necessary for everyday clinical chemistry work. When further information is needed by the reader I recommend the excellent texts in this bibliography.

Inorganic Ions and Water Balance

The roles of water and electrolytes in the body are diverse and intertwined. Water is the universal solvent capable of making solutions of sodium chloride, calcium sulfate, potassium phosphate, and other nonelectrolytes such as creatinine and urea. Water provides the medium in which the chemical and enzymatic reactions of the body can occur; water's ionization properties affect enzymes, proteins, amino acids, and lipids. The electrolytes maintain osmotic pressure, control fluid volumes in the various fluid compartments, maintain body pH and participate as cofactors in many enzymatic reactions.

Electrolytes are characterized by their electrical charges. Those electrolytes having positive charges are called cations, while those having negative charges are called anions. Electrolytic compounds, when dissolved in water, will dissociate into their respective ionic forms. If an electrical current is applied across this solution, the cationic substances will migrate toward the cathode and the anionic substances will migrate toward the anode. For example, if sodium chloride is dissolved in water, it will dissociate into a positively charged sodium ion and a negatively charged chloride ion. If an electrical current is then applied to the solution, the sodium ions will migrate to the cathode and the chloride ions will migrate toward the anode. The other electrolytes in solution will behave in a similar manner. The major electrolytes, their chemical symbols, the reference values in milliequivalents (mEq/L), and their reference values in International Units (SI) are listed in Table I.

Since the human body must maintain electrical neutrality, there must be an equal number of positive and negative charges. This electrical neutrality does not mean that there will be an acid-base neutrality or any specific pH. It simply means that the number of positive charges equals the number of negative charges. It is important that the measurement of electrolytes be expressed in the appropriate terms to signify this electrical neutrality. If electrolytes are measured in terms of the number of milligrams per deciliter, it may appear as though the number of electrical charges are unequal. Electrolytes, therefore, must be expressed in terms of milliequivalents per liter. Milliequivalents per liter are determined in the following manner:

1. 1 milliequivalent is 1/1,000th of an equivalent.

2. An equivalent weight is the atomic weight of an element divided by its value.

TABLE 1

SUMMARY OF ELECTROLYTES; THEIR SYMBOL AND REFERENCE RANGES

Electrolyte	Symbol	mEq/L	SI(mmoles/L)
Sodium	Na+	135–148	135–148
Potassium	K+	3.5–5.3	3.5–5.3
Calcium	Ca++	4.6–5.5	2.3–2.8
Magnesium	Mg++	1.3–2.1	0.7–1.1

Anions	Symbol	mEq/L	SI9mmoles/L)
Bicarbonate	HCO_3^-	21–28	21–28
Chloride	Cl^-	98–106	98–106
Phosphate	HPO_4^-	approx 2	– –
Sulfate	SO_4^-	approx 1	– –
Organic Acids	$OrgAc^-$	approx 6	– –
Proteins	Pr^-	approx 16	– –

Problem: If a calcium level is determined to be 8.5 mg/dl, we can convert to mEq/L in the following manner:

Step 1: Convert mg/dl to mg/L

$$\frac{8.5 \text{ mg}}{100 \text{ ml}} \times \frac{1{,}000 \text{ ml}}{1 \text{ liter}} = 85 \text{ mg/L}$$

Step 2: Determine the equivalent weight of calcium atomic weight = 40; valence of calcium = 2

$$\text{equivalent weight} = \frac{\text{atomic weight}}{\text{VALENCE}} = \frac{40}{2} = 20 \text{ (for calcium)}$$

Step 3: Determine milliequivalents per liter

$$mEq/L = \frac{mg/L}{\text{equivalent weight}} = \frac{85 \text{ mg/L}}{20} = 4.25 \text{ mEq/L}$$

Recently, there has been growing interest in expressing all laboratory data in SI units. SI units are the units of the International System of Units. The SI unit for electrolytes is millimoles per liter (mmol/L). The SI units for the major electrolytes are found in Table 1.

WATER BALANCE

In an average adult, water represents 60–70% of the total body weight. Intracellular fluid constitutes approximately 40% of the body weight while the remaining 25% due is intracellular fluid. Extracellular fluid may be further divided into interstitial fluid (which bathes the cells) 20%, and plasma water, 5%. To understand fluid movement between these compartments, we must discuss diffusion, hydrostatic pressure, and osmotic pressure.

Table 2 shows that the three major fluid compartments have differences in their compositions. This is partly due to the semipermeable membranes that separate them. The cell membranes between the interstitial and intravascular fluid compartments are selectively permeable allowing water and only some solutes free passage. There are several forces which control the passage of water, nutrients, wastes, and ions across cell membranes. One such force is simple diffusion. This is the process by which a solute may spread throughout a solution. Molecules or ions in a solution are in constant motion and consequently bump into each other. Diffusion can occur across a membrane only if that membrane is permeable to certain ions or molecules. Oxygen enters the blood via the lungs and diffuses into the cells at the capillary beds.

TABLE 2

ELECTROLYTE COMPOSITION OF SERUM, INTERSTITIAL FLUID, AND INTRACELLULAR FLUID

		SERUM	INTERSTITICAL FLUID	INTRACELLULAR
Cations (mEq/L)	Total	155	154	187
	Na+	142	145	10
	K+	5	4	135
	Ca++	5	3	2
	Mg++	3	2	40
Anions (mEq/L)	Total	155	154	187
	Cl^-	104	116	5
	HCO_3^-	27	27	10
	$HOP_4^=$	2	3	83
	$SO_4^=$	1	2	14
	$OrgAc^-$	5	5	
	Pr^-	16	1	75

Osmosis is the movement of fluid through a selectively permeable membrane. This is demonstrated in Figure 1.

FIGURE 1

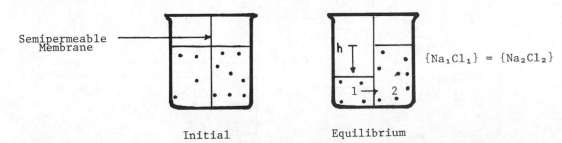

Semipermeable Membrane

$\{Na_1Cl_1\} = \{Na_2Cl_2\}$

Initial   Equilibrium

Figure 1 represents two different NaCl concentrations separated by a membrane permeable only to water. Water will flow across this semipermeable membrane causing an equilibrium to exist between the NaCl concentrations of their respective sides. (The subscripts refer only to the two sides of the membranes.) After osmosis, the concentration of salt solution on both sides of the membrane is the same. Two forces are created by osmosis as illustrated in Figure 1. At equilibrium, the height of the column of solution 2, h, counter balances the tendency of the water to flow from solution 1 to solution 2. This force which causes water to flow from a solution of higher concentration to one of lower concentration is called osmotic pressure. The unequal flow of water into solution 2 has caused the height of the column to rise and its weight to increase proportionately. The force of the weight per area is called hydrostatic pressure and is represented by h. Hydrostatic pressure equals osmotic pressure and they are always applied in opposition to one another. In the body, hydrostatic pressure is created by the pressure exerted by the heart and the elasticity of the blood vessels. In Figure 1, the osmotic pressure is created by the semipermeable membranes which are permeable to water, but impermeable to salt. Hydrostatic pressure causes water to flow from the plasma to the interstitial space. Osmotic pressure is greater in the plasma than in the interstitial fluid thus causing a greater movement of water from the interstitial fluid to the plasma. At the arterial side of the capillary bed, the hydrostatic pressure is greater causing a net flow of water from the plasma to the interstitial fluid. Conversely, at the venous side the osmotic pressure is greater causing water to move from the interstitial fluid to the plasma. The movement of fluid between interstitial and intracellular fluid compartments depends solely on osmotic pressure because the hydrostatic pressure remains constant.

The presence of proteins in body fluids complicates the diffusion of ions across semipermeable membranes. The cellular membranes in the body are permeable to water, sodium, chloride, urea, and glucose.

Table 2 demonstrates that proteins add approximately 16 mEq/L of anionic charge in plasma and 75 mEq/L in intravascular fluid. Just to maintain electrical neutrality, the diffusion of ions will have to be unequal to offset the effects of the non-permeant proteins. Albumin is the major protein contributing to the osmotic effect of plasma. Albumin represents slightly less than half of all plasma proteins, has the lowest molecular weight of the major plasma proteins, and at a pH 7.4 has 18 negative charges per molecule.

To unravel this confusion let's consider the Gibbs-Donnan Law which states that the product of the concentration of the diffusible ions in one compartment is equal to the product of the concentration of diffusible ions in the other compartment. If we go back to our example of osmosis and add protein to one compartment, we can see the difference protein makes.

This time consider that the volumes are fixed and the membrane is nonelastic. To preserve neutrality, Na^+ and Cl^- ions must diffuse unequally until equilibrium is reached (Figure 2).

FIGURE 2

INITIAL			EQUILIBRIUM	
Na^+ 15	Na^+ 15		Na^+ 10	Na^+ 20
Cl^- 15	Cl^- 0		Cl^- 10	Cl^- 5
	Pr^- 15			Pr^- 15

The presence of protein on one side will cause the (Na_2^+) to be greater than (Na_1^+) and the (Cl_2) is less than (Cl_1). At equilibrium, each compartment has achieved electrical neutrality, but the uneven distribution of diffusible ions has produced an electrical potential across the membrane. This potential could be explained by the Nernst Equation.

The osmotic pressure produced by proteins plays an important part in the body's

maintenance of water balance. Decreases in the plasma proteins due to either inadequate intake, synthesis, or excessive loss cause a decreased osmotic pressure which
sends more fluid into the interstitial spaces. This condition is known as edema. Increased hydrostatic pressure brought about by back pressure of a failing heart, from
thrombotic closure of veins, or from compression of veins by tumors can also increase
the flow of fluid into the interstitial space by increasing hydrostatic pressure. This
increased flow of water into the interstitial space will lower the osmotic pressure of
the interstitial fluid causing water to flow into the cells. Edema becomes a self
limiting process. When a sufficient rise occurs in the interstitial fluid increased
hydrostatic pressure will block further fluid movement. The concentrating plasma's
osmotic pressure rises enough to also stop further water movement. When the plasma
fluid is lost due to acute blood loss, the plasma protein concentration rises, osmotic
pressure rises, and fluids are pulled from the interstitial spaces into the plasma.
To complete equilibrium, the osmotic pressure of the interstitial fluid is raised by
the outflow of water thus drawing water from the cells.

There are no laboratory tests which measure the loss or gain of body fluids. The
hematocrit, serum total protein, urea nitrogen, urine or serum osmolality are often
helpful but never diagnostic. Disturbances in the body fluids usually accompany illness. A patient who weighed 175 pounds yesterday may weight 185 pounds today because
of excess fluid volume. Although we can detect volume losses or gains of body fluids
through secondary laboratory testing, we must be constantly aware of its effects.
The chief sources of fluids are through ingestion of liquids and solids and the oxidation processes of metabolism. Normal fluid losses occur through the gastrointestinal
tract, the lungs, the skin, and the kidneys. Knowledge of fluid intake and fluid loss
is important in assessing fluid volume imbalances.

Conditions associated with fluid volume deficit are: vomiting, diarrhea, surgical
drainage, internal pooling (ileus), renal disease, severe burns, fevers, diabetes
insipidus, diuretic administration, and hypoadrenocorticism (Addison's disease).
Typical laboratory test results from a fluid volume deficient patient include an
elevated hematocrit and total protein; urea nitrogen (BUN) elevated more than creatinine; urine/plasma osmolality ratio greater than 1; and the urine sodium less than
20 mEq/L. The physiological response begins with a decreased osmotic pressure of the
intracellular fluid. This increased loss of extracellular fluid causes it to become
hypertonic to the intracellular fluid, resulting in fluid movement from the cells to
the plasma. The posterior pituitary gland secretes antidiuretic hormone (ADH) which
increases the reabsorption of water at the renal distal tubules.

It is possible to overhydrate the fluid compartments. If a person drinks an excessive amount of water or if a large volume of fluid is given intravenously, over-
hydration can occur. In this case, the physiologic response would be to step up
urine output by decreasing the effects of ADH. Excessive water intake may lead to
water intoxication where the tissues become saturated with fluid. Other causes of
increased fluid volume are cardiac failure, cirrhosis, and nephrotic syndrome. Laboratory findings usually include hyponatremia and hypochloremia. The urea nitrogen is
usually normal unless the patient has renal disease. An interesting sidelight is
that water intoxication occurs in starvation. A person on a restricted diet will not
vary in total body weight for the first week or two due to the fact that the oxidation
of body fat produces water. With continued food deprivation, the water will be lost
through the kidneys. It is possible to overhydrate the fluid compartments. When the
healthy individual ingests large quantities of water the kidneys eliminate the excess.
In individuals with renal disorders, the kidneys may not excrete the excess fluid
and the tissues may become saturated.

OSMOLALITY

The addition of electrolytes, small solutes (such as glucose and urea), and colloids (proteins) to water alter its colligative properties. The freezing point, boiling point, vapor pressure, and osmotic pressure are properties of solutions which are dependent on the <u>number</u> of particles present. Measurement of any of these can be related to the concentration of particles per unit volume of solvent. The addition of solute depresses the freezing point and boiling point. For the clinical labora-tory, the measurement of freezing point depression is the most accessible.

When 1 mole of nonionic solute containing 6.023×10^{23} particles (Avogadro's num-ber) is added to 1 kilogram of water, the freezing poing is lowered by 1.858°C. One mole of glucose in solution will depress the freezing point 1.858°C. When one mole of NaCl is added to water, the freezing point is lowered by almost twice that amount. If we examine 100 particles of that 1 molar NaCl, we would expect the ideal behavior to occur as follows:

$$100 \text{ NaCl} \rightarrow 100 \text{ Na}^+ + 100 \text{ Cl}^- \qquad \text{(or 200 particles)}$$

One mole of NaCl provides twice the number of particles to the solution than does 1 mole of glucose, and therefore lowers the freezing point twice as much.

We can see then that for compound ions (NaCl, $CaCl_2$), we must account for the ions resulting by dissociation. Actual measurements of freezing point depression and osmolality of a 1 molar NaCl do not verify that the freezing point is depressed 3.716°C (2 x 1.858°C). The difference between the theoretical and actual freezing point depression is the osmotic coefficient (ϕ). Instead of the ideal behavior of:

$$100 \text{ NaCl} \rightarrow 100 \text{ Na}^+ + 100 \text{ Cl}^-$$

we see:
$$100 \text{ NaCl} \rightarrow 86 \text{ Na}^+ + 86 \text{Cl}^- + 14 \text{ NaCl} \text{ (or 186 particles)}$$

When the NaCl molecules dissolve into solution, not all of them break up into ions. The anticipated number of ions (100 Na^+ and 100 Cl^-) does occur, but are not inde-pendently expressed due to the concentration of the ions and their electric charge interferences. The difference we saw was:

$$186 \text{ particles/200 particles} = 0.93 = \phi$$

If we pull the effects of the number of ions (n) and the osmotic coefficient (ϕ) to-gether with 1.858°C, we can calculate the freezing point depression in the following manner:

$$\phi \times n \times 1.858°C = \text{freezing point depression}$$

If we consider the molar concentration of a substance, we can calculate the osmolality

$$\phi \times n \times \text{molar concentration} = \text{osmole}$$

Therefore, 1 molar NaCl depresses the freezing point

$$0.93 \times 2 \times 1.858°C = 3.34$$

and has an osmole of

$$0.93 \times 2 \times 1 \text{ mole} = 1.86 \text{ osmole or } 1860 \text{ mosmole}$$

FIGURE 3

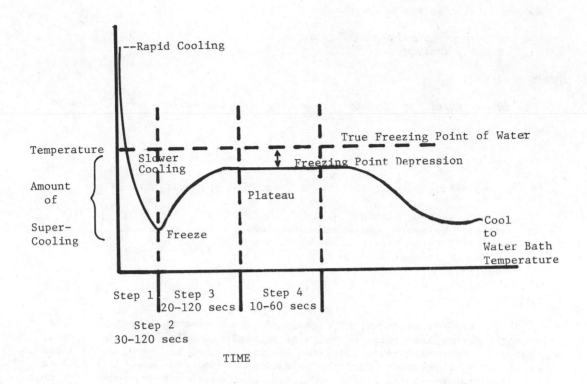

TIME

Method of Analysis: A sample of serum or urine is centrifuged twice to eliminate any particulate matter. A specific volume of sample is placed in a glass tube in the osmometer and supercooled to a point below the true freezing point of water. (Illustrated in Step 1 of Figure 3). Because plasma or urine will not freeze at 0°C, the solution must be supercooled. Once supercooled, any movement will cause instantaneous freezing. In osmometry, a vibrating rod is used to "shock" the supercooled solution causing it to freeze. Once a temperature plateau is reached and the solution is frozen, the temperature is measured and the freezing point depression is calculated.

Reference Value:

Serum: 290 - 300 mOSm/Kg H_2O

Urine (random specimen):   300-900 mOsm/Kg H_2O

Ratio: $\dfrac{\text{urine osmo}}{\text{serum osmo}}$ (Random)   1.0 - 3.0

Ratio: $\dfrac{\text{serum Na}}{\text{serum osmo}}$ 0.43 - 0.50

It is more useful to measure serum and urine osmolality together than each separately. A random urine specimen of 900 or greater mOsm/Kg H_2O represents good renal concentrating ability.

URINE

Low osmolalities may be indicative of:

    chronic progressive renal failure
    diabetes insipidus

SERUM

Low osmolalities (hypotonicity resulting from low sodium) may occur after:

    surgery
    congestive heart failure
    hepatic failure with ascites

High osmolalities (hypertonicity) may occur as a result of:

    chronic wasting disease
    methanol poisoning and other poisonings
    severe diabetes mellitus
    trauma or illness
    dehydration

Electrolytes

    Although oxygen, hydrogen, nitrogen, and carbon make up almost all of the total
body weight, other inorganic ions such as potassium, sodium, chloride, calcium, and
magnesium are important to the body and easily measured in the clinical laboratory.
These elements are present mainly as salts, and in solution are fully ionized. Sodium
is the chief extracellular cation. Chloride and bicarbonate represent the chief extracellular anions. Magnesium and potassium are the chief intracellular cations while
phosphates, sulfates, and proteins comprise the intracellular anions. These ions contribute chiefly to the control of osmotic pressure and are often used as an indirect
measurement of water balance. Care must be taken in the interpretations of any or
all of the inorganic ions. A 125 mmol/1 (mEq/L) sodium concentration can be misleading. The low sodium could be due to the dilutional effect of excessive water administration or artifactual hyponatremia, secondary to hyperglycemia. Elevated glucose
levels cause hyperosmolality which causes fluid movement from the intracellular to the
extracellular fluid compartment. This fluid movement can result in depressed sodium
levels. Another case of artifactual hyponatremia occurs with lipemic specimens. The
elevated triglycerides create a situation where there is a decreased aqueous phase
for sodium and therefore, the serum sodium concentration is artificially low. Whether
artifactually produced or a true representation of total body stores, the concentrations must be carefully examined.

    Sodium represents the major cation of the extracellular fluid. Daily intake of
dietary sodium is usually in the form of sodium chloride and the amount usually is
reflective of the individual intake of the person. The average daily requirement of
sodium chloride for adults is approximately six grams. Sodium is absorbed into the
bloodstream from the small intestine by an active transport mechanism which requires
glucose. Sodium shows a renal threshold of 110-130 mmol/1. When the sodium levels
fall below 110 mmol/1, all the sodium filtered by the glomerulus is reabsorbed. Sodium added to plasma through dietary or intravenous means, is quickly mixed with the
body pool of exchangeable sodium. About 50-60% of this exchangeable pool is found in
the plasma and interstitial fluid. The remainder is found in bone, tendon, and car-
tilage. It must be remembered that over half of the total body sodium is found in
bone, and only 1/3 of that sodium is available as exchangeable sodium.

Sodium is responsible for controlling the water balance between the fluid compartments. Perhaps this is because sodium does not easily cross cell membranes. Once across the membrane, it is rapidly returned to the extracellular fluid by an active process requiring adenosine triphosphate (ATP). Therefore, regulation of sodium concentration is regulation of extracellular fluid volume. Two important fluid conditions are summarized in Figure 4.

FIGURE 4

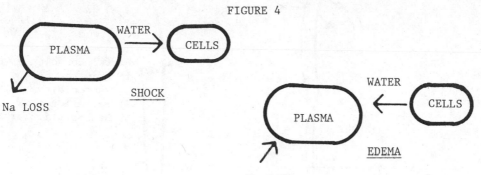

REFERENCE RANGE: 135-145 mmol/L

CONDITIONS ASSOCIATED WITH ABNORMAL SODIUM VALUES

HYPONATREMIA

When the loss of sodium begins to exceed the replacement, serum sodium concentrations will decrease.

Severe polyuria.
Metabolic acidosis: the kidneys exchange sodium for hydrogen ions.
Addison's disease: decrease secretion of aldosterone which is responsible for sodium retention.
Severe diarrhea: increased loss of sodium in feces and decreased sodium absorption.
Kidney diseases: where the sodium absorption is interrupted.

HYPERNATREMIA

Hypernatremia does not always imply an increase in total body sodium. Dehydration is the most common cause of hypernatremia. If the dehydration is "isotonic", the sodium measurement will be of little help because water and salt are lost in equal proportions.

Hyperadrenalism (Cushing's disease)
Severe dehydration
Certain types of brain injuries
Diabetic coma after therapy with insulin
Excessive administration of sodium salts
Kidney disease

PHYSIOLOGY OF THE KIDNEY

Kidney filtration and selective reabsorbtion regulate sodium metabolism. Present theories state that 90-98% of the filtered sodium is reabsorbed by active transport. Urine formation is illustrated in Figure 5.

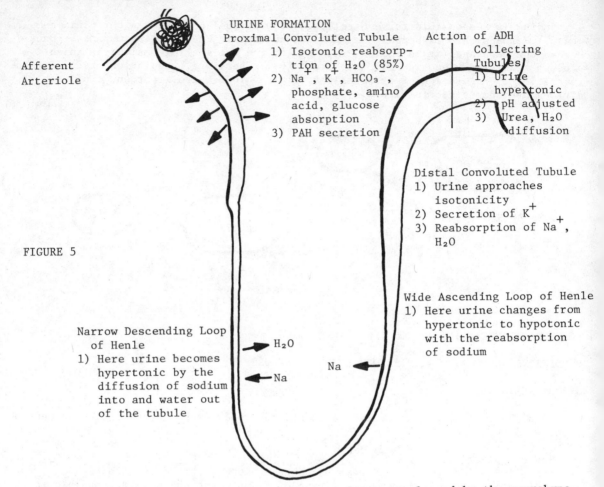

URINE FORMATION

Proximal Convoluted Tubule
1) Isotonic reabsorption of H_2O (85%)
2) Na^+, K^+, HCO_3^-, phosphate, amino acid, glucose absorption
3) PAH secretion

Afferent Arteriole

Action of ADH
Collecting Tubules
1) Urine hypertonic
2) pH adjusted
3) Urea, H_2O diffusion

Distal Convoluted Tubule
1) Urine approaches isotonicity
2) Secretion of K^+
3) Reabsorption of Na^+, H_2O

FIGURE 5

Wide Ascending Loop of Henle
1) Here urine changes from hypertonic to hypotonic with the reabsorption of sodium

Narrow Descending Loop of Henle
1) Here urine becomes hypertonic by the diffusion of sodium into and water out of the tubule

H_2O

Na

Na

Antidiuretic hormone (ADH) or vasopressin is a hormone released by the neurohypophysis in response to low plasma volumes. ADH works at the distal convoluted tubule of the nephron increasing the tubule cell's permeability to water. The hyperosmolality caused by the low plasma volume is corrected with the retention of water. Lack of ADH causes diabetes insipidus and nephrogenic diabetes insipidus. With the increased reabsorption of water, the urine composition becomes concentrated.

When serum sodium concentration falls, fluid moves from the extracellular to the intracellular compartment. The body cannot tolerate this situation for long. Aldosterone is the major sodium-retaining steroid: it is secreted by the adrenal cortex in response to ACTH, the renin-angiotension system of hyperkalemia. The aldosterone secretion is usually inversely proportional to the concentration of sodium. The major intermediary in aldosterone synthesis and secretion is reninangiotensin. The juxtaglomeruli cells in the walls of the afferent arterioles secrete renin, a proteolytic enzyme. Renin acts on renin substrate or angiotensinogen to form angiotensin I. The inactive peptide angiotensin I, is then acted upon by a converting enzyme to produce angiotensin II which stimulates the release of aldosterone. Aldosterone causes potassium to be exchanged for sodium in the distal convoluted tubule. One can see hypokelemia as a sympton of primary aldosteronism.

Methods are now available to provide accurate measurements of aldosterone, renin activity, angiotensin I, and angiotensin II.

Causes of increased aldosteronism:

Primary aldosteronism

> adrenal cortex adenoma
> carcinoma
> nodular hyperplasia

Secondary aldosteronism

> hyponatremia
> potassium loading
> generalized edema
> hypertension
> renal ischemia
> pregnancy and estrogen containing medications.

Aldosterone assays may be performed on plasma or urine. All 24-hour urines for aldosterone assay should be analyzed for creatinine to verify a total 24-hour collection. The total creatinine may be below the reference range, but should not vary daily by more than 10-15%. The urine should be analyzed for sodium. Sodium values less than 30 mmol/l suggest decreased sodium secretion and a falsely elevated aldosterone.

POTASSIUM

Potassium's unique biologic role is ambivalent. On the one hand, excessive potassium (hyperkalemia > 7.5 mmol/l) can cause: (a) muscle irritability due to exertable and slowly repolarized membranes; (b) respiratory and myocardial alterations; and (c) a characteristic peaking of the T wave in electrocardiographs. With proper renal function, these hyperkalemic traits do not occur. On the other hand, low potassium levels (hypokalemia) can also induce: (a) changes in muscle irritability because the membrane is harder to excite with the electrical potential elevated; and (b) a characteristic depression of the S - T segment and flattening of the T wave in electrocardiographs.

The body has no effective way of preserving potassium. When sodium levels fall below 110 mmol/l, sodium is completely reabsorbed. Potassium does not exhibit such a threshold. The total body potassium levels are not great and the kidneys cannot conserve potassium. Consequently, hypokalemia can occur rapidly when a person is on a low potassium diet. When the cells are deficient of potassium, the potassium is replaced by either sodium or hydrogen ions. For every 2 potassium ions lost, 3 sodium ions enter the cell. If hydrogen ions replace potassium, the hydrogen ions enter at a 1 to 3 ratio. Hypokalemia is practically synonymous with alkalosis. Alkalosis results from low extracellular H^+ concentration. Hydrogen ions must be conserved by the kidneys. Potassium ions are excreted as a result of sodium ion absorption.

Bananas, meat broths, skim milk, boiled meats, oranges, and tomatoes are excellent sources of potassium. Such foods should not be consumed by dialysis patients.

Potassium is filtered by the glomerulus and normally completely reabsorbed at the proximal tubule. The distal tubules actively secrete potassium in competition with hydrogen ions. According to the acid-base balance of the body, cortisol and aldosterone levels, intercellular potassium levels, and the metabolic state of the renal tubular cells, either potassium or hydrogen ions are exchanged for sodium ions. In acidosis, potassium is conserved and H^+ excreted, whereas in alkalosis potassium is preferentially excreted.

Most of the total body store of potassium is held intracellularly. The concentration of potassium within the erythrocytes is approximately 20 times that of plasma. This is an important fact to the clinical chemist because hemolysis can falsely elevate the plasma K concentration. If whole blood is allowed to stand uncentrifuged for long periods of time, potassium will leak from the erythrocytes to the plasma producing an aritifical hyperkalemia.

REFERENCE RANGE: 3.5 - 5.0 mmol/L

CONDITIONS ASSOCIATED WITH ABNORMAL VALUES

HYPOKALEMIA

Dietary

anorexia
low sodium diets
malnutrition
starvation

Renal Loss

primary aldosteronism
excessive use of diuretics (thiazide mercurial, alone or with ammonium chloride)

Protracted Vomiting

Infusions of solutions that are potassium free

Cirrhosis

Treatments with large doses of ACTH or cortisol

Surgery

Diabetes (treatment of diabetic acidosis without potassium supplements can lead to hypokalemia,   Once insulin is administered and glucose starts to enter the cells, potassium will follow).

HYPERKALEMIA

Renal shutdown

Artificial hyperkalemia due to

prolonged contact of cells and serum
gross hemolysis

METHODS OF ANALYSIS

Sodium and potassium have been assayed by (1) chemical methods (sodium: Albanese and Lein--uranylacetate precipitation; potassium: Lochhead and Purcell-sodium cobaltinitrite precipitation) by (2) neutron activation (3) atomic absorption (4) flame photometry, and (5) ion selective electrodes. At this time flame photometry is the method most widely used in the clinical laboratory. Ion selective electrodes present the possibility of a bright future. The ion-selective electrodes measure ion activity which must then be converted to concentration. Disease states with altered protein concentrations have shown differences in sodium and potassium determinations when assayed by ion-selective electrodes. As with any method, selection, accuracy, precision, and ease of operation must dictate the method of choice. Currently, flame photometry meets those guidelines for the clinical laboratory.

Heparinized plasma is the specimens of choice for sodium and potassium. Serum has replaced heparinized plasma in today's laboratory partly due to convenience. But, heparinized plasma offers speed in specimen processing and fibrin free specimens. Potassium levels in plasma are 0.1 to 0.7 mmol/L lower than serum, most probably due to the potassium released by platelets in the clotting process. After collection, specimen should be processed as soon as possible in order to minimize potassium leakage from enythrocytes.

CALCIUM

Calcium is the most versatile of the inorganic ions for calcium:

--provides the chemical foundation of teeth and bones

--acts as a cofactor in the coagulation cascade and many enzymatic reactions

--with ATP, calcium plays an important role in the transfer of other inorganic ions across cell membranes

Calcium metabolism is closely linked to phosphate metabolism. Most of the body's total supply of calcium and phosphorous are found in bone in the form of calcium fluorophosphate apatite while lesser amounts are found in the extracellular fluid and various tissues. Of the 1,000 - 2,000 g of calcium present in the adult body, only 1.0% is available as exchangeable calcium which aids in meeting extracellular demands. The calcium requirements for an individual is widely varied. Milk, cheese, butter and certain vegetables and meats are good sources of calcium. Calcium absorption into the body takes place in the upper portion of the intestine. Parathyroid hormone (PTH) and 1,25 dihydroxycholecalciferol control calcium absorption. An acid pH insures maximal absorption of calcium whereas an alkaline pH decreases the absorption rate.

Calcium is present in serum in three forms:

nondifussible protein-bound   45%

diffusible free

    ionized   50%
    complexed   5%

Most of the calcium that is protein bound is carried by albumin, however globulin also plays a role. A 1g/dl drop in albumin will cause a concurrent 1mg/dl drop in serum calcium levels. The patient with low albumin and low calcium level will not exhibit tetany because the biologically active calcium (ionized) is unaffected by serum total protein concentrations. Complexed, diffusible, free calcium is calcium bound to citrates, phosphates, bicarbonates, or sulfates; these also exert biological activity. Although protein concentrations do not affect diffusible calcium, acidosis increases diffusible calcium, where alkalosis decreases.

Numerous factors affect the level of calcium in serum. Some important factors are summarized in Table 3.

TABLE 3

FACTORS CONTROLLING SERUM CALCIUM LEVELS

CONTROLLING FACTORS	STRUCTURE	SITE OF ORIGIN	EFFECT
Parathyroid hormone (PTH) regulates the concentration of ionic calcium in extra-cellular fluids	Polypeptide hormone two forms: 1) C terminal: has no bio-logical activity, but longer half life 2) intact or N-terminal has short half life. The N term-inal is used to measure acute changes in PTH whereas C terminal reflects chronic changes	Parathyroid gland	1) mobilizes calcium from bone 2) increases the synthesis of 1.25 dihydroxycholecalciferol 3) increases renal absorption of calcium and decreases the reabsorption of phosphorus
Calcitonin (thyrocalci-tonin) antagonistic to PTH	Polypeptide hormone	c-cells of thyroid glands	1) inhibits bone reabsorption of calcium 2) increases renal excretion of phosphates
Vitamin D compounds Calciferol and cholecalciferol	Sterol, fat soluble	liver/kidney	1) increases intestinal ab-sorption of calcium 2) increases resorption of calcium from bone

The calcium concentrations in serum will parallel the protein levels, due to Ca+ binding to transport proteins. Calcium and phosphate exhibit a reciprocal relationship.

REFERENCE VALUE: 9.2 - 11.0 mg/dl

CONDITIONS ASSOCIATED WITH ABNORMAL VALUES

HYPERCALCEMIA

Hyperparathyroidism
Multiple myeloma
Vitamin D intoxication
Lymphoma and Leukemia
Carcinoma (most frequently breast cancer)
Laboratory error: hemoconcentration
Technical error due to prolonged tourniquet application
Hyperproteinemia

HYPOCALCEMIA

Newborns
Hypoparathyroidism
Vitamin D deficiency
Renal failure
Hypoproteinemia
Pregnancy
Steatorrhea
Acute pancreatitis
Laboratory error: plasma with calcium chelating anticoagulant used as specimen

Diagnosis of hypercalcemia or hypocalcemia, as with any diagnosis, relies on a careful history, physical examination, and a careful selection of laboratory tests. The differential diagnosis of the causes of hypercalcemia is important. If untreated, hypercalcemia can lead to calcification of renal tubules, renal calculi, neuromuscular alterations and death. Hypoparathyroidism can lead to low PTH levels low calcium levels accompanied by paresthesias, muscle cramps, and tetany. Hypocalcium does not always lead to tetany. Tetany symptoms are not present in people having both low albumin and low calcium levels because the ionized calcium level is unaffected. Renal failure patients exhibit low calcium levels because the kidneys are unable to respond to PTH, but the acidosis associated with renal disease favors the ionization of calcium and as a result, symptoms of hypocalcemia are rarely seen.

METHODS OF ANALYSIS

CLARK-COLLIP METHOD

Calcium is precipitated by ammonium oxalate. The precipitate, calcium oxalate, is washed with dilute ammonium hydroxide to remove impurities. Dilute sulfuric acid is added to convert the calcium oxalate to oxalic acid which is then titrated with standard potassium permanganate.

O-CRESOLPHTHALEIN COMPLEXONE METHOD

Technician (SMA 12/60): The sample stream is mixed with 0.125N HCl to release protein-bound calcium. The stream is dialyzed against a 0.125N HCl recipient stream to which is added cresolphthalein complexone with 8-hydroxyquinoline, and diethylamine. 8-hydroxyquinoline eliminates magnesium interference. The final reaction mixture is read at 580 nm.

Other methodologies include:

1. Atomic emission

2. Atomic absorption spectrophotometry

3. Ion selective electrodes

4. EDTA titration with calcium indicator

IONIZED CALCIUM

Ionized calcium is a term that has come to mean the free, unbound calcium ions that are physiologically active. Little technical literature is available as to the clinical usefulness of ionized calcium. However, preliminary work does agree that ionized calcium levels do reflect the functional status of the patient's calcium metabolism better than total calcium determinations.

Elevated ionized calcium levels may result in:

   1. Hyperparathyrodism
   2. PTH producing tumors

Low ionized calcium may cause:

   1. Hypoparathyroidism: conditions with low total proteins and low calcium usually show normal ionized calcium concentrations.

METHODS OF ANALYSIS

The calcium ion-selective electrode is the method of choice. For this analysis serum, collected in the fasting state, is the preferred specimen. One manufacturer recommends whole blood specimens, but whatever the specimen used, pH changes must be avoided because pH changes affect the equilibrium between bound and free calcium. If serum is used, it should be drawn into a vacutainer tube, placed on ice, allowed to clot, and centrifuged with the stopper in place.

Reference ranges are dependent on the methodology used.

The ionized calcium level may be approximated by the following formula based on the nomogram by McLean and Hastings describing the relationship of Ca and total protein at pH 7.35 and 25°C.

$$\text{mgCa}^{++}/dl = \frac{6\{\overset{\text{mg/dl}}{\text{calcium}}\} - \overset{\text{g/dl}}{\text{protein}}/3}{\text{protein} + 6}$$

This formula does not account for changes in pH or in alterations of total protein constituent concentrations. Calcium does not bind uniformly to all proteins in the same manner. Therefore any change in the pH or protein concentration will invalidate this formula.

MAGNESIUM

Magnesium plays an essential role in the metabolism of both carbohydrates and proteins, but acting as a coenzyme for such enzymes as phosphatases, carboxylases, transphosphorylases and hexokinases.

Furthermore, magnesium is essential in the maintenance of the macromolecular structure of DNA and RNA. Magnesium is absorbed predominantly in the small intestine and it is second in abundance to potassium as a intracellular cation. Little is known about magnesium regulation but PTH and aldosterome are involved. About half of the total body store of magnesium is present in bone. Of the remaining 50%, 45% may be found intracellularly and 5% extracellularly.

Magnesium is present in nearly all foods and consequently, deficiencies rarely occur in well-fed individuals. However, hypomagnesium is clinically more significant and frequent than hypermagnesium. Causes of hypomagnesiumemis are listed below.

REFERENCE VALUE: 1.4 - 2.3 mmol/L

CONDITIONS ASSOCIATED WITH ABNORMAL CHLORIDE VALUES

HYPOMAGNESIUMEMIA

> Malabsorption
> Severe diarrhea
> Bowel fistulas
> Gastrointestinal lavage
> Acute pancreatitis
> Digitalis intoxication
> Diuretic therapy
> Chronic dialysis
> Magnesium free intravenous fluids

Hypermagnesemia is rarely encountered in a patient with normal kidney function. It may be caused by renal failure, acute diabetic acidosis, Addison's disease, severe dehydration, or ingestion of excessive amounts of magnesium containing antacids.

METHODS OF ANALYSIS

Serum levels of magnesium do not accurately reflect the total body store because serum levels do not fall below 1.0 mmol/L until 25% of cellular magnesium is lost. The method of choice for the analysis of magnesium is atomic absorption spectroscopy. Other methods such as flame photometry, fluorescence spectrophotometry, spectrophotometry of dye-lake combinations (tital yellow) or other magnesium indicator compounds should only be used when an atomic absorption method is not available. Specimen for magnesium analysis should be hemolysis free.

OTHER ESSENTIAL ELEMENTS

Not long ago, elements other than sodium potassium, chloride, calcium, phosphorus, and magnesium were considered "trace elements." Crude methods were available for their measurement. Improved methods of analysis have shown that iron, zinc, copper, manganese, chromium, cobalt, molybdenum, iodine, selenium, tin, nickle, fluorine, and vanadium are essential elements. Most are necessary cofactors in enzymatic reactions. Fluorine aids in the prevention of dental caries, iodine is important in thyroid metabolism, and the importance of iron, zinc, copper, manganese and lead are summarized in Table 4. Cobalt is structurally important to vitamins.

ANIONS

In most clinical laboratories, the only plasma electrolytes that are measured are sodium, potassium, chloride, and total CO_2 content. These four are generally taught together as a unit which is in some respects, a mistake. The cations Na, K and the anions (Cl, CO_2) are never in equilibrium. There are too many other inorganic ions adding charges. The concentration of undetermined anions can be calculated by:

TABLE 4

ELEMENT	REFERENCE VALUE	PHYSIOLOGICAL ROLE	ELEVATIONS SEEN IN	DECREASES SEEN IN	METHODS OF ANALYSIS
Iron	75-175 mg/dl	constituent of hemoglobin, myoglobin, and various enzymes	1. hemolytic anemias 2. lead poisoning (other decreased RBC formation diseases) 3. necrotic hepatitis (↑ release of Fe from stores) 4. hemochromatosis (↑Fe absorption)	1. infections 2. neoplasia 3. arthritis 4. dietary: insufficient intake 5. increased physiological need (pregnancy) 6. chronic hemorrhage	1. atomic absorption (lacks sensitivity) 2. most assays require three steps a. release of ion from proteins b. reduction Fe^{+3} to Fe^{+2} c. reaction of Fe^{+2} with a chromogen such as ferrozine, thiocyanate, and sulfonated bathophenamthzoline
Zinc	55-150 mg/dl	cofactors of many enzymes including carbonic anhydase, alkaline phosphatase and alcohol dehydrogenase	1. increased uptake associated with industrial exposure, chunks from galvanized cans, children's toys	nonspecific decreases associated with cirrhosis (alcoholic), oral contraceptives, sickle cell anemia; low zinc levels have been associated with impaired taste perceptions	Atomic absorption spectroscopy
Copper	25-43 mg/dl	cofactors of enzymes required for synthesis of hemoglobin	pregnancy cirrhosis thyrotoxicosis	Wilson's disease hypoproteinemia Menkes kinky hair syndrome	Atomic absorption spectroscopy

TABLE 4 (continued)

ELEMENT	REFERENCE VALUE	PHYSIOLOGICAL ROLE	ELEVATIONS SEEN IN	DECREASES SEEN IN	METHODS OF ANALYSIS
Manganese	0.08-0.26 mg/dl	cofactor of enzymes important in lipid metabolism	industrial over-exposure		atomic absorption spectroscopy; malachite green decolorization
Lead	normal 0-50 mg/dl toxic above 80 mg/dl		seen in children from eating lead-containing paint or plaster industrial over-exposures		atomic absorption spectroscopy colorimetic diphenylthiocarbazone

$$Na - (\{Cl\} + (CO_2)) = \text{undetermined anions}$$

The difference is usually 5-15 mEq/L.

There are many cases when this difference will not fall within the range. The anion difference should be calculated as:

$$(Na^+ + K^+ + 2Ca^{++} + 2Mg^{++}) - (Cl + CO_2 + Protein + Organic\ acids + Phosphate + Sulfate)$$

Despite the fact that Na, K, Cl, and total CO_2 are assayed as a unit, other inorganic ions should be taken into account especially the anions and cations which affect the Na, K, Cl and CO_2 concentrations.

CHLORIDE

The chloride concentration usually parallels the sodium concentration. Chloride usually decreases when sodium decreases. However, this may not always be the case especially when acid-base changes occur. In this case, chloride concentrations will reflect the changes in bicarbonate concentrations. Chloride is the major extracellular anion. The intracellular chloride concentration is small. The daily chloride requirement is unknown. Serum chloride and H^+ are used by the parietal cells of the stomach to produce hydrochloric acid. Low serum chloride concentrations occur in conditions causing excessive gastric juice loss.

The most important role of chloride is evidenced in the chloride shift. When red cells become oxygenated in the lungs, chloride leaves the cells. When hemoglobin releases O_2 and the red cells take up CO_2, chloride enters the red cells. This exchange is referred to as the chloride shift. The chloride shift also occurs when the pH of the extracellular fluid becomes alkaline. Further discussion on the chloride shift can be found in the CO_2 section of this chapter.

The measurement of chloride in sweat is important in the diagnosis of cystic fibrosis.   Infant cystic fibrosis patients excrete up to five times the reference values of chloride. Ion-selective electrodes are used to measure sweat chloride that has been produced by the introduction of pilocarpine into the skin by electrical stimulation.

REFERENCE VALUES FOR SWEAT CHLORIDE: non-diseased up to 35 mmol/L
                                       borderline 35 to 75
                                       affected 75 and above

REFERENCE VALUES FOR SERUM CHLORIDE: 96-110 mmol/L

CONDITIONS ASSOCIATED WITH ABNORMAL CHLORIDE VALUES

HYPERCHLOREMIA	HYPOCHLOREMIA
Nephritis	Addison's disease
Prostatic obstruction	Diabetes
Eclampsia	Intestinal obstruction
Hyperventilation	Uremia
Hypoproteinemia	Vomiting
	Non-fasting specimen
	Hypercorticoadrenalism

METHODS OF ANALYSIS

COULOMETRIC

Cotlove chloridometer: Serum is added to a dilute nitric acid solution. A silver rod is placed in the solution. When an electrical current is applied across the solution Ag^+ are released. As the chloride and silver ions react the resistance of the solution decreases and eventually the decrease in resistance causes a timer to stop the Ag^+ generation. Time is related to the concentration of chloride ions.

FERRIC-MERCURIC THIOCYANATE

Chloride ions combine with mercuric thiocynante with the release of SCN^-. The exact reactions and products have not been defined but it is believed that ferric ions (Fe^{+3}) combine with SCN^-. This complex is measured spectrophotometrically.

SCHALES AND SCHALES TITRATION METHOD

Chloride ions in a protein free filtrate react with mercuric nitrate. Once all the chloride has reacted to form mercuric chloride, the addition of excess mercuric nitrate causes a change to occur in the color indicator diphenylcarbazene.

PHOSPHATE

Phosphate is the major intracellular anion. The netabolism of phosphorus inversely follows that of calcium: as calcium decreases phosphous usually increases. Phosphate, measured on the clinital laboratory as inorganic phosphorus, is present in all foods. It is absorbed with calcium in the upper small intestine. Excessive intake results in increased excretion by the kidneys. Acid-base regulation and renal efficiency affect the urinary output of phosphorus. Phosphorus is present in the body in two forms: inorganic and organic phosphates.

REFERENCE VALUE: 2.5 - 4.5 mg/Cl

CONDITIONS ASSOCIATED WITH ABNORMAL-PHOSPHORUS VALUES

HYPERPHOSPHATEMIA

    Hemolysis
    Children (usually slightly elevated)
    Renal failure uremia
    Acidosis
    Dietary: increased uptake
    Vitamin D poisoning
    Bone healing

HYPOPHOSPHATEMIA

    Excessive use of antacids
    Vitamin D deficiency
    Renal tubular disease

METHODS OF ANALYSIS

Most of the methods involve the use of molybdenum blue.

1. TECHNICON: serum is dialyzed into a recipient stream to which is added acid molyb-
    date and stannous chloride-hydrazine.

2. SULFATE: the resultant color is measured at 660.

3. FISKE—SUBBAROW: a trichloroacetic acid protein free filtrate is added to a moly-
    bdenum solution to form phosphomolydic acid which is reduced to a blue colored
    complex. The resultant color is measured spectrophotometrically.

CARBON DIOXIDE

The total CO_2 present in venous or arterial blood is present as bicarbonate, car-
boxic acid, and carbamino compounds (CO_2 bound to proteins). The CO_2 measured in a
set of electrolytes reflects the total venous CO_2 content which is a measure of all
forms of CO_2 in the plasma. Most of the CO_2 exists as bicarbonate and, therefore, the
total CO_2 usually reflects the bicarbonate ion concentration.

FIGURE 6

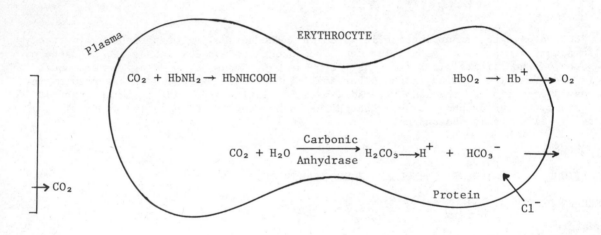

The CO_2 produced by the oxidation of carbohydrates, fats, and proteins diffuses
across the cell wall and into the plasma. In the plasma, some CO_2 will dissolve and
some will become hydrated to H_2CO_3. Since this is a very slow reaction, most of the
CO_2 will enter the erythrocyte. Upon entry, carbonic anhydrase catalyzes the hydration of CO_2.

$$CO_2 + H_2O \longrightarrow H_2CO_3$$

The remaining CO_2 will be bound to plasma proteins. Deoxygenated hemoglobin binds
to CO_2 more easily than does oxygenated hemoglobin.

H_2CO_3 dissociates. The formation of H_2CO_3 lowers the pH of the erythrocyte fluid
while the deoxygenation of hemoglobin tends to raise the pH. Therefore, the H+ pro-

duced by $H_2CO_3 \rightarrow HCO_3^- + H^+$ is accepted by HbO_2 to form $Hb^- + O_2$. The net result is no pH change. These reactions are referred to as the isohydric shift (or a shift in which the concentration of H^+ remains essentially the same).

Normally, carbonic acid dissociates into bicarbonate and hydrogen ions, i.e.,

(1) $$H_2CO_3 \;\rightarrow\; HCO_3^- + H^+$$

According to the Mass Law Equation:

(2) $$\frac{\{H^+\}\,\{HCO_3^-\}}{\{H_2CO_3\}} = K$$

For convenience of pH determinations, equation (2) can be rearranged to:

(3) $$\{H^+\} = \frac{K\,\{H_2CO_3\}}{HCO_3} \qquad \frac{K\,\{H_2CO_3\}}{\{HCO_3\}}$$

Taking the logarithum of both sides the following results:

(4) $$\log\{H^+\} = \log K + \log\{H_2CO_3\} - \log\{HCO_3^-\}$$

then by multiplying by -1:

(5) $$-\log\{H^+\} = -\log K - \log\{H_2CO_3\} + \log\{HCO_3^-\}$$

Definition $-\log\{H^+\} = pH$ and $-\log K = pK$, thus equation (5) becomes:

$$pH = pH + \log\frac{\{HCO_3^-\}}{\{H_2CO_3\}} \qquad pK + \log\frac{\{HCO_3^-\}}{\{H_2CO_3\}}$$

Both plasma and erythrocyte fluid contain H_2CO_3 and HCO_3^-. As H_2CO_3 dissociates and HCO_3^- rises inside the erythrocyte, an imbalance results between plasma HCO_3 and erythrocyte HCO_3. Due to the Gibbs-Donnan Effect, the plasma $\{HCO_3^-\}$ must be greater. Consequently, this imbalance causes the erythrocytes HCO_3^- to enter the plasma until the ratio HCO_3 plasma/HCO_3 erythcocyte has been <u>corrected</u>. Plasma chloride ions enter the erythrocyte to preserve electrical neutrality. This sequence of events is referred to as the chloride shift.

The physiological importance of CO_2 ties in the role bicarbonated carbonic acid play in the pH balance of the body. The Henderson-Hasselbalch equation is a help in understanding the alterations of body pH and the compensatory mechanisms in the body. Normally, HCO_3^-/H_2CO_3 is 25/1.25 or 20/1. The pK of bicarbonate/carbonic acid at body pH is 6.1. Thus pH is $pH = 6.1 + 1.3 = 7.4$.

$$pH = pH + \log\frac{\{HCO_3^-\}}{\{H_2CO_3\}}$$

$\{H_2CO_3\}$ is actually a measure of dissolved CO_2 which includes the small amount of undissociated carbonic acid. It is equal to $\alpha \times pCO_2$ where α is the solubility coefficient of CO_2 and is equal to 0.03. $pH = pK + \log\dfrac{\{HCO_3^-\}}{.03 \times pCO_2}$

Equation (6) can be used for all weak acids and their salts, therefore:

$$pH = pK\ acid + \log\frac{\{A^-\}}{\{HA\}}$$

If we consider: $CO_2 + H_2O \rightarrow H_2CO_3 \rightarrow HCO_3 + H^+$ and the effects of the addition of acids and bases, we can see how the body effectively uses these buffers to maintain a narrow pH range.

An acid is a substance that liberates hydrogen ions (H^+). In diabetic acidosis, acetoacetic acid and B-hydroxybutyric acid accumulate. The dissociation of these acids produce H^+. The H^+ will combine with bicarbonate to form:

$$HCO_3^- + H^+ \rightleftharpoons H_2CO_3$$

The body's response to the additional H^+ and H_2CO_3 is twofold: (1) a change in PCO_2 ($H_2CO_3 = .03 \times pCO_2$) and (2) a decrease in pH. Pulmonary ventilation increases. Hyperventilation reduces the concentration of CO_2 thus restoring the HCO_3^-/H_2CO_3 ratio to 20/1. An important point here is that although the HCO_3/H_2CO_3 ratio may be restored, the concentration of both is low. The reduction in pH causes acidification of the urine, which begins when H_2CO_3 dissociates in the renal tubule cell. H^+ is exchanged for Na^+ in the glomerular filtrate. The glomerular filtrate has essentially the same concentration HCO_3^- as the plasma. With the increased H^+ in the filtrate and the body's added need for HCO_3^-, the kidneys reabsorb the filtered bicarbonate with greater efficiency. The exact mechanism is unknown, but has been postulated to include the following: $HCO_3^- + H^+ \rightleftharpoons HHCO_3 \rightleftharpoons H_2CO_3 \rightleftharpoons H_2O + CO_2$.

The increased CO_2 tension causes CO_2 to diffuse into the renal tubule cell. The increased CO_2 reabsorption helps to restore the HCO_3^-/H_2CO_3 ratio by increasing the concentration of HCO_3^-. Under normal circumstances, reabsorption of bicarbonate occurs when the plasma HCO_3 concentration drops below 24-28 mmol/L. An excess of bicabonate reduces its reabsorption resulting in an alkaline urine. As HCO_3^- is reabsorbed, plasma Cl^- is lost to the urine.

If a base (defined as a substance that accepts hydrogen ions) is added to plasma, it will react with H_2CO_3 directly to form water and bicarbonate. This occurs as follows($H_2CO_3 + OH^- \rightarrow HCO_3 + HOH$. An excess of bicarbonate or a deficit of H_2CO_3 results in an alkaline pH. To conserve H_2CO_3, the respiratory mechanism decreases. Hypoventilation conserves H_2CO_3 thus helping to balance the altered HCO_3^-/H_2CO_3 ratio. The resulting increase in PCO_2, however, tends to increase ventilation resulting in hyperventilation. Thus, hypoventilation is not an effective compensatory mechanism for decreased H_2CO_3. The renal compensatory mechanism is slow but much more effective. In this case there is a decreased H^+ - not exchange. and a decreased reabsorption of bicarbonate. Although the lungs attempt to conserve H_2CO_3, the kidneys attempt to eliminate the excess HCO_3^- and consequently the HCO_3^-/H_2CO_3 ratio returns to normal.

Laboratory measurements of CO_2 do not reflect the acid-base status of intercellular or extracellular fluid. Hydrogen ion excesses or deficits do not occur without a concommitant anion change (Cl^-, SO_4^-, lactate); a cation exchange (Na^+, K^+); or a CO_2 alteration. For this reason, CO_2 measurements and electrolyte measurements are done to determine acid-base status.

Acid-base disturbances are classifed as:

1. Metabolic acidosis   3. Respiratory acidosis

2. Metabolic alkalosis   4. Respiratory alkalosis

ACID/BASE DISTURBANCES

Metabolic imbalances are primarily due to an excess (alkalosis) or deficit (acidosis) of bicarbonate. The concentration of bicarbonate ions is determined by renal function. The term respiratory imbalance is indeed a misnomer. The imbalance usually reflects the depth of ventilation. Respiratory imbalances are primarily concerned with an excess (acidosis) or deficit (alkalosis) of carbonic acid.

Establishing strict criteria for the four imbalances is an impossible task. Several authors have attempted nanograms and other charts to correlate laboratory pH, pCO_2, HCO_3^- findings with the four acid-base imbalances. Two often though two conditions are superimposed on the other, or the body has attempted a compensatory action making correlation impossible. Whenever any of these acid-base imbalances exists, the body attempts to restore a normal pH. If the restoration is complete enough to bring the pH between 7.35-7.45, then it is said that the condition is fully compensated. If, despite the compensatory mechanisms, the pH stays abnormal (below 7.35, or above 7.45) the condition is said to be partially compensated. It is difficult to find a perfect case of either of the four imbalances. Generalized conditions and compensatory mechanisms are disussed below.

METABOLIC ACIDOSIS

Metabolic acidosis is an altered physiologic state where:

1. The body pH is less than 7.35

2. HCO_3^- is low either due to its combination with inorganic acid or to its excessive loss (i.e., diarrhea)

3. There is acid excess and the acid is not carbonic acid.

There are three types of metabolic acidosis.

1. Those associated with increased unmeasured ions (i.e., $Na^+ - (Cl^- + CO_2) > 17$)

    lactic acidosis
    diabetic ketoacidosis
    renal failure
    drug, ingestion (salicylate, methyl alcohol)

2. Metabotic acidosis with normal measured ions (i.e., $NA^+ - (Cl^- + CO_2) = 12\pm3$) generally cause:

    diarrhea
    fistulas
    renal tubular disease
    carbonic anhydrase inhibitors

3. Hyperchloremia is the third type of metablic acidosis which may be due to

    severe diarrhea
    ingestion of ammonium chloride

BODY COMPENSATORY ACTION TO METABOLIC ACIDOSIS

BUFFERING ACTION: the excess H^+ will combine with HCO_3^-.

RESPIRATORY ACTION: the drop in body pH will stimulate respiration. Hyperventilation decreases the pCO_2 thus decreasing the H_2CO_3 to balance the HCO_3^-/H_2CO_3 ratio.

RENAL ACTION: increased excretion of acid; increased reabsorption, increased ammonia production.

EXPECTED LABORATORY FINDINGS DUE TO METABOLIC ACIDOSIS:

pH	acidic
pCO_2	normal, slightly decreased
HCO_3^-	low

LABORATORY FINDINGS AFTER COMPENSATION:

pH	slightly acidic to normal
pO_2	markedly reduced
$HCO_3^=$	low

ALTERATION OF HENDERSON-HASSELBALCH EQUATION:

$$\frac{HCO_3^-}{H_2CO_3} = \frac{12mEq/L}{1.2mEqL} = \frac{10}{1}$$

$$pH = pK + \log \frac{HCO_3^-}{H_2CO_3}$$

$$pH = 6.1 + \log \frac{10}{1}$$

$$pH = 6.1 + 1.0 = 7.10$$

METABOLIC ALKALOSIS

Metabolic alkalosis is an altered physiologic state where

1. The body pH is above 7.45

2. HCO_3 is elevated

3. There is a deficiency of H^+ either due to an accumulation of base or the loss of H^+

CAUSES

--diuretic therapy
--nasogastric suction resulting in excessive loss of stomach HCl
--potassium loss (i.e., Cushing Disease)
--excessive alkali administration
--excessive mechanical hyperventilation

COMPENSATORY ACTIONS

Action of buffers: excess base reacts with H_2CO_3

Respiratory Action: the increased pH depresses the respiratory system resulting in retention of CO_2. One would expect this hypoventilation to correct the imbalanced HCO_3^-/H_2CO_3 ratio but in metabolic alkalosis the respiratory compensation is the least efficient of all the compensatory mechanisms. Apparently the stimuli of increased pCO_2 is stronger than the increased pH stimuli and hyperventilation occurs.

Renal: decreased $Na^+ - H^+$ exchange, decreased ammonia production, and decreased reabsorption of bicarbonate occurs.

Expected laboratory findings:

pH	Basic
Pco_2	normal or slightly elevated
HCO_3^-	elevated

Alteration of Henderson-Hasselbalch Equation Due to Metabolic Alkalosis:

$$\frac{HCO_3^-}{H_2CO_3} = \frac{36 \text{ mEq12}}{1.2 \text{ mEq12}} = \frac{30}{1}$$

$$pH = pK + \log \frac{HCO_3^-}{H_2CO_3}$$

$$pH = 6.1 + \log 30$$

$$pH = 6.1 + 1.48$$

$$pH = 7.58$$

RESPIRATORY ACIDOSIS

Respiratory acidosis is an altered physiologic state where:

1. The body pH is less than 7.35

2. There is CO_2 accumulation

3. Pco_2 is elevated

CAUSES

--emphysema and other parenchymal lung diseases
--Guillain-Barre syndrome and other neuromuscular disorders
--obesity
--depression of respiratory cycle by drugs or sleep
--chronic heart failure and other cardiac disorders resulting in decreased
    blood flow

COMPENSATORY ACTIONS

BUFFERING ACTION: the excess H^+ from the carbonic acid is buffered by hemoglobin and proteins.

RESPIRATORY ACTION: the lungs attempt to hyperventilate to eliminate the excess CO_2. Many of the causes of respiratory acidosis relate to a decreased efficiency in the respiratory function and in this case, the respiratory compensatory action, is ineffective.

RENAL ACTION: the kidneys respond to respiratory acidosis the same as they do to metabolic acidosis, but it must be remembered that renal compensation is slower than respiratory compensation. Acute compensation is most often respiratory in function, while chronic compensation is accomplished by the kidneys.

EXPECTED LABORATORY FINDINGS

pH	acidic
P_{CO_2}	elevated
HCO_3	slightly elevated

AFTER COMPENSATION

pH	normal, slightly acidic
P_{CO_2}	elevated
HCO_3^-	markedly elevated

ALTERATION OF HENDERSON-HASSELBALCH EQUATION

$$\frac{HCO_3^-}{H_2CO_3} = \frac{24}{1.84} = \frac{13}{1}$$

$$pH = pK + \log \frac{HCO_3^-}{H_2CO_3}$$

$$pH = 6.1 + \log 13$$

$$pH = 6.1 + 1.11$$

$$pH = 7.21$$

RESPIRATORY ALKALOSIS

Respiratory alkalosis is an altered physologic acid/base state where

1. The body pH is greater than 7.45

2. CO_2 excretion exceeds CO_2 production

3. There is a low P_{CO_2}

CAUSES

--increased ventilation
--fever
--hysteria
--salicylate poisoning
--hepatic coma
--anemia
--pulmonary fibrosis

COMPENSATORY ACTION

RENAL ACTION

The kidneys respond as they do in metabolic alkalosis--by excreting bicarbonate. There is also a concommitant lactic acid production which reduces the bicarbonate concentration.

EXPECTED LABORATORY FINDINGS

pH   alkaline
P_{CO_2} low
HCO_3^- normal or slightly decreased
(lactic acid   elevated)

ALTERATION OF H–H EQUATION

$$\frac{HCO_3^-}{H_2CO_3} = \frac{24}{0.6} = \frac{40}{1}$$

$$pH = pK + \log \frac{HCO_3}{H_2CO_3}$$

$$pH = 6.1 + \log 40$$

$$pH = 6.1 + 1.6$$

$$pH = 7.70$$

CO_2 METHODS OF ANALYSIS

Specimen: heparinized plasma separated as soon as possible is the preferred specimen.

NATELSON MICROGASOMETER OR MODIFICATIONS THEREOF

CO_2 liberation is accomplished by agitating the sample and adding acid. The CO_2 produced exerts pressure against the fixed volume of the reaction chamber. The difference in pressure is a measure of the total CO_2 content.

TECHNICON METHODOLOGIES

Buffered phenolphthalein: CO_2 is liberated by an acid diluent and is trapped in a gas-liquid phase separator or the CO_2 is dialyzed with the use of CO_2 permeable membranes into a weakly buffered phenolphthalein solution. The loss of color in the phenolphthalein solution is measured at 550 mm.

P_{CO_2} ELECTRODE METHOD

Serum is mixed anaerobically with HCl which liberates CO_2. The P_{CO_2} of this mixture is related to the total CO_2 content of the sample.

VAN SLYKE NANOMETRIC ANALYSIS METHOD

CO_2 is liberated by lactic acid and measured nanometrically. This method is a favorite topic of conversation with older "techs", but has fallen into disuse due to the hazards of handling mercury.

ORGANIC ACID ANIONS

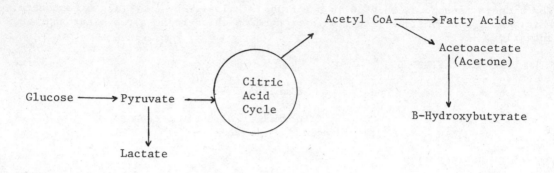

Pyruvate is an intermediary product of glucose metabolism. Pyruvate represents a crossroad in glucose metabolism: it can be reconverted to glucose, reduced to lactate, transaminated to alanine, or combined with Co Enzyme A to form acetyl Co A which can enter the citric acid cycle or lipid metabolism cycles. During episodes of anaerobic conditions, lactate (lactic acid) is produced. Exercise is the most familiar example of oxygen deprivation at the tissue level. Both lactate and pyruvate concentrations will rise, normally in a 7/1 lactate/pyruvate ratio. Under conditions of severe cellular oxidative process deterioration, lactate accumulates at a faster rate. This condition is seen in late stages of shock, diabetic coma without ketosis, and various terminal stages illnesses.

SPECIMEN COLLECTION

Blood specimens collected for pyruvate _must_ be done without a tourniquet, or the tourniquet should be released after the puncture and blood allowed to circulate 2 minutes before the specimen is drawn.

Protein free filtrates must be prepared immediately with perchloric acid. This mixture is stable for a week at 4°C.

METHOD OF ANALYSIS

An accepted method of analysis is to use the reaction
$$\text{lactate} + \text{NAD} \underset{}{\overset{\text{LD}}{\rightleftharpoons}} \text{pyruvate} + \text{NADH} + \text{H}^+$$

which occurs naturally in the body. The equilibrium here lies to the left but the addition of excess NAD at pH 9.0–9.6, and taking the pyruvate out from the reaction by combining it with hydrazine, this reaction can be made to go to the right.

PYRUVATE

The measurement of pyruvate utilizes the reverse reaction, remembering that natural equilibrium is to the right at pH 7.5.

KETONES: ACETOACETATE

Acetoacetate, β-hydroxybutyrate, and acetone are referred to as ketone bodies. Normal fat metabolism produces small amounts of ketones. When the body is deprived of glucose and is required to use fatty acids as a source of energy, ketone bodies accumulate at a faster rate. Acetoacetate is converted to both acetone and β-hydroxybutyrate. The proportions vary and the most popular method of analysis (Acetest) reacts with both acetoacetate and acetone.

KETONEMIA

Decreased carbohydrate intake

Starvation
Digestive disturbances
Vomiting

Decreased utilization of carbohydrates

Diabetes

METHODS OF ANALYSIS ACETAST (Ames)

The Acetest tablet contains glycine, sodium nitroprusside, disodium phosphate, and lactose. The acetoacetate and acetone react with sodium nitroprusside to form a purple color. For serum determinations, the tablet should be crushed to minimize false low results. Serial dilutions can be prepared to provide a semiquantitative estimation of the ketone bodies.

Another method is Gerhardt's test which is based on the reaction of acetoacetate with ferric chloride to produce a red-wine color. Salicylates, phenol, and antipyune give similar reaction colors. This test has been replaced by the Acetest antipyrine.

Nonprotein Nitrogen

Nonprotein nitrogen substances is a collective term that covers the heterogenous product of body metabolism. This group includes: urea, creatinine, creatine, uric acid, amino acids, nucleotides, polypeptide, glutathione, and others. Urea, creatinine, and uric acid are commonly used to measure renal function. These three "renal indicators" are at best insensitive. The large reserve of the kidneys to perform adequately in the face of huge nephron damage makes these tests insensitive.

UREA

Urea (commonly referred to as BUN, blood urea nitrogen)

BUN is the waste product of protein and amino acid catabolism. It is formed in the liver from CO_2 generated by the metabolic processes and NH_4 produced by amino acid deamination. BUN's chemical formula is NH_2CONH_2. An elevated BUN will be seen:

1. When protein catabolism is accelerated as in starvation, infection, and post-operative states, or

2. When the enzymes of the urea cycle are stimulated as occurs with a diet rich in protein. Low BUN's are seen when the patient is in negative nitrogen balance as occurs in conditions favoring anabolism, i.e., low protein diets. For these reasons BUN is not a good measure of renal function.

REFERENCE RANGE: 10-20 mg/dl

CONDITIONS ASSOCIATED WITH ABNORMAL BUN VALUES

ELEVATED	DECREASED
Nephritis	Acute liver destruction
Intestinal obstruction	Pregnancy
Urinary obstruction	High fluid intake
Cardiac failure	Poor nutrition
Dehydration	
Uremia	

METHODS OF ANALYSIS

DIACETYL MONOXIME

Acidic diacetyl monoxime reacts with urea in the presence of heat and thiosemi-carbozide. The absorbance of the resultant yellow chromagen is measured at 540 mm.

UREASE

Urea is enzymatically cleaved by urease to form two moles of NH_4 and one of CO_2:

$$Urea + H_2O + H^+ \xrightleftharpoons{Urease} 2NH_4^+ + CO_2$$

Measurement of either by-product can be related to the concentration of urea. A technical note about urease methodologies: NaF plasma is not an acceptable specimen because fluoride inhibits urease.

CREATININE

Creatinine is an end product of muscle metabolism. Creatine phosphate, creatine, and creatinine form a triad as shown below.

$$creatine \xrightleftharpoons{CK} creatine\ phosphate$$
$$\searrow \qquad \swarrow$$
$$creatinine$$

Both creatine and creatine phosphate are converted to creatinine at a steady daily rate of about 2% per day. Creatine phosphate is a reserve for energy in the muscles. Creatine is synthesized in the liver and pancreas from the three amino acids: arginine, glycine, and methionine. Creatinine is excreted by the kidneys at a fairly steady rate. A common practice of assessing 24 hours urine collections should be viewed with caution. Many studies have shown that individual variations may be as great as 0.8 d/day. The fairly constant production of creatinine by the tissues makes creatinine a better assessor of renal function than BUN.

REFERENCE RANGE: SERUM CREATININE: males 0.9 - 1.5 mg/dl
                                       females 0.8 - 1.2 mg/dl

                   SERUM CREATINE: males 0.17 - 0.50 mg/dl
                                       females 0.35 - 0.93 mg/dl

                   URINE CREATININE: males 1.0 - 2.0 g/day
                                       females 0.8 - 1.8 g/day

METHODS OF ANALYSIS

JAFFE REACTION

   Creatinine reacts with alkaline picrate to form an amber colored chromagen. The absorbance of the chromagen is measured at 505 mm. Creatine is measured by converting it to creatinine with either the addition of heat or acid. Creatinine measurements before heat or acid addition subtrated from those after represent the creatine concentration. Acetoacetate, acetone, barbiturates, phenol sulfonaphthalein, and protein interfere with the Jaffe reaction. Lloyd's reagent, an aluminum silicate, is sometimes used to absorb out those substances which interfere with the Jaffe reaction.

   The ratio of BUN to creatinine is used to add sensitivity to these tests as renal function indicates. Normal functioning kidneys usually show a 10:1 BUN/creatine ratio in the serum. In conditions where urea is diminished (low protein diet) there will be a decreased BUN/creatinine ratio. Oddly enough renal dialysis patients show a decreased BUN/creat ratio because BUN is more readily dialyzed than creatinine. Prerenal causes of azotemia (conditions associated with inadequate blood flow to the kidneys, i.e., dehydration or shock) will show a BUN creatinine ratio greater than 15:1.

URIC ACID

   Uric acid is an end product of purine-nucleoprotein catabolism. Uric acid is produced by the breakdown of purines and nucleo proteins from tissue sources (endogenous) and the metabolism of foodstuffs. Elevated uric acid levels are seen in one or any combination conditions:

   1. Increased dietary intake of purines

   2. Increased biosynthesis of endogenous purines

   3. Decreased renal excretion

   4. Decreased endogenous destruction of urates

   Uric acid cannot be used solely as an indicator of renal function because there are many other diseases that cause elevations. Gout is the best known condition which causes an elevated uric acid.

REFERENCE RANGE: male 3.5 - 7.2 mg/dl
                     female 2.6 - 6.0 mg/dl

CONDITIONS ASSOCIATED WITH ABNORMAL URIC ACID VALUES

                     Gout
                     Lead poisoning
                     Hyperparathyroidism
                     Hypertension
                     Diabetic acidosis
                     Polycythemia
                     Toxemia of pregnancy
                     Dietary (increased intake of purines, i.e.,
                              sweetbreads, liver)
                     Leukemia (increased breakdown of purines)

DECREASED

    Xanthinurea
    Fanconi's syndrome
    Acromegaly

METHODS OF ANALYSIS

PHOSPHOTUNGSTIC ACID

    Phosphotungstic acid is reduced by uric acid to a blue phosphotungstite complex. The absorbance of the resultant chromagen is measured at 660 nm.

URICASE

    Uric acid displays an absorbance peak at 290-293 nm. As uricase destroys uric acid there is a decrease in absorbance that can be related to the concentration of the uric acid.

Carbohydrates

    Carbohydrates, particularly glucose, play an important role as the chief fuel supplier for the body processes. The energy that is necessary for much of the molecular synthesis and metabolic processes of the cells is provided by the metabolism of glucose. Therefore, the level of circulating carbohydrates in the serum, and particularly the levels of glucose available to the cells, is of vital interest.

    There are two major pathologic problems associated with the circulating levels of carbohydrates: diabetes and hypoglycemia. In diabetes the serum glucose levels rise due to insufficient levels of active insulin. While in hypoglycemia the serum glucose levels drop due to the presence of too much insulin. Both of these conditions may result in debilitating and/or fatal complications for those people who have these disorders. Although other disorders involving carbohydrates other than glucose do occur, the emphasis in this section will be placed on the monosaccharide glucose.

    D-glucose is a six carbon (hexose) monosaccharide with an aldehyde functional group. D-glucose is usually depicted in one of the following ways:

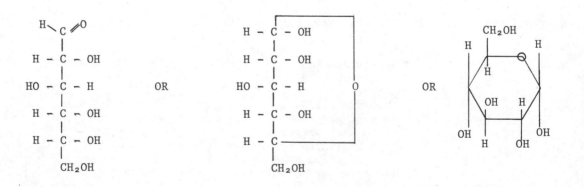

D-glucose, like many other carbohydrates exists in two anomeric forms, α-D-glucose and β-D-glucose. The majority of the circulating glucose is in the β-D-glucose form. This is of importance because these anomers do not have identical physical properties. The enzymatic methods utilized in the measurement of circulating glucose level are specific for the β-D-glucose form. In addition, in alkaline media, the aldehyde group of glucose can chemically rearrange and dissociate a carboxyl group yielding a nega- tively charged enol anion molecule with a double bond. The resulting molecule serves as an active reducing substance. This reducing property of glucose formed the basis for most of the earlier methods of glucose determination, however, these non-specific reducing tests are generally considered outdated since the enzymatic methods currently available are far more sensitive and specific for glucose.

METABOLISM

The human body acquires glucose from several sources, including monosaccharides, disaccharides, and polysaccharides. The monosaccharides most frequently ingested are glucose and fructose. Common food sources of glucose and fructose include fruits and honey. The disaccharides most commonly ingested are lactose (glucose + galactose) maltose (glucose + glucose), and sucrose (glucose + fructose). Common food sources of the disaccharides include milk products (lactose), starchy vegetables (maltose), and common table sugar (sucrose). The polysaccharides most frequently ingested are starch (amylose) and glycogen. Common food sources of starch include vegetables and grains. Whatever the source, once ingested the disaccharides and polysaccharides are enzymatically cleaved in the small intestine to the monosaccharide units: glucose, fructose, and galactose. In the small intestine, the monosacchatides are absorbed by an active cellular process, or diffusion and transported to the liver. Glucose, fructose, and galactose are removed from the circulation by the hepatic cells and im- mediately phosphorylated. The fate of the monosaccharides depends totally upon the body's immediate needs. The sugars could be converted to glycogen and stored, meta- bolized through Kreb's cycle for immediate energy, or converted to keto acids, amino acids, fats, or proteins.

The liver plays a major role in the regulation of blood glucose levels. The liver accomplished this major task in one or more of the following ways: (1) by release of absorbed glucose for the cells immediate energy needs; (2) by conversion of non-car- bohydrate substances, such as amino acids, to glucose (glucogenesis); (3) by conversion of excess glucose into glycogen for storage (glycogenesis); or (4) by breaking down stored glycogen to glucose (glycogenolysis). One or more of these processes may be occuring simultaneously to provide the necessary levels of circulating glucose for the cells energy requirements. After a meal, the liver releases the glucose that is im- mediately needed, and converts the remainder into glycogen for storage and maintenance of normal levels during fasting states. In diabetes, there is increased glycogenoly- sis taking place in the liver as well as the degradation of fatty acids by β-oxidation. In hypoglycemia there is increased glycogenesis taking place in the liver.

Insulin is closely related to the metabolism of glucose in that it facilitates the entrance of glucose into the extrahepatic cells, increases glucose oxidation, and pro- motes glycogenesis. Glucose is used by all cells of the body, however, only cardiac and skeletal muscles are capable of storing glycogen. Insulin increases the permea- bility of the body's cells to glucose facilitating glucose transfer through cell mem- brances. This results in a decreased blood glucose level. Insulin is a polypeptide chain of 51 amino acid residues which is synthesized and continuously secreted by the beta cells of the islets of Langerhans in the pancreas. In diabetes, where there is a lack of active insulin, the entrance of glucose into the tissue cells is decreased, glucose oxidation is slowed and glycogenolysis is increased. Fat metabolism is also increased with a resultant ketogenesis. In hypoglycemia, where there is an over- abundance of active insulin, all of the normal activities of insulin will be increased resulting in a marked reduction of the serum glucose levels. Other endocrine hormones also effect the blood glucose level. Thyroid hormones stimulate glycogenolysis; growth hormone from the anterior pituitary counteract the action of insulin and elevate the blood glucose level. Epinepherine, most frequently produced by stress, promotes glycogenolysis and elevated the glucose level. Glucagon, secreted by the alpha cells of the pancreas stimulates glycogenolysis.

Methods of Glucose Determinations

Glucose was among the first of the chemical constituents of blood to be determined analytically. The initial methods for the determination of blood glucose levels were based on the principle that glucose in a hot alkaline medium would reduce copper ions. The copper reduction methods, which include the Benedict's test, the Somogyi-Nelson test, the Folin-Wu test, and most recently the neocuprine tests, are for the most part considered obsolete. A later adaptation of this principle, the alkaline ferricyanide method, utilizes iron instead of copper, with the ferricyanide ions being reduced to the ferrocyanide ions. This procedure, as with the copper reduction methods is now considered to be obsolete. These methods, for the most part, have been replaced by the enzymatic procedures which have been shown to be far more sensitive, specific, and reliable. Another method employing o-toluidine is still in use, though to a limited degree. The o-toluidine method is based on the principle that glucose, in a hot acetic acid solution, will react with o-toluidine to form a glycosylamine and its corresponding Schiff base resulting in a green color which is measurable at 630 nm. This method is relatively easy to perform, is inexpensive, and does not require sophisticated equipment, but in general may also be considered outdated.

There are, at present, three enzymatic procedures that are available for use in the determination of serum glucose levels: the glucose oxidase, hexokinase, and glucose dehydrogenase methods.

GLUCOSE OXIDASE

This method is based on the principle that glucose oxidase catalyzes the oxidation of glucose to form gluconic acid and hydrogen peroxide. The hydrogen peroxide that is formed reacts with a peroxidase and a chromagen receptor resulting in an oxidized chromagen receptor with a color that is spectrophotometrically measured. The first step in this procedure is extremely sensitive and specific, however, the second step is not specific. Any strong reducing substance may compete with the chromagen receptor resulting on falsely decreased glucose levels. One glucose analyzer, the Beckman Glucose Analyzer (Beckman Instruments Inc., Fullerton, CA 92634) has overcome the problem of the second step of the reaction by utilizing an electrode that measures the amount of oxygen consumed in the first step of the reaction. This combination of the enzyme glucose oxidase and the oxygen electrode provides a rapid, highly specific, and highly sensitive method for the determination of glucose.

HEXOKINASE METHOD

The hexokinase methods are, like the glucose oxidase methods, two step procedures.

$$\text{Glucose} + \text{ATP} \xrightarrow{\text{hexokinase}} \text{glucose-6-phosphate} + \text{ADP}$$

$$\text{Glucose-6-phosphate} + \text{NAD} \xrightarrow{\text{G-6-PD}} \text{6-phosphogluconate} + \text{NADH} + \text{H}^+$$

The first step is the phosphorylation of glucose, utilizing hexokinase and ATP, to produce glucose-6-phosphate and ADP. The second step is the oxidation of the glucose-6-phosphate by NAD, in the presence of glucose-6-phosphate dehydrogenase, to produce glucose-6-phosphogluconate and NADH + H$^+$. As the NADH is produced, it is measured by the spectrophotometer at 340 nm. This procedure is highly sensitive and specific, however, it does require a spectrophotometer that is capable of ultra-violet measurement, 340 nm.

GLUCOSE DEHYDROGENASE METHOD

The glucose dehydrogenase method is the newest of the enzymatic procedures for glucose determinations. It is based on the principle that glucose is dehydrogenated by glucose dehydrogenase in the presence of NAD to yield gluconolactone and NADH. The production of NADH is measured spectrophotometrically at 340 nm and is directly proportional to the amount of glucose present in the sample. As in the other enzymatic procedures, a mutarotase is used to convert the α-D-glucose to the β form. This method has a distinct advantage over the other enzymatic procedures in that it is a one step procedure that is highly specific and highly sensitive for glucose.

GLUCOSE TOLERANCE TESTS

In the past, the glucose tolerance test has been used rather extensively for the diagnosis of mild or latent diabetes and for the detection of hypoglycemia. This test is based on the administration of a specific amount of glucose, orally or parenterally, with serial determinations of the blood glucose levels at specific periods of time, usually one half hour, 1 hour, 2 hour and 3 hours after the administration of the measured amount of glucose had been ingested. Simultaneous measurement of urine glucose levels are performed specifically for the detection of renal glycosuria.

Much debate has centered around the usefulness of the glucose tolerance test. Many say the test should only be performed on ambulatory patients, that a 40g per m^2 of surface area dose of glucose should be given, and that the patient should be on a high carbohydrate diet three days in advance of the test. I tend to agree with these points. There are, however, many variables left that cannot be controlled: the specific tension or anxiety level of the patient at the time of the test, the state of the patient's activity level, drugs including oral contraceptives, and the presence of a variety of diseases. As in the case of any other clinical test, the greater the number of variables, the less reliable the results. When the number of variables for glucose tolerance testing are considered, the results of a glucose tolerance test must be carefully used. Many other alternatives have been offered for the detection of mild or latent diabetes including: three or more fasting glucose levels about 140 mg/dl; a fasting blood sugar of greater than 180 mg/dl; and two hour post-prandial blood sugar determinations.

GLYCOSYLATED HEMOGLOBIN DETERMINATIONS

Most recently, the measurement of glycosylated hemoglobins has been advocated as the test of preference in the determination of the state of control of diabetic patients. The determination of hemoglobin A$_{1c}$ levels provides the clinician with insight relating to the long term control of patients with diabetes mellitus. Glycosylated hemoglobins are formed by the binding of glucose and adult hemoglobin (HbA). This results in a fast moving hemoglobin that may be separated by chromatographic and ion exchange procedures from other hemoglobins. Normally, approximately 6-9% of the adult hemoglobin is glycosylated while in the diabetic, 12-21% of the adult hemoglobin may be glycosylated. Glycosylation of hemoglobin takes place as the result of the binding of hemoglobin A to a hexose moiety during the 120 day life span of the RBC. This is an irreversible reaction. Unlike the traditional glucose determination which look at a momentary state of control or uncontrol in glucose metabolism, the determination of glycosylated hemoglobin provides a picture of the state of control over a two to three month period, thereby providing the clinician with a fairly accurate measure of the state of control of the diabetic patient. Moreover, this test may provide data concerning the suspected "mild diabetic" in that it provides long term information rather than momentary glances at the patients glucose levels.

Glycosylated hemoglobin assays do have their promise: they are independent of the patient's cooperation, it is independent of the time of day, and may provide a better bridge between laboratory data and metabolic control than a single glucose level. The major drawbacks include: it does not reflect acute insulin changes, nor does it ever reflect hypoglycemia, and is difficult to interpret in the presence of hematological abnormalities to the RBC. This test may well be the test of the future with regards to the detection, diagnosis, and treatment of diabetes mellitus.

D-XYLOSE AND GALACTOSE TOLERANCE TESTS

In addition to the glucose determinations, there are at least two other carbohy-drates that are of clinical interest, namely D-xylose and galactose. The D-xylose test is a test for the diagnosis of malabsorption wherein a measured amount of D-xylose is administered orally and the excretion of D-xylose in the urine is determined. Galactose is of clinical importance in the estimation of liver function. The galac-tose tolerance test is based on the principle that a measured dose of galactose, ad-ministered orally, will be converted by the liver to glycogen. If there is a liver disorder which prevents this from occuring, excess amounts of galactose will appear in the patients' urine.

INSULIN ASSAY

In the past, the determination of serum insulin levels was performed by in vitro biological methods. Since this time, insulin levels have been determined by radio-immunoassay procedures. The assay of serum insulin levels appears to be of value in the ultimate diagnosis of diabetes. There is, however, some concern about the find-ings since there have been intraindividual differences reported.

Proteins

Proteins are the basic structural and functional biochemicals most commonly asso-ciated with life. They are extremely specific biochemicals, having different chemical arrangements depending on the task required of the specific protein. Proteins are used by the human body as structural components, catalytic biochemicals, immune bio-chemicals, clotting factors, and transportation mechanisms.

CHEMISTRY

Proteins are biochemicals made up of varying numbers and sequences of alpha-amino acids. The specific function or action of the protein is established by the number, sequence, and chemical bonding structure of the particular protein. Over 100 amino acids have been discovered, however, only approximately 20 are found with any degree of frequency in human proteins. These twenty (most common amino acids) are:

1.	Aspartic acid	11.	Cysteine
2.	Glutamic acid	12.	Methionine
3.	Asparagine	13.	Tryptophan
4.	Glutamine	14.	Glycine
5.	Lysine	15.	Alanine
6.	Arginine	16.	Valine
7.	Histidine	17.	Leucine
8.	Serine	18.	Isoleucine
9.	Threonine	19.	Phenylalanine
10.	Tyrosine	20.	Proline

The specific action of the protein is determined by its primary, secondary, and tertiary structure. The primary structure of a protein is determined by the number and sequence of amino acids in the protein chain. The secondary structure of the protein is determined by the hydrogen bonds formed by the protein resulting in helices. The tertiary structure of the protein is determined by the ultimate hydrophilic action of the various amino acids in the chain resulting in a definitive and sp-cific three dimensional structure.

The basic structural unit of proteins is the alpha amino acid. They combine with one another to form peptide chains. The amino acids are those chemicals that contain both an amino group and a carboxylic acid group on the same molecule. The amino group is a basic group having a positive charge, while the carboxylic acid group is an acidic group having a negative charge. Molecules that exist in this form naturally are called zwitterions. Zwitterions are capable of assuming either a cationic or anionic form, depending on the pH of the solution in which they are found. Therefore, they are capable of acting as buffers. Amino acids combine to form peptide chains by chemically reacting with each other to form the peptide bond. This occurs when the amino group of one amino acid reacts with the carboxyl group of another amino acid resulting in the classic peptide bond. The basic chemical reaction occurs as follows:

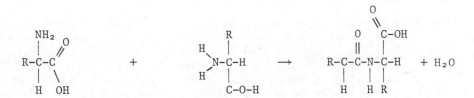

As the chain progresses to grow, the resulting molecule assumes an amphoteric property which is the basis for one of the methods of protein determination, the net positive or negative electrical charge.

Chains of amino acids that contain less than 40 amino acids are referred to as polypeptides while those that contain 40 or more amino acids assume the properties of proteins.

Proteins may be separated and classified by several methods, all of which have something to do with the chemical or physical nature of the proteins. The separation of proteins (and classification of proteins) may be based on the presence or absence of prosthetic groups, their solubility in salt solutions or dehydrating agents, their differences in size, volume, shape, molecular mass, or net surface electrical charge. The most widely used methods for the separation and identification of proteins in the clinical laboratory utilize the difference in net surface electrical charge, and the immunochemical properties of the individual proteins.

Methods

The methods most commonly utilized for the determination of proteins depends, for the most part, on what type of information about the serum proteins the clinician is most interested in. That is to say whether the physician is interested in knowing the total amount of protein in the serum, the ratio of albumin to globulin, the specific distribution of the various groups of proteins, or the lack of, or increase in, a specific serum protein. If the clinician is interested solely in the amount of protein circulating, then a total protein determination will be performed, usually by the biuret method. If the clinician is interested in the ratio of the albumin level to the globulin level, then a total protein determination will be performed, and an albumin level, usually by a dye binding technique, will be performed. If the clinician is concerned with the specific distribution of the various groups of proteins then an electrophoretic procedure will be performed. If the clinician is interested in the increase or decrease of a specific protein, then an immunoelectrophoretic procedure will be performed.

THE BIURET METHOD

The biuret method of protein determination is by far the most widely used method for the determination of total serum protein. The biuret reaction gets its name from the reaction that occurs between cupric ions and the organic chemical known as biuret. The reaction takes place between the cupric ions and carbonyl and imine groups of polypetide compounds, yielding a violet colored complex. The greater the amount of protein present in the sample, the more intense the color that is formed. The biuret method has become the most widely used method for total protein determination because it is simple to perform, inexpensive, rapid, accurate, and does not require the use of highly sophisticated expensive equipment.

REFERENCE RANGE: 6.0-8.0 g/dl

DYE BINDING METHODS FOR SERUM ALBUMIN

The dye binding methods for the determination of the serum albumin levels are based on the propensity of proteins, particularly albumin, to react with anionic colored dyes. Some colored dyes, such as methyl orange, bromcresol green, and HABA, bind tightly to albumin with a resulting spectrophotometrically different color than the free dye. These methods are widely used in both the manual and automated methods for the determination of the serum albumin levels. These methods have the same basic advantages as the biuret method in that they do not require the use of esoteric expensive equipment, are simple, rapid, inexpensive, and accurate. The combined use of the biuret method and one of the albumin binding techniques allows the clinician to evaluate the ratio of albumin to globulin.

ELECTROPHORETIC PROCEDURES

As previously mentioned, the amphoteric nature of proteins provides a means for the separation and quantitation of specific protein fractions. Fractionation of the proteins is accomplished by placing the fluid containing the proteins on a semi-solid medium, in a solution of specific pH, and applying an electrical current through this solution. Because of the differences in net surface electrical charges the protein will migrate to either the anode or cathode. At a pH of 8.6, all proteins are electronegative and will migrate to the anode. The rate of migration will be dependent upon the net surface electrical charge, the ionic strength of the buffer, the adsorptive capacity of the media, and in the case of gel media, the pore size of the media. The media employed in protein electrophoresis range from paper and cellulose actetate to starch and polyacrylamide gels. Probably the most popular medium for routine protein electrophoresis is the cellulose acetate medium. Cellulose acetate is easy to handle, provides clear separation of the protein fractions, and is easily cleared (made transparent) for optical scanning. Routine electrophoresis provides for the separation of the serum proteins into approximately six fractions: Albumin, alpha-1-globulins, alpha-2-globulins, beta-1-globulins, beta-2-globulins, and gamma globulins. Each of these fractions contains one or more specific proteins. The albumin band is composed of albumin. The alpha-1-globulin band contains: alpha-1-anti-trypsin, alpha-1-lipoprotein, and Orosomucoid. The alpha-2-globulin band contains: alpha-2-macroglobulin, haptoglobin, and pre-beta-lipoprotein. The Beta-1-globulin band contains: Transferrin, hemopexin, and beta-lipoprotein. The beta-2-globulin band is only obtained in fresh serum specimens and has as its only constituent, beta-1-c, a complement fraction. The gamma-globulin fraction contains the immunoglobulins, IgG, IgM, IgA. These specific protein bands are detected and quantitated by staining the medium after the electrical current has been applied to the medium, with one of the following dyes: Ponceau S., Amido black 10B, Lissamine green, or Nigrosin, followed by spectrophotometric scanning or elution.

IMMUNOELECTROPHORETIC PROCEDURES AND IMMUNODIFFUSION TECHNIQUES

These methods combine the electrophorectic properties of proteins with the specific immunochemical properties of proteins. All, some, or any one specific protein may be fractionated by these methods since they employ the separation available with electrophoresis, and the specificity of the antigen-antibody reaction. These procedures allow for the specific fractionation of individual protein constituents within specific electrophoretic bands. These procedures allow for the differentiation of approximately 20 or more protein fractions. In addition to the procedures mentioned, there are methods available for the specific fractionation of individual protein fractions based on one or more of the principles already mentioned.

CLINICAL SIGNIFICANCE

TOTAL PROTEIN HYPERPROTEINEMIA

Increase in the total serum protein concentration may be due to any of several states of dehydration, such as severe vomiting, diarrhea, Addison's disease, or diabetes; any one of the gammopathies of which multiple myeloma is the primary disease will generally show elevated total proteins. Decreases in the total serum protein concentration may be due to acute protein starvation, nephrotic syndrome, open wounds, burns, or excessive bleeding. All of the serum proteins are synthesized in the liver except the immunoglobulin. Liver diseases which cause a decreased protein synthesis capability will also lower the total protein. Examples are infectious hepatitis and cirrhosis.

ALBUMIN

Most commonly, water depletion, as in the case of the dehydration problems generally serves to raise the albumin levels along with the total protein levels. Hypoalbuminemia, on the other hand, is most commonly associated with nephrotic syndrome and liver disorders.

PROTEIN ELECTROPHORESIS

The various bands produced by protein electrophoresis may be increased or decreased by a variety of disorders. Below is a list of some of the disorders that may increase/decrease each of the particular bands.

ALBUMIN

Increased in: dehydration

Decreased in: acute infections, chronic infections, diabetes mellitus, renal disor-
               ders, hepatic disorders, myelogenous leukemia, lymphomas, macroglubu-
               linemia, myeloma, myxedema, rheumatoid arthritis, systemic lupus, and
               scleroderma

ALPHA-1-GLOBULIN

Increased in: diabetes mellitus, glomerulonephritis, and ulcerative colitis

Decreased in: hepatitis and scleroderma

ALPHA-2-GLOBULIN

Increased in: acute infections, diabetes mellitus, Hodgkin's disease, myxedema,
               nephrosis, rheumatoid arthritis, systemic lupus, and ulcerative colitis

Decreased in: hepatitis, and scleroderma

BETA-1-GLOBULINS

Increased in: hepatitis, macroglobulinemia

Decreased in: scleroderma and ulcerative colitis

BETA-2-GLOBULIN

Increased in: acute phase reactions

Decreased in: glomerulonephritis, systemic lupus, and other autoimmune disorders

GAMMA-GLOBULIN

Increased in: chronic infections, cryoglobulinemia, hepatic disorders, Hodgkins di-
               sease, macroglobulinemia, myeloma, and rheumatoid arthritis

Decreased in: lymphomas, nephorosis, scleroderma, and ulcerative colitis

TOTAL IMMUNOELECTROPHORETIC PROCEDURES AND IMMUNODIFFUSION TECHNIQUES

The increase or decrease of specific protein fractions may be determined by using
either immunoelectrophoresis or immunodiffusion. Immunoelectrophoresis (IEP) may be
performed as a screening procedure utilizing a polyvalent antiserum, or may be performed for the detection of specific protein fractions by utilizing specific antisera
for the protein fraction in question. Immunodiffusion, or more specifically radial
immunodiffusion (RID) utilizes agar gel or agarose gel plates implanted with specific
antisera for the quantitation of specific protein fraction levels. Most frequently
this procedure is used for the quantitation of the immunoglobulins IgA, IgG, and IgM.

Lipids

The lipids are relatively large organic compounds that are essentially insoluble in water and are soluble in non-polar substances such as ether and benzene. The lipids are most commonly found bound to proteins which allows them solubility in aqueous solutions of the body. Those lipids that are bound to proteins are referred to as lipoproteins. In addition to lipoproteins, other lipids of clinical significance include: cholesterol, carotene, fatty acids, triglycerides and vitamins A, D, E, and K. For purposes of brevity, this section will deal specifically with the fatty acids, cholesterol, tryglycerides, and the lipoproteins.

CHEMISTRY

FATTY ACIDS

The fatty acids are long carbon chains, which usually range from lengths of 16-24 carbon atoms, and are essentially all monocarboxylic acids. The fatty acids are often referred to as being saturated or unsaturated. These terms refer to whether or not the fatty acid chain contains double bonds. The greater the number of double bonds present in the chain, the more unsaturated the chain is said to be. The number of double bonds present is limited by the fact that the double bonds are usually separated by at least three carbons.

TRIGLYCERIDES

When three fatty acid chains are reacted with a molecule of glycerol, simple esters are formed between the hydroxyl groups of the glycerol molecule and the carboylic acid group of the fatty acids. The bulk of the triglycerides are found stored in the adipose tissue of the body.

CHOLESTEROL

Cholesterol is one of a group of substances known as sterols. Sterols are substances that have sterane (perhydrocyclopentanophenanthrene) as their skeleton structure.

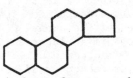

Perhydrocyclopentanophenanthrene (Sterane)

Cholesterol is often depicted in the following manner:

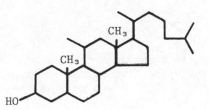

Approximately two-thirds of the body's cholesterol is found in the esterified form, that is as esters of fatty acids.

LIPOPROTEINS

The lipoproteins found in the body are generally classified as chylomicrons, VLDL (very-low-density-lipoproteins), LDL (low-density-lipoproteins), and HDL (high-density-lipoproteins). The chylomicrons and VLDL are composed primarily of triglycerides, while the LDL and HDL are composed primarily of cholesterol and cholesterol esters. The lipoproteins, like the proteins, differ in the net surface electrical charge, which makes it possible to separate them by electrophoresis.

METABOLISM OF LIPIDS

When lipids are ingested, they are emulsified by bile salts in the small intestine. Triglycerides are converted to fatty acids and monoglycerides which react with bile salts to form soaps, and are absorbed as such. Within the mucosal cells, the triglycerides and cholesteryl esters are reformed, and incorporated into chylomicrons. The chylomicrons enter lymphatic vessels, are transported to the blood stream by way of the thoracic duct, and are transported to the liver for degradation or biosysnthesis.

BETA-OXIDATION

Beta-oxidation is the term used for the process of the degradation of fatty acids for energy. In this process, long chain fatty acids are broken down at a rate of two carbon atoms at a time. These two carbon molecules are an intermediate substance known as acetyl CoA. Acetyl CoA is normally condensed with oxaloacetate to form citrate which continues through the tricarboxylic acid cycle for final oxidation.

KETOSIS

Whenever there is a disturbance in the metabolism of glucose, such as in starvation, excessive vomitting, diarrhea, or in diabetes, fatty acids stored in the adipose tissue are broken down to provide the energy normally acquired through the glucose metabolism. The fatty acids are broken down by beta oxidation as previously mentioned. However, since oxaloacetate is normally produced as the result of glucose metabolism and the glucose metabolism is impaired, the acetyl CoA that is produced by beta-oxidation accumulates. The accumulation of the acetyl CoA results in the condensation of two molecules of acetyl CoA to form an intermediate compound which reacts with another molecule of acetyl CoA to yield acetoacetic acid. As the acetoacetic acid accumulates, some of it decomposes to form acetone and CO_2, while more of it is reduced to form beta-hydroxybutyric acid. The accumulation of acetoacetic acid and beta-hydroxybutyric acid produces a metabolic acidosis known as ketosis. The entire process can be stopped by restoring normal glucose metabolism.

METHODS

FATTY ACIDS

The determination of fatty acids in serum is a complex and rather time consuming method. This procedure calls for the extraction of the fatty acids with heptane, followed by the stirring of the solution with nitrogen gas, followed by titration of the solution with sodium hydroxide.

REFERENCE VALUES: 0.30 to 0.90 mmol/l.

TRIGLYCERIDES

The estimation of serum triglyceride levels may be performed by enzymatic and flourometric techniques. There are two enzymatic procedures both of which involve the hydrolysis of the triglycerides and measurement of the liberated glycerol. The first method employs an alkaline solution (Potassium hydroxide) while the second method employs a lipase to hydrolyze the triglycerides. The subsequent sequence of reactions takes place with the alkaline hydrolysis method: the glycerol, along with ATP, in the presence of glycerol kinase to yield glycerol-3-phosphate and ADP. The ADP which is produced, along with PEP (Phosphenol pyruvate) reacts with pyruvate kinase to yield ATP and pyruvate. The pyruvate that is produced, along with NADH is reacted with lactate dehydrogenase to yield lactate and NAD. Ultraviolet spectrophotometric measurement of the decrease of the NADH is performed at 340 nm. The amount of the decrease in NADH is equivalent to the concentration of the glycerol present in the original sample.

The second method, employing the lipase for hydrolysis of the triglycerides has the following set of reactions taking place after hydrolysis: glycerol, along with ATP reacts with glycerol kinase to yield glycerol-3-phosphate and ADP; the glycerol-3-phosphate produced, along with NAD, in the presence of glycerol phosphate dehydrogenase yields dihydroxyacetone and NADH. The production of the NADH can be measured with ultraviolet spectrophotometry at 340 nm. The amount of NADH produced is directly proportional to the amount of glycerol present in the original sample. The fluorometric technique employs the use of the Hantzsch condensation reaction. This procedure calls for the hydrolysis of the triglycerides, followed by the oxidation of the glycerol to formaldehyde. The formaldehyde produced is then reacted with ammonium ions and acetyl acetone which results in the production of a fluorescent, yellow colored diacetyldihyrolutidine which may be measured fluorometrically. The amount of fluorescent compound produced being directly proportional to the amount of glycerol in the original sample.

CHOLESTEROL METHODS

Probably the most widely used method for cholesterol determination is the Liebermann-Burchard reaction. This method may be employed as a direct method or as an extraction method. In either case, the principle of the reaction is that cholesterol, as an alcohol will react with strong acids to produce colored derivatives. The reagent is composed of acetic acid, acetic anhydride, and sulphuric acid. The sulphuric acid is used as a dehydrating and oxidizing agent, while the acetic acid and acetic anhydride are used as solvents and dehydrating agents.

LIPOPROTEINS

The measurement of lipoproteins involves the fractionation of the serum lipoproteins and is best accomplished by electrophoresis. The electrophoresis of lipoproteins is essentially the same as for serum proteins, however, the electrophoresed strip is stained with a fat stain such as Oil-Red-O.

CLINICAL SIGNIFICANCE

FATTY ACIDS

An increase in the fatty acid level may be the result of hormonal activity, diabetes, starvation, or stress.

TRIGLYCERIDES

Elevation of serum triglyceride levels have been associated with primary hyper-lipidemias and with the hyperlipidemias that are secondary to other disease states. Increases in serum triglyceride levels have also been shown to be related to increased risk of arteriosclerotic heart disease.

CHOLESTEROL

Increased levels of serum cholesterol have been associated with a variety of dis-orders including: diabetes mellitus, hypothyroidism, nephrotic syndrome, hepatitis, and emotional stress. Elevations of serum cholesterol have also been associated with the increased risk of arteriosclerotic heart disease.

LIPOPROTEIN ELECTROPHORESIS

Lipoproteins are amphoteric substances which allows for their separation by electrophoresis. The bands produced are called the alpha-1 band, alpha-2 band, pre-beta band, the beta-1 band, and the beta-2 band. Normal sera contain an alpha-1 band of HDL lipoprotein and a beta-1 band of LDL lipoprotein. Other sera may contain VLDL, LDL, and HDL lipoproteins in each of the various bands, as well as VLDL chy-lomicrons at the point of origin. Lipoprotein electrophoresis is most often employed to classify the hyperlipoproteinemias and to identify abnormal lipoproteins. Through the work of Fredrickson and his co-workers, six inherited types of hyperlipoproteine-mias have been identified. The six types, and their patterns are:

Type I: Serum - has a creamy layer over a clear layer
           Cholesterol - elevated
           Triglycerides - elevated
           Electrophoretic pattern: heavy chylomicron band at the point of origin,
                                      with a faint beta and pre-beta band

Type IIa: Serum - clear
           Cholesterol - elevated
           Triglycerides - normal
           Electrophoretic pattern: no chylomicrons, with a heavy beta band

Type IIb: Serum - clear or faintly turbid
           Cholesterol - elevated
           Triglyceride - elevated
           Electrophoretic pattern: no chylomicrons, with a heavy beta and pre-beta
                                      band

Type III: Serum - faint creamy layer over a turbid layer
           Cholesterol - elevated
           Triglycerides - elevated
           Electrophoretic pattern: slight amount of chylomicrons at the point of
                                      origin, with a broad beta band

Type IV: Serum - turbid
           Cholesterol - normal or slightly elevated
           Triglycerides - elevated
           Electrophoretic pattern: no chylomicrons, with a heavy pre-beta band

Type V: Serum - has a creamy layer over a turbid layer
           Cholesterol - elevated
           Triglycerides - elevated
           Electrophoretic pattern: heavy chylomicrons at the point of origin, with
                                       a heavy pre-beta band

Types IIa, IIb, III, IV, and V, have all been shown to be associated with premature arteriosclerotic vascular disease.

Enzymes

CO_2 and H_2O combine very slowly when mixed in a test tube. Inside the erythrocyte, however, this action: $CO_2 + H_2O \rightarrow H_2CO_3$ occurs rapidly. Living organisms possess catalysts, enzymes, that increase the speed of chemical reaction.

Enzymes have been used by man ever since the production of cheese and alcoholic beverages began. But, it has only been within the last century that clinical enzymology has been used effectively in the diagnosis of disease states.

Plasma should be regarded as a recepticle for enzymes. Under normal homeostatis, there exists an activity gradient between cells and plasma. Tissue destruction and necrosis interrupts the energy which maintains the gradient and enzymes are released into the plasma. Damage to myocardial tissue releases several enzymes into the circulation: creatine kinase, aspartate aminotransferase, and lactate dehydrogenase.

Enzymes are defined as biological catalysts. A catalyst is any substance that accelerates a chemical reaction, yet remains chemically unaltered at the end of the process. If we look at a chemical reaction substrate (S) $\rightarrow$ Product (P), sufficient energy must be supplied to the environment from an outside source to raise the molecules of (S) to a transition state where a chemical bond can be made or broken and (P) formed. The energy required to bring (S) to a reactive state is called the activation energy. If we look at the same reaction with an enzyme, substrate enzyme product, several changes will be noted: (1) the reaction will occur at a more accelerated rate, (2) less activation energy will be required, and (3) the enzyme will not be consumed.

Enzymes are proteins. They are a linear sequence of amide bonds binding amino acids to produce an energetic environment. As are all proteins, they are arranged in four structural levels:

Primary: relating to the linear sequential combination of the 20 amino acids

Secondary: relating to the spiral configuration produced by hydrogen bonding
               imide (-N-) and carboxyl (-C-) groups of the amide bonds
                     H   O

Tertiary: relating to the special folding of the primary and secondary structures

Quartinary: relating to the subunit structures of the enzyme, i.e., two subunits of creatine kinase

Enzymes are labile and inactivated, if denatured. They range in molecular size from 10^4-10^6 daltons. Their unique amino acid sequences give them a unique chemical charge allowing them their own specific migration in electrophoresis chambers. Enzymes accelerate chemical reactions, altering the rate of reaction, but not the equilibrium constant. They not only increase the speed of reactions but they may also regulate the reaction.

DEFINITION OF TERMS

The protein portion of an enzyme is called the APOENZYME. Although many enzymes consist entirely of protein, some contain a nonprotein moiety. If this nonprotein part is firmly attached and cannot be dialyzed from the enzyme, it is referred to as a PROSTHETIC GROUP. Examples of prosthetic groups are vitamin B, nicotinamide, pyridoxine, ADP, and ATP. If the nonprotein part is easily dialysed it is referred to as a coenzyme. For ease of understanding, coenzyme is used to refer to both terms. Essentially there is no difference between the two, and both are required for catalytic activity. The apoenzyme and the coenzyme together are referred to as the HALOENZYME.

Enzymes were once classified by the substrate they acted upon. Many of those names still remain today (i.e., amylase: from AMYLUM meaning starch; -ase to denote enzyme). Much discussion exists as to establishing a universal enzyme nomenclature. The accepted nomenclature provides a systemic name and numerical code, and a working or practical name. The practical names usually are the trivial names that have become attached to the enzymes. The systemic name consists of two words: the first identifies the substrate, the second identifies the type of reaction with -ase tacked on the end (if two substrates are involved both are listed, separated by a colon). The numerical number usually begins with EC denoting Enzyme Commission, followed by four sets of numbers separated by periods.

The first number is related to the class:

    EC 1 OXIDOREDUCTASES: enzymes which catalyze electron transfer reactions

    EC 2 TRANSFERASES: enzymes which are involved in the transfer of functional
                            groups from a donor to an acceptor molecule

    EC 3 HYDROLASES: enzymes which catalyze the cleavage of C-O, C-N, or C-C
                            bonds

    EC 4 LYASES: enzymes which cleave C-O, C-N, C-C bonds by elimination,
                            leaving double bonds

    EC 5 ISOMERASES   enzymes which catalyze geometrical or structural changes

    EC 6 LIGASES   enzymes which catalyze the joining of two molecules

The second number refers to a subclass, the third a sub-subclass, and the fourth number is the specific serial number given to that enzyme within its sub-subclass.

COMMON ENZYMES MEASURED IN CLINICAL CHEMISTRY

1. OXIDOREDUCTASES

    Ceruloplasmin EC 1.16.3.1
    Lactate dehydrogenase (LD) EC 1.1.1.27
    Hydroxybutyrate dehydrogenase (HBD)

2. TRANSFERASES

Aspartate aminotransferase AST(SGOT) EC 2.6.1.1
Alanine aminotransferase ALT (SGPT) EC 2.6.1.2
Creatine kinase (CK) EC 2.7.3.2
Gamma glutamyl transferase (GGT) EC 2.3.2.2

3. HYDROLASES

Phosphatase, Acid (ACP) EC 3.1.3.2
Phosphatase, Alkaline (ALP) EC 3.1.3.1.
Cholinesterase (CHS) EC 3.1.1.8
Lipase (LPS) EC 3.1.1.3
Amylase (AMS) EC 3.2.1.1

4. LYASES

Aldolase (ALS)

5. ISOMERASES

Glucose phosphate isomerase

MODE OF ACTION

The exact mode of enzyme action is still unknown. It is thought that the enzyme and substrate must come in close contact with each other, combine to form enzyme-substrate complexes, and subsequently break apart to yield a product and free enzyme. Emil Fischer (1894) described this process as a lock and key combination. His theory appears to be accurate in that the enzyme's amino acid sequence, electrical charge, and special arrangement form a "lock" into which the "key" substrate fits. Every enzyme contains many potential chemically active areas, but catalytic activity appears to be confined to a specific area on the enzyme called the "active site".

It would be an oversimplification if we said that all enzymatic reactions proceed as such:

$$E + S \rightleftharpoons ES \rightleftharpoons P + E$$

Here, an enzyme combines with its substrate to eventually produce a product and free enzyme. Most enzymes have more than one substrate and catalyze reactions of the type $A + B \rightleftharpoons C + D$. But whether one substrate or two substrate reactions, the same basic kinetics occur.

In any given volume of serum, the amount of enzyme will have a finite number of active sites. If sufficient substrate is supplied, all the active sites of the enzyme present will become saturated. Further addition of substrate to the reaction will not enhance the rate at which the enzyme produces products. Under this condition, the following reaction occurs:

$$(1) \qquad E + S \underset{K_2}{\overset{K_1}{\rightleftharpoons}} ES \underset{K_4}{\overset{K_3}{\rightleftharpoons}} E + P$$

   Michaelis and Menton described an equation for a single substrate and a single product where an enzyme (E) combines with a substrate (S) to form a substrate enzyme complex (ES) which then gives a product (P) and free enzyme (E).   Graphically E + S   ES   P + E becomes

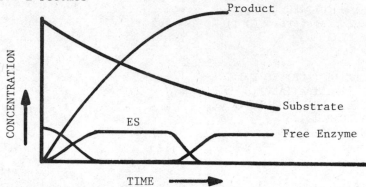

   Where products increase with respect to time, substrate decreases, free enzyme decreases, and ES increases until all of the substrate is bound to an enzyme and a plateau is reached where all of the enzyme present is bound to the substrate.

   Calculus provides a means of expressing rate.   In enzymatic reactions we are concerned with the rate of change of reaction velocity with respect to the concentration of the reactants. $\frac{d(ES)}{dt}$ express the rate of accumulation of ES for a given increment change in time. $\frac{-d(ES)}{dt}$ represents the rate of consumption of ES for a given increment change in time.   The negative sign expresses the disappearance of a reactant.

   From equation 1

(2)
$$E + S \underset{K_2}{\overset{K_1}{\rightleftharpoons}} ES \underset{K_4}{\overset{K_3}{\rightleftharpoons}} E + P$$

$$\frac{d\{ES\}}{dt} = K_1 \left(\{E_{Total}\} - \{ES\}\right) \{S\}$$

   The rate of accumulation of ES is influenced by the rate of free enzyme combining with the substrate.

(3)   The amount of free enzyme is defined as $\{E_{Total}\} - \{ES\}$

(4)
$$\frac{-d\{ES\}}{dt} = K_2 \{ES\} + K_3 \{ES\}$$

   The rate of disappearance of ES is influenced by the rate of ES breaking apart to become enzyme and substrate again, and the rate of ES breaking into products and free enzymes.

   At the steady state where the enzyme may be assumed to be saturated with substrate, the formation and disappearance of ES is equal, thus:

(5)
$$\frac{-d\{ES\}}{t} = \frac{d\{ES\}}{t}$$

and

(6) $K_1 (\{E\} - \{ES\}) \{S\} = K_2 \{ES\} + K_3 \{ES\}$

which simplifies to:

(7) $K_1 (\{E\} - \{ES\}) \{S\} + (K_2 + K_3) \{ES\}$

Michaelis and Menton described a constant, Km, which related the velocity constants K_1, K_2, K_3 as such:

(8) $$Km = \frac{K_2 + K_3}{K_1}$$

Thus rearranging equation 7

(9) $$Km = \frac{K_2 + K_3}{K_1} = \frac{\{S\} (\{E\} - \{ES\})}{\{ES\}}$$

By solving for {ES}

(10) $$\{ES\} = \frac{\{S\}\{E\}}{Km + \{S\}}$$

The breakdown of ES into product and free enzyme occurs at a rate determined by the concentration of the enzyme substrates complex. Measurements of either free enzyme or ES is not practical for the clinical laboratory, but the measurement of velocity is. The initial velocity of the reaction is defined as:

(11) $$V_{initial} = K_3 \{ES\}$$

At the initial stage of the reaction where the substrate concentration is highest and the product concentration is lowest, the enzyme exerts its maximal influence. Thus:

(12) $$V_i = K_3 \frac{\{S\} \{E\}}{Km + S}$$

Maximum velocity is reached when all of the enzyme is satuated with substrate, or when

(13) $\{E\} = \{ES\}$, therefore $V_{max} = K_3 \{E\}$

By substituting terms, equation 12 becomes

(14) $$V = \frac{\{S\}V_{max}}{Km + S}$$

If we theoretically allow the velocity to occur at one half the maximum velocity

$$1/2 = \frac{(S)}{K_m + S}$$

$$2S = K_m + S$$

$$S = K_m$$

The Michaelis-Menton Constant, K_m, reflects the rate at which substrate and enzyme combine and the stability of the enzyme substrate complex. It is also equal to the substrate concentration permitting the reaction to occur at a half maximal velocity. Vmax is characteristic for a given enzyme and reflects the rate of generation of product.

The Michaelis-Menton Constant, K_m, was originally believed to be a true equilibrium constant. Low K_m's were thought to indicate high affinities of enzyme for substrate and vice versa. However, recent research has shown that K_m is not a true equilibrium constant. By taking the reciprocal of equation 14 we obtain

(15)
$$\frac{1}{V} = \frac{Km}{Vmax\ \{S\}} + \frac{1}{Vmax}$$

This linear equation is referred to as the Lineweaver-Burk Equation, and is useful in the study of enzyme inhibition. Graphically the Lineweaver-Burk Equation becomes:

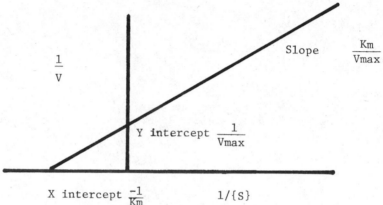

Enzyme inhibitions usually occur in two ways: specific and nonspecific. Nonspecific inhibition results from the denaturation of the enzyme, i.e., serum for acid phosphate not preserved at pH 4.9 will quickly result in the loss of catalytic activity. Specific inhibition is either competitive or noncompetitive. Trace metals are a common noncompetitive inhibiton. Heavy metals interfere with the coenzyme or other activitors of an enzyme. EDTA prevents blood clotting by noncompetitive inhibition: the calcium ions required for the activation of thromboplastin are bound by the EDTA and cannot be used in the reaction. A Lineweaver-Burk plot of a noncompetitive inhibited reaction would be similar to:

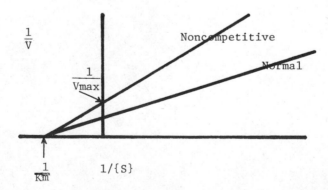

In noncompetitive inhibition the Vmax of the reaction decreases, while the K_m remains constant. The addition of more substrate to this system will not help because the active site of the enzymes has been altered and cannot accept substrate.

Competitive inhibition usually occurs when the inhibitor resembles the substrate. Malonic acid and succinic acid are structurally similar

$$HOOCCH_2CH_2COOH \qquad \text{succinic acid}$$
$$HOOCCH_2COOH \qquad \text{malonic acid}$$

and malonic acid is a strong competitive inhibitor of the oxidation of succinic acid by succinic dehydrogenase. In this case, the reaction is slowed down because some of the active sites are occupied by the inhibitor. The Vmax remains constant but the K_m increases as shown below by the Lineweaver-Burk plot.

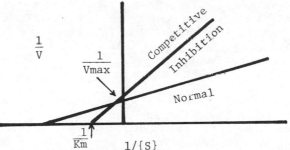

To achieve constant results in enzymatic assays, all the reactants must be of set, optimal concentrations. The concentration of the enzyme must be the only varying factor. Temperature, pH, and substrate are other important factors in enzymatic assays.

Reaction rates slow down with the lowering of temperature. Hibernating animals show a sharp drop in their basal metabolic rate during the cold winter months for this reason. Conversely, reaction rates increase with rising temperatures until a maximal rate is achieved. Temperatures beyond maximum result in decreased velocities and thermal denaturation of the enzyme. With few exceptions, the optimal activity of most enzymes is 35-55°C. A 10°C rise in temperature usually results in 50 to 100% rise in activity. One must be careful to use a manufacturer's kit at the specified temperature. The enzyme assay has been optimized at that temperature and kits designed for use at 30°C will show non-linear results at 37°C.

Salt linkages and hydrogen bonds between the side chains of the amino acids hold enzymes in their characteristic shape. The addition of H^+ and OH^- result in altered ionization of anionic and cationic groups which compose the salt linkages of both enzymes and substrates. Loss of these types of bonds result in an alteration of the three dimensional structural arrangement and concomitant loss in catalytic activity. Enzymes exert optimum activity over a very narrow pH range. pH is affected by temperature, nature of the buffer, and substrate. These variables must also be kept constant to insure a stable optimal pH in the assay medium. Most enzymes have an optimum pH close to neutrality (pH 7) although acid phosphatase requires a pH 4.8 environment and pepsin a pH of 2.5.

By definition, enzymes are catalysts and are not, therefore, consumed during the reaction. Once the enzyme-substrate complex breaks apart to form product and free enzymes, that enzyme is free to catalyze the modification of another substrate molecule. Enzymes have been recorded to modify 6 to 17,000,000 molecules of substrate per minute. If an excess of substrate is available, the rate of the reaction will be proportional to the amount of enzyme present.

$$V = \frac{\{S\}\ Vmax}{Km + \{S\}}$$ can be graphically shown as:

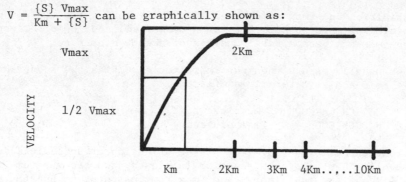

As the substrate concentration increases, the velocity of the reaction will approach Vmax. Remembering that K_m is one half the substrate necessary to allow the reaction to proceed at Vmax, $2K_m$ must represent the substrate concentration at Vmax. As the substrate concentration indeed does increase above $2K_m$, no further velocity change is noted. It is on this "plateau" that (1) the enzyme is saturated with substrate, (2) the velocity of the reaction is constant, (3) zero order kinetics is reached, and (4) kinetic measurements are taken to measure enzyme activity. Usually a substrate concentration of 10 K_m is chosen in enzymatic assays to ensure that Vmax is obtained.

If a person runs by us on the street, we can visually estimate his speed by comparing him to a stationary object. In enzymatic assays, we measure the change in absorbance with respect to time and convert to enzyme units. The preferred method of determining the absorbance change is by kinetic or time rate methods, where several measurements are taken over an increment of time. Some assays require only an initial reading and an endpoint reading. Several hazards lie in this method: the enzyme could be inhibited and the resultant enzyme value falsely low, or the enzyme concentration could be elevated, but due to substrate depletion, the value reported as falsely low. Most enzyme assays are a multienzyme system with the eventual reduction of nicotinamide adenine dinucleotide, NADH, which absorbs light at 340 nm while its oxidized form NAD^+ shows minimal absorption at 340 nm. Creatine kinase (CK) is usually assayed in the following reaction sequence:

Reaction 1:   Creatine phosphate +   ADP $\xrightleftharpoons{\text{CK}}$ ATP + Creatine
           (Substeate 1)   (Coenzyme)   Product   Product

Reaction 2:   Glucose   +   ATP $\xrightleftharpoons{\text{Glucose Hexokinase}}$ Glucose-6-phosphate +   ADP
           (Substrate)   Coenzyme   Product   Product

Reaction 3:   Glucose-6-phosphate +   NAD $\xrightleftharpoons{\text{C-6PDH}}$ 6-phosphogluconate + NADH
                           Coenzyme   Product   Product

Notice how the product from Reaction 1 becomes the substrate for Reaction 2, and the product of Reaction 2 feeds Reaction 3. ADP as a product in Reaction 2 insures adequate supplies for Reaction 1. This use of the products of one reaction as substrate for the next also insures that none of the reverse reactions occur. (The production of NAD in the course of the reaction results in an increase in absorbance which can be related to the initial CK activity in the serum.)

Conversion of absorbance change to enzyme units such as International Units per liter (U/L) is made with:

$$U/L = \frac{\Delta A/\text{min} \times 1000 \times RV \times T \times 1000}{6.2 \times 10_3 \times SV}$$

RV = reaction volume in ml

SV - sample volume in ml

6.2×10^3 = molar absorbtivity of NADH of 340 nm

T = temperature conversion factor for enzyme activity other than that temperature of the assay.

The thousands are conversion factors, one to convert mole substrate/min/ml to International Units, and the other to convert millimoles to micromoles.

Some enzymes have near absolute specificity for a given substrate, while others exhibit broad specificity. The substrate must have a specific chemical bond that can be attacked by the enzyme and usually has a functional group that properly aligns the chemical bond for attachment with the enzyme. Enzyme specificity is exhibited by muscle lactate dehydrogenase which will catalyze only L-lactate and not D-lactate. Lipase exhibits a broad specificity catalyzing the hydrolysis of fats and carboxylic acid esters.

Some enzymes appear as multiple forms in different organs of the body. These different molecular forms of an enzyme are called isoenzymes and exhibit differences in physical, biochemical, and immunological properties. These isoenzymes possess the same active site, but it is believed that the remainig protein structure differs in amino acid sequence. The altered amino acid sequence results in complete molecules of different electric charges, thus allowing the isoenzymes to be separated by electrophoresis. Creatine kinase is an important enzyme for the diagnosis of myocardial infarction. The three isoenzymes of creatine kinase are made up of combinations of two different kinds of polypeptide chains, each of molecular weight of 50,000 daltons. The B chain (B for brain or nervous tissue) and M chain (M for skeletal muscle) have different amino acid sequences and composition. The BB (CK_1) isoenzyme migrates the closest to the anode, the MM (CK_3) migrates the least, and the hybrid, MB (CK_2) migrates in the middle. Recent literature has also suggested that there are possibly other variant CK isoenzymes than the three just named. The isoenzymes differ significantly in the Vmax and K_m.

It was discovered that many enzymes became inactive when they were dialyzed and reacquire their catalytic activity when they were recombined with the dialysate. The dialysate was found to contain a thermostable, dialyzable compound later called coenzyme. A coenzyme assists the enzyme by either accepting the group being cleaved or by contributing a group for synthesis. Currently, much discussion centers around the use of exogenous pyridoxal-5'-phosphate (P-5-P) in the assay of aspartate transaminase. P-5-P acts as a coenzyme, accepting the amino group from L-aspartate to form an enzyme-substrate-P-5-P complex. P-5-P then transfers the amino acid group to the substrate oxoglutarate to form oxalacetate.

$$\text{L-aspartate and oxoglutarate} \underset{\text{P-5-P}}{\overset{\text{AST}}{\rightleftharpoons}} \text{oxalacetate and L-glutamate}$$

Serum deficient in P-5-P due to nutritional deficiences, exhibits low AST values especially in dialysis patients. Addition of P-5-P to the assay medium is believed to "activate" the aspartate transaminase (AST) that is there, but that would not be activated due to the endogenous deficiency of P-5-P.

Metal ions also act as activators of enzymes. The kinases (i.e., creatine kinase, CK) require the presence of magnesium. Amylase requires chloride; the blood clotting enzymes, calcium; pyruvate kinase requires both magnesium and potassium; the peptidase, zinc and manganese. N-acetylcysteine, an activator of creatine kinase, as other

TABLE 5

SUMMARY OF CREATINE KINASE ASSAYS

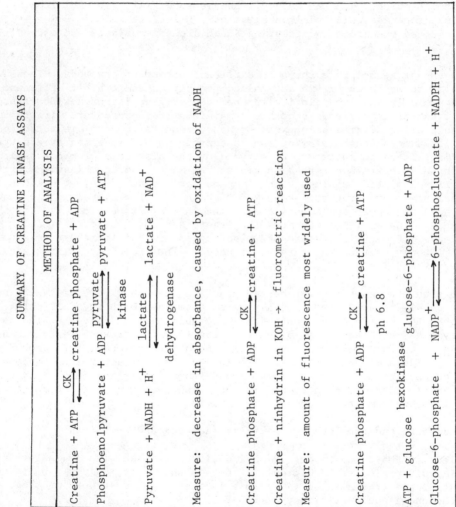

METHOD OF ANALYSIS

Creatine + ATP $\xrightarrow{\text{CK}}$ creatine phosphate + ADP

Phosphoenolpyruvate + ADP $\xrightarrow{\text{pyruvate kinase}}$ pyruvate + ATP

Pyruvate + NADH + H$^+$ $\xrightleftharpoons{\text{lactate dehydrogenase}}$ lactate + NAD$^+$

Measure: decrease in absorbance, caused by oxidation of NADH

Creatine phosphate + ADP $\xrightarrow{\text{CK}}$ creatine + ATP

Creatine + ninhydrin in KOH → fluorometric reaction

Measure: amount of fluorescence most widely used

Creatine phosphate + ADP $\xrightarrow[\text{ph 6.8}]{\text{CK}}$ creatine + ATP

ATP + glucose $\xrightarrow{\text{hexokinase}}$ glucose-6-phosphate + ADP

Glucose-6-phosphate + NADP$^+$ $\rightleftharpoons$ 6-phosphogluconate + NADPH + H$^+$

TABLE 5 (continued)

ISOENZYME	SPECIMEN OF CHOICE: STORAGE	COFACTORS	INHIBITORS
CK is a dimer	Serum or heparined plasma	Mg^{++}	Heavy metal ion citrates
CK₁ (BB) primary sources nervous tissue	Preservation of activity is subject to much controversy. CK should be assayed within 4 hours at room temperature or stored at 4°C for 6–8 hours	Cystine Kinase	Fluorides L-thyroxine Uric acid Adenylate
Other prostate thyroid intestine kidney	Frozen for 2–3 days		

CK₁ (BB) primary sources nervous tissue

Mg^{++}

Cystine Kinase

Heavy metal ion citrates
Fluorides
L-thyroxine
Uric acid
Adenylate

TECHNICAL NOTES FOR ASSAYS

THIOL COMPOUNDS

The addition of N-acetyl cysteine to the substrate mixture appears to "reactivate" the enzyme.

DILUTIONS

Dilution of high CK sera into the assay range of the procedure results in an apparent increase in CK activity. Inactivated serum appears to be the best dilutent for those specimens requiring dilution.

HEMOLYSIS

Should be avoided. The addition of RBC adenylate kinase causes a side reaction of 2ADP → ATP + AMP. Some manufacturers include AMP to act as a competitive inhibitor for this side reaction.

CK₂ (MB) primary source cardiac muscle

Other diaphragm esophagus uterus

CK₃ (MM) primary source skeletal muscle and all other tissue except nervous tissue activators, alters the spacial arrangement of the enzyme to insure proper enzyme-substrate alignment. Metal ions help to link the enzyme to the substrate or an enzyme to a coenzyme. They also aid in the transfer of electrons.

Millions of enzymatic reactions occur in the body every day which control vital processes that if left unchecked, would be disastrous. These processes usually occur in multienzymatic systems where one enzyme produces a product that is catalyzed by another enzyme.

$$A + E_1 \rightarrow B + E_2 \rightarrow C + E_3 \rightarrow D + E_4 \rightarrow P$$

inhibitor

The end product of this sequence is usually inhibitory to the first enzyme. This effector can have a negative effect and inhibit further activity by the first enzyme. In this way, enzymatic systems control themselves.

Enzymes are a complex analyte for the clinical chemist. Rarely do two manufacturer's kits duplicate patient values. Several contradicting theories exist regarding the proper assay mediums for enzymes. This whole section spells confusion unless the clinical chemist takes the time to understand the basics of enzymology and test each kit to insure zero-order kinetics (a reaction solely dependent on enzyme concentration) is being achieved in his laboratory.

CREATINE KINASE (CK)

ADENOSINE TRIPHOSPHATE: CREATINE N-PHOSPHOTRANSFERASE

EC 2.7.3.2.

Creatine kinase catalyzes the reversible reaction:

$$\text{creatine} + \text{ATP} \underset{\substack{\text{Mg}^{++} \\ \text{pH6.7}}}{\overset{\substack{\text{pH9.0} \\ \text{CK}}}{\rightleftharpoons}} \text{creatine phosphate} + \text{ADP}$$

The equilibrium is dependent upon pH and the reverse reaction occurs faster than the forward reaction. CK is found in a variety of tissues, predominantly in skeletal tissue, myocardial tissue, and nervous tissue, but also in the prostate, thyroid, kidney, and intestine. CK is a dimer composed of subunits M and B. CK_1 or BB, is found primarily in nervous tissue; the hybrid, CK_2 or MB, is found primarily in myocardial muscle and CK_3 or MM is found in skeletal muscle. CK_1 moves fastest toward the anode.

Serum for CK analysis should be stored at 0-5°C if the assay cannot be done immediately. The enzyme deactivation is thought to be due to the unfolding of the enzyme structure. The addition of thiol compounds to the assay medium appears to restore the lost activity. Popular thiol compounds are N-acetylcysteine, 2-mercaptoethanol, and 1-thioglycerol.

Creatine kinase was first used in the diagnosis of muscular dystrophies and other myopathies. But the electro phoretic separation of CK isoenzymes has popularized the use of CK-2 (MB) as an indicator of myocardial damage. The presence of CK-2 in concentrations greater than 6% and 10 U/L usually indicates a damaged myocardium. CK-2 appears 4-6 hours after chest pain and peaks at 18-24 hours. CK-2 is seen in these non-cardiac diseases: muscular dystrophies, severe skeletal muscle trauma, Reye's Syndrome, and polymyosites. CK-2 is also seen in post-open heart surgery patients, carbon monoxide poisoning, myocarditis, and coronary insufficiency. It would seem then, that the presence of CK-2 is not enough to diagnose myocardial infarction, but when combined with a flipped $LD_1 > LD_2$ the specificity increases. It is this author's experience that the most important use of CK_2 is to show that it does not appear within 48 hours, thus ruling out myocardial infarction.

CK_3 (MM) is most abundant in skeletal muscle and normal serum contains 100% CK_3 (MM). CK_1 (BB) rarely is seen in serum. It is an enzyme that does not cross the blood brain barrier. CK_1 has been seen following central nervous system surgery, breakage of blood-brain barrier, malignant hyperpyrexia, bowel infarctions, and some types of malignant tumors.

REFERENCE RANGE

Males: 12-65 U/1 at 30°C
Females: 10-50 U/1 at 30°C

CONDITIONS ASSOCIATED WITH ABNORMAL CREATINE KINASE

ELEVATED

Myocardial infarction
Polymyositis
Crush injuries
Muscular dystrophy
Cerebral infarctions
Delirium tremens
Hepatic coma (effects on other tissues)

CONDITIONS WHERE CK IS WITHIN THE REFERENCE RANGE

Acute hepatitis
Obstructive jaundice
Hemolytic anemias

ARTIFICIAL ELEVATIONS

Frequent IM injections
Following brief periods of exercise
Pregnancy (baby's kicking)

LACTATE DEHYDROGENASE (LD)

L-lactate: NAD oxidoreductase

EC 1.1.1.27

Lactate dehydrogenase catalyzes the reversible oxidation of lactate to pyruvate:

$$\text{Lactate} + \text{NAD}^+ \underset{\text{pH } 7.4-7.8}{\overset{\substack{\text{pH } 8.8-9.8 \\ \text{LD}}}{\rightleftharpoons}} \text{Pyruvate} + \text{NADH} + \text{H}^+$$

TABLE 6

SUMMARY OF LACTATE DEHYDROGENASE ASSAYS

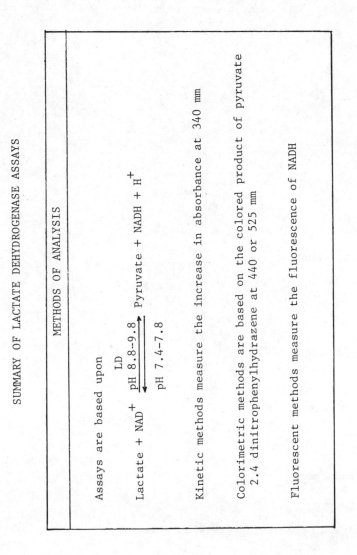

METHODS OF ANALYSIS

Assays are based upon

$$\text{Lactate} + NAD^+ \underset{\text{pH } 7.4-7.8}{\overset{\text{LD} \quad \text{pH } 8.8-9.8}{\rightleftharpoons}} \text{Pyruvate} + NADH + H^+$$

Kinetic methods measure the increase in absorbance at 340 mm

Colorimetric methods are based on the colored product of pyruvate
2.4 dinitrophenylhydrazene at 440 or 525 mm

Fluorescent methods measure the fluorescence of NADH

TABLE 6 (continued)

SUMMARY OF LACTATE DEHYDROGENASE ASSAYS

ISOENZYME	SPECIMEN OF CHOICE: STORAGE	COFACTORS	INHIBITORS
LD is a tetramer	SERUM	NAD	Mercuric ions
LD (HHHH) heart kidney	Conflicting date for storage	Postulated need for zinc	p-chloromer-curibenzoate
LD_2 (HHHM)	Room temperatures for up to 10 days		
LD_3 (HHMM) spleen leukocytes	Some suggest 4°C for up to 4 weeks		borate
			oxalate
			EDTA
			urea
LD_4 (HMMM) liver skeletal muscle			
LD_5 (MMMM) liver skeletal muscle			

(Electrophoretic mobility: ANODE — MOBILITY — ELECTROPHORETIC — CATHODE)

TECHNICAL NOTES FOR ASSAYS

HEMOLYSIS

RBC contains up to 150 times more LD than serum.

TURBID OR ICTERIC SERA

May have to be assayed on dilution to produce an initial absorbance acceptable for the assay reaction.

The total activity of LD in serum is very non-specific. All human tissues contain LD. The specificity of LD is enhanced when the five isoenzymes of lactate dehydrogenase are electrophoretically fractionated. Each of the five isoenzymes are considered tetramers containing various combinations of two subunits, M and H. The H type is found primarily in aerobic tissues such as myocardial tissue and erythrocytes, where the accumulation of lactate cannot be allowed. Conversely, the M subunit is found predominantly in anaerobically metabolic tissues such as skeletal muscle. The isoenzymes of LD are as follows: LD_1 (HHHH or H_4) LD_2 (HHHM or H_3M) LD_3 (HHMM or H_2M_2) LD_4 (HMMM or H_1M_3) LD 5 (MMMM or M4). LD_1 possesses the fastest mobility towards the anode.

The LD isoenzymes are currently used in the diagnosis of myocardial infarctions. In myocardial infarction LD_1 and LD_2 will show the greatest elevations. Normally, LD_2 is found in greater concentration than LD_1. Following myocardial infarctions, LD_1 rises higher than LD_2 resulting in a "flipped LD pattern" with $LD_1 > LD_2$. The presence of CK-MB and a flipped LD are considered laboratory evidence of myocardial damage. Eighty percent of myocardial infarction patients will show flipped LD ($LD_1 > LD_2$) 48 hours after the onset of the infarction. Care must be taken to avoid hemolysis of serum for LD isoenzymes because hemolysis associated with both in vivo causes (prosthetic heart values, hemolytic anemia, and pernicious anemia) and in vivo causes (difficulty in venipuncture, prolonged contact of serum with the clot) can show a flipped $LD_1 > LD_2$ isoenzyme pattern.

Total lactate dehydrogenase measurement is done in fluid other than serum but its usefulness is suspect. Total LD is elevated greated than 50 U/L in cerebrospinal fluid in patients with subarachnoid hemorrhage and cerebrovascular thrombosis and hemorrhage. Bacterial meningitis may show an elevated total LD, whereas viral meningitis does not. LD may be helpful in other fluid analyses. Transudates show a total LD less than 550 U/L whereas exudates show greater levels. A pleural fluid with a markedly elevated LD is consistent with neoplastic involvement of the pleura.

REFERENCE RANGE

Total LD: 95-200 U/L at 30°C (Pyruvate → Lactate)

LD_1 25-31% of total
LD_2 38-35% of total
LD_3 17-22% of total
LD_4 5-8% of total
LD_5 3-6% of total
C_sf total LD: 7-30 U/L at 30°C (P→L)

DISEASES ASSOCIATED WITH ABNORMAL LD

ELEVATIONS

Myocardial infarction
Hepatitis
Cirrhosis
Infectious mononucleosis
Obstructive jaundice
Hemolytic anemias
Pulmonary infarction
Congestive heart failure
Muscular dystrophy

AMINOTRANSFERASES
Aspartate Aminotransferase (AST)
Glutamate Oxalacetate Transaminase (SGOT)
EC 2.6.1.1

Alanine Aminotransferase (ALT)
Glutamate Pyruvate Transaminase (SGPT)
EC 2.6.1.2

The aminotransferases catalyze the interconversion of amino acids and α oxoacids by transferring amine groups. The specificity of the enzyme results from the amino acid which serves as the donor of an amine group. Pyridoxal-5'-phosphate serves as a cofactor for both enzymes accepting the amine group and transferring it to the resulting product. The aminotransferases are found in serum, bile, Csf and saliva, also in heart, liver, skeletal muscle, kidney, pancreas, spleen, lung, and erythrocyte tissues.

Aspartate Aminotransferase (AST)

Aspartate Aminotranferase Catalyzes

$$\text{L-aspartate} + \alpha\text{-oxoglutarate} \underset{\text{P-5-P}}{\overset{\text{AST}}{\rightleftharpoons}} \text{oxalacetate} + \text{L-glutamate}$$

AST is found in many tissues: cardiac, hepatic, skeletal muscle, kidney, brain, pancreas, spleen, and lung. Diseases associated with any of these tissues result in elevations of AST.

For many years AST has been used in the diagnosis of acute myocardial infarction. Elevated AST usually begins to rise 10-12 hours after an infarction, peaking by 48 hours. The current use of creatine kinase and LD totals and isoenzymes have made AST a redundant enzyme and many hospitals have discontinued its use as a "cardiac enzyme".

REFERENCE RANGE

(without P-5-P activation) 6-25 U/L at 30°C
(with P-5-P activation)   12-29 U/L at 30°C

Alanine Aminstransferase

Alanine aminstransferase catalyzes:

$$\text{L-alanine} + \alpha\text{-oxoglutarate} \underset{\text{P-5-P}}{\overset{\text{ALT}}{\rightleftharpoons}} \text{pyruvate} + \text{L-glutamate}$$

ALT is found in the same tissues as is AST. However, ALT's higher concentration in hepatic tissue than in myocardial tissue has led to its use as a hepatic enzyme. In liver diseases, ALT appears to be less sensitive than AST because more extensive damage to liver tissue must occur before ALT aises. Slight elevations of alanine aminotransferase are seen in myocardial infarctions. The ratio of AST/ALT has been used to add greater differential diagnostic force to the measurement of both enzymes rather than relying on just AST. The ratio AST/ALT is particularly helpful when the activity of both enzymes is less than 500 units.

TABLE 7

SUMMARY OF ALT/AST ASSAYS

METHODS OF ANALYSIS

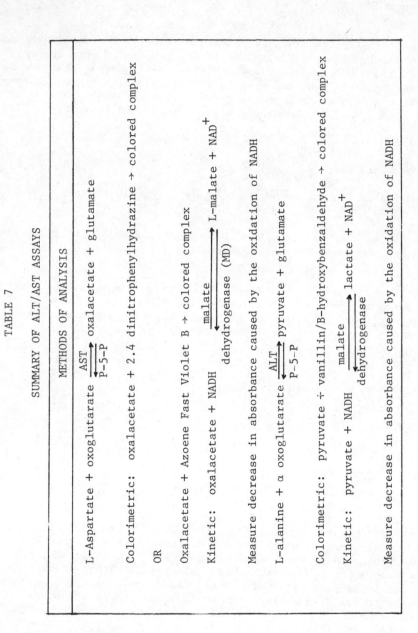

L-Aspartate + oxoglutarate $\xrightleftharpoons[P-5-P]{AST}$ oxalacetate + glutamate

Colorimetric: oxalacetate + 2.4 dinitrophenylhydrazine → colored complex

OR

Oxalacetate + Azoene Fast Violet B → colored complex

Kinetic: oxalacetate + NADH $\xrightleftharpoons[\text{dehydrogenase (MD)}]{\text{malate}}$ L—malate + NAD$^+$

Measure decrease in absorbance caused by the oxidation of NADH

L-alanine + α oxoglutarate $\xrightleftharpoons[P-5-P]{ALT}$ pyruvate + glutamate

Colorimetric: pyruvate + vanillin/β-hydroxybenzaldehyde → colored complex

Kinetic: pyruvate + NADH $\xrightleftharpoons[\text{dehydrogenase}]{\text{malate}}$ lactate + NAD$^+$

Measure decrease in absorbance caused by the oxidation of NADH

TABLE 7 (continued)

SPECIMEN OF CHOICE	COFACTORS	INHIBITORS
SERUM	Pyridoxal-5'-phosphate	Mercury
STORAGE	(P-5'-P)	Cyanide
4°C for 1-3 days		
Frozen for longer periods		

TECHNICAL NOTES FOR ASSAYS

1. Side reactions occasionally occur at an elevated rate. Patients with parenchymal liver disease show elevated glutamate dehydrogenase which consumes oxoglutarate and NADH if ammonia is present.

2. Hemolysis must be avoided. RBC contain 10-15 times more transaminases than serum.

3. Turbid or icteric sera must be run on dilution or against a dichromate blank.

AST/ALT ratio and some hepatic—biliary diseases:

	RATIO
Acute hepatic neurosis	<1
Intrahepatic cholestasis	<1
Infectious mononucleosis	<1
Acute epidemic hepatitis	<1
Extra hepatic obstruction	>1
Cirrhosis	>1
Metastatic carcinoma	>1
Myocardial infarction	>1
Progressive muscular dystrophy	>1

REFERENCE RANGE: 6-21 U/L at 30°C

CONDITIONS ASSOCIATED WITH ABNORMAL AST AND ALT

ELEVATIONS

Hepatitis
Infectious mononucleosis
Cirrhosis
Obstructive jaundice
Crush injuries
Myocardial infarctions
Pulmonary infarction
Cerebral infarction
Toxemia of pregnancy
Drugs: salicylates in large doses; opiates

DEPRESSED

Pregnancy and renal dialysis patients

ALKALINE PHOSPHATASE (ALP)

Orthophosphoric acid monoester phosphohydrolase
EC 3.13.1

Acid Phosphatase (ACP)

Orthophosphoric acid monoester phosphohydrolase
EC 3.1.3.2

The phosphatases hydrolyze organic phosphate esters with the formation of an alcohol and a phosphate ion.

$$
\begin{array}{cc}
& \text{ALP } \{OH^-\} \\
O & \text{ACP } \{H^+\} \qquad\qquad\qquad O \\
\| & \qquad\qquad\qquad\qquad\qquad \| \\
R - O - P - OH \rightleftharpoons R\text{-}OH + HO - P - OH \\
| \qquad\qquad\qquad\qquad\qquad\qquad | \\
OH \quad \pm H_2O \qquad\qquad\qquad OH
\end{array}
$$

There are two types of phosphatases: alkaline phosphatase which has pH optimum of 8-10.2; and acid phosphatase with optimal activity at pH 4-7.

Alkaline Phosphatase

Alkaline phosphatase is a non-specific enzyme that hydrolyzes phosphate esters in an alkaline medium. ALP is inert in serum and is also found in urine, feces, lymph, sweat, and breast milk. The liver, bones, and intestines are the organs associated with the enzyme. Its body function is not well understood, but the enzyme is found at the cell membrane and is believed to aid in the transfer of metabolites across cell walls. It is produced by osteoblasts and other cells of the bone, by cholangiola epithelium, intestinal mucosa, human placenta, and certain cancerous tissues.

Alkaline phosphatase is a nonspecific enzyme which is elevated in a variety of disorders. It is useful in evaluation of calcium and phosphate metabolism, metabolic bone diseases, space occupying lesions of the liver, and obstruction of the biliary system.

Eight or more isoenzymes have been identified but rarely are more than 3-4 found in one individual. Electrophoretic migration occurs anode to cathode: liver-bone-intestine-placental-regan. Regan is an isoenzyme found in many patients with cancer. Alkaline phosphatase isoenzymes have been separated by inhibition techniques. The heat-fractionated alkaline phosphatase test is based on the heat lability of the bone isoenzyme. Serum is heated at 56°C for 15 minutes and then assayed for the enzyme. If more than 30% activity remains after heating, the elevation was thought to be liver alkaline phosphatase. If less than 20% activity remained, it was thought to be of bone origin. Normals have 15-30% remaining. Intestinal alkaline phosphatase also has beat stability and interferes with the test. Many laboratories are replacing this test with gamma glutamyltransferase which is elevated in liver disease but not in bone disorders.

Artificial alteration of alkaline phosphatase activity is seen in newborns and prepubertal individuals where skeletal alkaline phosphatase is elevated. Pregnancy, especially during the last trimester, artificially elevates the ALP. ALP is lowest in the fasting state, rising slightly in the post-prandial individual.

REFERENCE RANGE: 30-105 IU/L

CONDITIONS ASSOCIATED WITH ABNORMAL ALP

ELEVATED ALP

    Hepatobiliary

        Obstructive jaundice
        Biliary fibrosis
        Space occupying lesions
        Viral hepatitis
        Intrahepatic cholestasis
        Infectious mononucleosis

    Bone

        Paget's disease

    Rickets

    Osteomalacia

       Hyperparathyroidism
       Metastatic Bone Disease
       Fractures

DEPRESSED ALP

     Cretinism
     Malnutrition
     Metabolic Disease Hypophosphatasia
       (autosomal recessive tract with skeletal deformities caused by impaired
       mineralization of bone)

The methodologies used for ALP measurements are summarized in Table 4.

Acid Phosphatase

    Acid phosphatase hydrolyzes phosphate esters in an acid medium. It is an extremely labile enzyme in serum which has a pH 7.3. Serum for ACP analysis must be preserved with a citrate tablet to lower the pH to 5.0 in order to stabilize the enzyme. ACP is found in the prostate gland, liver, muscle, RBC, platelets, kidneys, spleen, and stomach tissue. Semen is also rich in ACP and acid phosphatase determination on vaginal washings are frequently done in suspected rape cases.

    Clinically, ACP is useful in the diagnosis of metastasized prostatic carcinoma. The prostatic isoenzyme is elevated in prostatic carcinoma with metastasis and is not in other disorders that clinically resemble prostatic carcinoma. ACP is also useful in monitoring therapy.

    The isoenzymes of acid phosphatase are not clinically useful. Specimen source and pH of electrophoresis buffers make the assay too variant. Historically, the significant distinction needed is that between prostatic ACP and all other forms. The chemical L-tartrate inhibits prostatic acid phosphatase and not the other forms. Recently, the use of thymolphthalein monophosphate as a "specific" substrate for prostatic acid phosphatase has gained acceptance.

REFERENCE VALUES: 2.5–11.7 U/L

CONDITIONS ASSOCIATED WITH ABNORMAL ACP

ELEVATIONS

    Prostatic ACP

       Prostatic carcinoma with metastases

    Total ACP

       Gaucher's disease
       Nieman-Pick's disease
       Myelocytic leukemia
       Viral hepatitis
       Hyperparathyroidism and multiple myeloma with bone involvement
       Malignant invasions of bone

TABLE 8

PHOSPHATASES: ALKALINE PHOSPHATASE (ALP)/ACID PHOSPHATASE (ACP)

METHODS OF ANALYSIS	SPECIMEN OF CHOICE	COFACTOR	INHIBITORS
BESSY/LOWRY/BROCK P-nitrophenylphosphate $\xrightarrow[\text{Mg}^{++}]{\text{ALP}}$ p-nitrophenol (yellow product) pH 10.3 P-nitrophenylphosphate $\xrightarrow[\text{pH 4.8}]{\text{ACP}}$ p-nitrophenol	Serum of heparinized plasma STORAGE ALP may increase in activity if left in a warm room. ACP is extremely unstable and must be stabilized using disodium citrate within one hour of serum separation	Magnesium	Calcium Phosphate ions Oxalate EDTA Citrate Ammonium hydroxide Borate fluoride
KING/ARMSTRONG phenylphosphate $\xrightarrow[\text{pH 9.6}]{\text{ALP}}$ phenol + phosphate ion phenylphosphate $\xrightarrow[\text{5.0}]{\text{ACP}}$ phenol + phosphate ion phenol + antipyrine → colored complex Reported as a King-Armstrong unit which is defined as the milligrams of phenol liberated by 100 ml of serum under the conditions of the assay.	TECHNICAL NOTES FOR ASSAYS 1. RBC contains large amounts of ACP and hemolyzed sera should be avoided. 2. Control sera containing acid phosphatase should also be stabilized with citrate. The use of diluents to produce clinical significant CO_2 values produces an alkaline medium in which ACP is extremely labile. 3. Reported that palpation of prostate during exam causes elevated ACP results.		
BODANSKY METHOD Glycerophosphate $\xrightarrow[\text{pH 5.0}]{\text{ACP}}$ phosphate + glycerol Glycerophosphate $\xrightarrow[\text{pH 8.8}]{\text{ALP}}$ phosphate + glycerol Measure amount of phosphate Reported as a Bodansky unit which is defined as the amount of ACP which will liberate 1 mg of phosphorus/dl under the conditions of the assay.			

The methodologies used for the measurement of acid phosphatase are the same as those used for alkaline phosphatase except an acid medium is used and tartrate is added to differentiate between total and prostatic acid phosphatase. Thymolphthalein monophosphate is used for prostatic acid phosphatase and is summarized with the other methods in Table 4.

5' NUCLEOTIDASE (5'N)
5' RIBONUCLEOTIDE PHOSPHOHYDROLASE
EC 3.1.3.5

5' Nucleotidase hydrolyzes nucleoside 5'-phosphates (AMP, ademylic acid) releasing inorganic phosphate. The enzyme is principally found in the bile duct epithelium and any disease process that results in bile flow obstructions will raise serum 5'N levels. 5N is sometimes used to differentiate obstructive jaundice (↑ALP, ↑↑5N) from hepto-cellular jaundice (ALP↑ , 5N normal-sl↑), and hepotobiliary (↑ALK, ↑5N) from osseous disease (↑ALK, Normal 5'N).

LIPASE

Lipase works at the surface of emulsified fats and the aqueous phase. Its activity is dependent on the amount of exposed surface area of fats and the presence of bile salts. Lipase is found in the pancreas, stomach, intestine, white blood cells, fat cells, and milk. Pancreatic lipase must be differentiated from other related, but distinct enzymes (carboxylic ester hydrolase EC 3.1.1.1., aryl-ester hydrolate EC 3.1.1.2, and lipoprotein lipase EC 3.1.1.34) to insure strict specificity in lipase assays.

The complexity of lipase measurements make it a less popular test than amylase. Lipase rises more slowly than amylase levels in acute pancreatitis, usually peaking by the fourth day after onset. Lipase is less sensitive than amylase but provides a confirmatory role when positive. A normal lipase with an elevated amylase suggests salivary gland involvement and an elevated lipase in a patient with the mumps strongly suggests pancreatic involvement.

REFERENCE RANGE: 28-280 U/L

CONDITIONS ASSOCIATED WITH ABNORMAL LIPASE VALUES   (have same clinical significance as amylase)

ELEVATED

    Acute pancreatitis
    Perforated duodenal ulcers
    Intestinal obstruction
    Acute cholecystitis
    Cirrhosis
    Multiple sclerosis
    Renal insufficiency (spurious elevations)

AMYLASE

    α 1,4,-glucan-4-glucanohydrolase, E.C.3.2.1.1.

Amylase is a hydrolytic enzyme which catalyzes the splitting of polysaccharides with an α 1.4 glucoside link such as amylase, amylopectin, and glycogen. Amylase is found in liver, kidney, and muscle. However, the most important sources are the

TABLE 9

SUMMARY OF LIPASE ASSAYS

METHODS OF ANALYSIS	SPECIMEN OF CHOICE	COFACTOR	INHIBITORS
	Serum	Activated by bile salts, ionized calcium	Hemoglobin Quinine Heavy metals
TURBIDIMETRIC Emulsions of fat lipase free fatty acids (triglyceride) Measurement: as the lipase hydrolyzes the micelles of fat, the milk substrate solution clears, thus the change in turbidity can be related to enzyme activity.	STORAGE Relatively stable, 3 weeks at 4°C. Bacterial contamination results in increase of lipase activity.		
CHERRY AND CRANDALL 50% emulsion olive oil lipase free fatty acid pH 7.0 Measurement: titration of fatty acid with NaOH, using phenolphthalein	TECHNICAL NOTES FOR ASSAYS 1. Care must be taken to prepare a substrate of reproducible, stable emulsions from lot to lot.		

pancreas and salivary glands. The pancreas and salivary glands provide most of the normal serum amylase. Amylase is synthesized in the endoplasmic reticulum of acinar cells. There is no known function of α-amylase in serum.

Elevated α-amylase values usually mean one of two things: (1) there has been a pancreatic ductal obstruction with continued acinar cell production of the enzyme and (2) there has been disruption of the acinar cells and ductal apparatus. Acute pancreatitis is usually indicated by abdominal pain and α-amylase is an important laboratory test in these situations. Many times, a normal amylase rules out pancreatitis. However, massive hemmorhagic pancreatic necrosis and chronic pancreatitis result in almost total acinar cell destruction so that no amylase is produced.

Amylase is cleared by the kidneys at a rate of 3 ml/hr. Urine amylase may be more helpful when serum levels are normal or equivocally elevated. The urine amylase rises before serum and remains elevated longer. Amylase/creatinine ratio is sometimes used to "correct" amylase excretion when renal function is impaired. One serum and one urine collection is required, and both must be assayed for amylase and creatinine. The amylase/creatinine ratio is determined by the following formula:

$$\text{AMS/creat ratio (\%)} = \frac{\text{urine amylase}}{\text{serum amylase}} \times \frac{\text{serum creatinine}}{\text{urine creatinine}} \times 100.$$ Normal ratios are

2-3%. The ratio is elevated in acute pancreatitis and depressed in renal insufficiency. An elevated serum amylase and depressed amylase/creatinine ratio suggests macroamylasemia. Amylase sometimes binds to proteins, especially globulin, forming a complex too large to be filtered by the glomerulus. Clinically, patients with macroamylasemia show no symptoms.

At least seven amylase isoenzymes have been identified but as of yet little use has been found for their routine separation.

REFERENCE RANGE: 60-180 SOMOGYI UNITS

CONDITIONS ASSOCIATED WITH ABNORMAL AMYLASE VALUES

ELEVATION

    Acute pancreatitis
    Carcinoma of the head of the pancreas
    Perforation of gastric ulcer
    Mumps
    Acute injury to spleen
    Renal disease with impaired renal function
    Drugs: morphine, codeine, meperidine

DEPRESSIONS

    Cirrhosis of liver
    Carcinoma of liver
    Abscess of liver
    Hepatitis
    Acute alcoholism
    Toxemia of pregnancy
    Administration of glucose will lower the serum amylase

The methodologies used for the measure of α-amylase are summarized in Table 6.

TABLE 10

SUMMARY OF α-AMYLASE ASSAYS

METHODS OF ANALYSIS	SPECIMEN OF CHOICE	COFACTORS
ENZYMATIC	Serum	Chloride
Starch $\xrightarrow{\text{amylase}}$ maltose and glucose	Urine, duodenal aspirate	Ions
Maltose $\xrightarrow{\alpha\text{-glucosidase}}$ 2-glucose	STORAGE 4°C	Calcium
Glucose + O_2 $\xrightarrow{\text{glucose oxidase}}$ gluconolactone + H_2O_2 measure consumption of O_2		
SACCHAROGENIC (measure reducing substances formed)		
Starch $\xrightarrow{\text{amylase}}$ maltose + glucose (potato, corn)		
DYE-LABELED (split products form colored water soluble complex)	TECHNICAL NOTES FOR ASSAYS	
Amylose or Amylopectin $\xrightarrow[\text{bound to dye}]{\text{amylase}}$ colored reaction	1. Urine specimen should be timed: 2, 4, 6, 24 hour specimens.	
AMYLOCLASTIC (measure decrease in substrate)		
Chronometric: time required to completely hydrolyze all the starch present in the assay.		
Amylometric: measure starch remaining after a certain increment of time. Iodine is reduced by starch to form a colored complex.		

ALDOLASE (ALS)

D-fructase-1.6-diphosphate

EC 4.1.2.13

Aldolase catalyzes the splitting of fructase 1.6-diphosphate to glyceraldehyde-3-phosphate and dihydroxyacetone phosphate. Aldolase is found in all cells of the body with highest concentrations in skeletal muscle. Erythrocytes contain an abundance of this enzyme and hemolysis must be avoided.

Methods of analysis for aldolase are based on the rate of product of the trioses glyceraldehyde-3-phosphate and dehydroxyacetone phosphate and the resultant compounds react with dinitrophenylhydrazone. Primarily, aldolase is used in the study of muscle disease; aldolase and creatine kinase levels will rise before overt clinical symptoms appear. Muscle aldolase has virtually 100% specificity for fructose 1.6 diphosphate and none for fructose 1-phosphate while liver aldolase is equally active against both. Distinction can be made between the two; and if it is not, then aldolase values can be confusing in the patient with liver damage.

REFERENCE RANGE: 1.0-7.5 U/L at 30°C

CONDITIONS ASSOCIATED WITH ABNORMAL RESULTS

ELEVATED

    Skeletal muscle diseases

        Muscular dystrophy
        Multiple sclerosis

    Carcinomatosis
    Crush injuries
    Granulocytic leukemia
    Hepatitis
    Lead intoxication

CHOLINESTERASE

ACYLOCHOLINE ACYL-HYDROLASE

EC 3.1.1.8

Plasma cholinesterase hydrolyzes acetylcholine. Acetylcholine is produced at nerve endings and helps to transmit nerve impulses. Cholinesterase destroys acetylcholine so that additional impulses may be sent. There are two enzymes with this "cholinesterase" activity: pseudocholinesterase (EC.3.1.1.8) which is found in the liver, pancreas, heart, white matter of the brain, and serum; and red cell cholinesterase (EC 3.1.1.7) which is found in the erythrocytes, spleen, grey matter of the brain, and nerve cell endings.

There are clinical situations where cholinesterase activity is significant. Succinyldicholine (Suxa methonium) used in surgery is hydrolyzed by cholinesterase. Patients with low cholinesterase levels cannot quickly metabolize the drug and

COLLATION OF LABORATORY DATA FROM PATIENT WITH MYOCARDIAL DAMAGE

	CK (150 IU/L)	AST (40 mU/ml)	ALT (37 IU/L)	LD (225 mU/ml)	CK ISOENZYMES	INTERPRETATION	LD	INTERPRETATION
Upper limits of Normal								
Admission	60	25	15	120	ALB CK-3	Normal	LD1 2 3 4 5	Normal
Admission plus 8 hours	1620	220	25	510	CK-2 ALB CK-3	15% CK-2 85% CK-3		CK-2 present, LD2>LD1
Admission plus 24 hours	1279	190	30	950	ALB CK-2 CK-3	5% CK-2 95% CK-3		LD1>LD2 with positive CK2 lab. evidence of myocardia infarction
Admission plus 48 hours	428	100	40	865	ALB CK-3	Elevation of CK-3 only		LD1>LD2 still "flipped"

FIGURE 7

experience a prolonged period of apnea in recovery. Dibucaine or fluoride numbers are usually measured and they are the percent inhibition of cholinesterase experienced in the presence of these compounds. Organic insecticides such as Parathion, Sarin, and tetraethyl pyrophosphate in toxic amounts can inhibit red cell cholinesterase to a point where death results.

REFERENCE RANGE: 2.2-5.0 U/ml at 25°C.

DIAGNOSTIC APPLICATIONS OF ENZYMES

Changes in the enzymes creatine kinase and lactate dehydrogenase isoenzymes and total enzymatic activity are the most helpful laboratory tests in the diagnosis of myscardial infarction. Careful observation of Figure 7 shows that the CK rises 4-6 hours post myocardial infarction (MI), peaks at 24-36 hours and returns to normal in 2-4 days.

The LD rises 12-24 hours post MI, peaks at 3-5 days, and returns to normal in 12-14 days.

The AST rises 6-12 hours post MI, peaks at 24-48 hours, and returns to normal in 4-7 days.

The ALT remains essentially normal.

The isoenzyme pattern for CK shows the appearance of CK-2 (MB) at a percentage greater than 6% and a quantitative value greater than 10 IU/L. The later "flipping" of LD_1 and LD_2 further documents a MI. The LD_5 elevation is probably due to liver congestion brought about by poor blood flow which is secondary to the MI. As the blood flow returns to normal this congestion clears and LD_5 diminishes.

Diseases and their associated liver enzyme alterations are summarized in Figure 8. Diseases which damage hepatocytes tend to show striking elevations in AST and ALT, with greater ALT than AST values. Characteristically LD_4 and LD_5 are elevated in LD isoenzyme patterns of these patients. When intra-hepatic cholestasis occurs, ALP shows marked elevations. GGT is a sensitive marker for both biliary tree obstructions and liver neophasms. In cirrhosis one would expect to see the characteristic beta-gamma bridging on protein electrophoresis.

Hepatitis is a viral disease which affects the liver. It is caused by viral agents (such as Eptein-Barr virus, cytomegalovirus, adenovirus, and the entecovirus), hepatitis A virus, hepatitis B virus, and other agents which to date are referred to as NonA, NonB hepatitis. Hepatitis A (HAV, hepatitis A virus) or infectious hepatitis is spread by oral or parenteral infection, usually by contaminated food or water. The hepatitis A virus (HAV) is found in the blood between 4-6 weeks, during the icteric

FIGURE 8

ENZYME CASE STUDIES IN LIVER DISEASES

	TOTAL PROTEIN 6.0–8.0 g/dl	ALBUMIN 3.5–5.0 g/dl	BILI 0.2–1.0 mg/dl	ALP 30–105 mU/ml	LD 100–225 mU/ml	AST 8–40 mU/ml	ALT 6–21 30°C U/L	GGT 8–37 30°C U/L	5N 2–17 37°C U/ml
VIRAL HEPATITIS	8.4	3.8	5.9	149	585	621	357	71	25
BILIARY OBSTRUCTION	6.2	3.8	3.1	192	156	78	65	314	28
GILBERT'S DISEASE	6.5	4.0	4.2 (direct–0.2 indirect–4.0)	55	21	21	10	14	10
HEAPTITIS (anicteric)	8.1	3.8	0.9	300	410	610	310	45	35
TUMOR SPACE OCCUPYING	7.5	3.6	0.6	375	390	76	48	681	25

IgG anti-HAV peaks at 10-12 weeks then declines. The presence of IgM HAV INDI-
CATES AN ACTIVE INFECTION WHEREAS IgG HAV INDICATES A PREVIOUS EXPOSURE TO THE HEPATI-
TIS A VIRUS.

The hepatitis B virus (or serum hepatitis) is associated with hepatitis acquired
through the contact with blood components. Laboratory personnel are forever conscious
of serum spillage and aerosols that can spread the hepatitis B virus. The incubation
period of hepatitis B is 50-150 days and infection is usually parenteral. There are a
number of antigenically related components in hepatitis B: surface antigen (HB_sAg);
core antigen (Hb_cAg); E antigen (HB_eAg) and the complete infectious virus (HB virus
previously known as the Dane Particle). The HB_sAg appears transiently in the serum
with the components appearing:

COMPONENT	APPEARS	PEAKS
HB_sAg	7-16 weeks	9 weeks
anti-HBc	9 + weeks	20-24 weeks
anti-HBs	20 + weeks	26-30 weeks
HbcAg	8-16 weeks	

The persistance of HBsAg indicates a carrier state. The appearance of anti-Hbc
correlate well with a complete immune response.

Hepatitis antigens and antibodies are measured by radioimmunoassay (coated beads,
third generation testings where two antibodies are used), hemagglutination, hemagglutination inhibition, or immunoelectrophoresis.

Bilirubin

Bilirubin is the waste produce of hemoglobin. After 120 days, red blood cells are
taken from the peripheral circulation. The reticuloendothial cells of the spleen,
liver and bone marrow separate the hemoglobin from the red cells and enzymes (containing heme) into a heme portion containing iron and a globin portion. The globin
is returned to the amino acid pool; the heme portion, a porphyrin complex, is broken
down releasing the iron to the total body iron stores and converting the remaining
portion to bilirubin. Bilirubin enters the peripheral circulation where it is bound
to albumin. This form of bilirubin is called the unconjugated or indirect bilirubin--
it is water insoluble, alcohol soluble.

Once at the cellular membrane of a hepatocyte, the bilirubin molecule enters the
cell. Failure of this transport mechanism is referred to as Gilbert's disease. Once
inside the hepatocyte, bilirubin is combined with glucuronic acid to form bilirubin
diglucuronide. Faulty conjugation here is referred to as Crigler-Najjar Disease:--
(hyperbilirubinemia in newborns results from the immaturity of the enzyme system
that results in the conjugation of bilirubin at this step.) Bilirubin diglucuronide
is called conjugated or direct bilirubin; it is water soluble which makes it suitable
for excretion.

Once conjugated, the bilirubin is transported to the bile canaliculi where it
passes into the intestines. Faulty transport at this level is called Dubin-Johnson
disease. Bacteria in the small intestine break down the bilirubin to urobilinogen.
Some of the urobilinogen is reabsorbed into the blood stream and is carried back to
the liver where it is either oxidized back to bilirubin, re-excreted, or excreted by
the kidneys. The urobilinogen that remains in the intestines becomes urobilin when
exposed to light.

Disorders in bilirubin metabolism occur when (1) there are increases in bilirubin production (hemolytic anemia); (2) hepatic cells are damaged and cannot process bilirubin (viral hepatitis, toxic hepatitis, cirrhosis, or by drugs such as chlorpromozine and organic arsenicals; or (3) a blockage of the excretion route of bilirubin (carcinoma in biliary free). Each disorder has either an elevation of direct, indirect, or both forms of bilirubin.

SUMMARY OF ELEVATIONS OF DIRECT AND INDIRECT BILIRUBIN AS REALTED TO DISEASE STATES
ELEVATIONS OF INDIRECT BILIRUBIN

Hemolytic States: excessive amount of bilirubin that the liver cannot completely process

Gilbert's Disease: defective transport from plasma to hepatocyte

Crigler-Najjar Disease: inability to conjugate bilirubin (neonates express a lack of the enzyme required for this conjugation step and show a jaundice early in life similar to Crigler-Najjar Disease

ELEVATIONS OF DIRECT BILIRUBIN

Primary hepatocellular damage (viral hepatitis, toxic hepatitis, alcoholic hepatitis, cirrhosis: hepatocytes lose their ability to remove bilirubin from plasma. Both direct and indirect are elevated in near equal amounts

Dubin-Johnson Disease: defective transport of direct bilirulin from hepatocyte to the bile canaliculus

Obstructions to Biliary Tree (stores, carcinoma, choledocholithiosis): bilirubin cannot pass into the bile and eventually backs up into serum

There are three widespread methods of analysis for bilirubin: Jendrassik and Grof, Evelyn-Malloy, and spectrophotometry.

JENDRASSIK-GROF

The Jendrassik-Grof adaptation for the Technicon continous flow instrument dilutes the serum with sodium acetate and caffeine-sodium benzoate before the addition of diazo reagent (sodium nitrate and sulfanilic acid), ascorbic acid, and tartrate buffer. A blank channel is included which contains all the reagents except the diazo. The absorbance is read at 600 nm.

EVELYN-MALLOY

Bilirubin is coupled with diazo reagent (sodium nitrate and sulfanilic). In the Jendrassik-Groff procedure alkaline tartrate is added to produce a purple color. The Evelyn-Malloy method measures the purple color initially formed by the reaction of diazo and bilirubin. Direct bilirubin is water soluble and reacts within one minute with the diazo.

Methanol is then added to release the indirect, alcohol-soluble bilirubin. A second reading is taken at 30 minutes at 540 mm for the total bilirubin.

SPECTROPHOTOMETRIC

We present the spectrophotometric assay only as a useful assay for total bilirubin in neonates. Yellow pigments in adult plasma such as lipochromes caratinoids, and drugs interfere with bilirubin's absorption peak at 460 mm. Many commercial instruments are available that relate absorbance at 460 mm to concentration. A dual wavelength is often used to negate the interference of hemoglobin.

Procedural Technical Points: (1) dilutions should be made with distilled water because saline interferes with the diazo coupling reaction; (2) bilirubin is extremely light sensitive; and (3) spectrophotometric assays must not be used for neonates that have been transfused with adult blood.

BIBLIOGRAPHY AND RECOMMENDED READINGS

Batsakis, J. G., Briere, R. O., Markel, S. F. *DIAGNOSTIC ENZYMOLOGY*. 1970. The American Society of Clinical Pathologists. Chicago.

Beeler, M. F. *INTERPRETATIONS IN CLINICAL CHEMISTRY*. 1978. The American Society of Clinical Pathologists. Chicago.

Campbell, J., Sanderson, J. A. *AMINOTRANSFERASES AND PLP ACTIVATION*. 1979. The Dow Chemical Company. Indianapolis.

Christensen, H. N., Palmer, G. A. *ENZYME KINETICS*. 1967. W. B. Saunders Company. Philadelphia.

Davidsohn, I. and J. B. Henry (Editors). *TODD-SANFORD CLINICAL DIAGNOSIS AND MANAGE-MENT BY LABORATORY METHODS*. Sixteenth Edition. 1979. W. B. Saunders Company. Philadelphia.

"Diabetes in the 1980's". *DIAGNOSTIC MEDICINE*. March-April 1980. Volume 3 Number 2. 31-52.

"Effects of Drugs on Clinical Laboratory Tests". *CLINICAL CHEMISTRY*. April, 1975. Volume 21. Number 5.

Fuller, J. B. *SELECTED TOPICS IN CLINICAL CHEMISTRY*. 1972. The American Society of Clinical Pathologists. Chicago.

Galen, R. S. "Isoenzymes and Myocardial Infarction". *DIAGNOSTIC MEDICINE*. February 1978. Volume I. Number 1. 40-52.

Goldberg, D. M. (Editor). *ANNUAL REVIEW OF CLINICAL BIOCHEMISTRY*. Volume I. 1980. John Wiley and Sons. New York.

Halstead, J. A. (Editor). *THE LABORATORY IN CLINICAL MEDICINE*. 1976. W. B. Saunders Company. Philadelphia.

Henry, R. H., Winkelman, J. W., and Cannon, D. C. (Editors). *CLINICAL CHEMISTRY PRINCIPLES AND TECHNIQUES*. Second Edition. 1974. Harper and Row Publishers. Haggerstown, Maryland.

Raphael, S. S. (Senior Author). *LYNCH'S MEDICAL LABORATORY TECHNOLOGY*. Volume I. Third Edition. 1976. W. B. Saunders Company. Philadelphia.

Tietz, N. W. (Editor). *FUNDAMENTALS OF CLINICAL CHEMISTRY*. Second Edition. 1976. W. B. Saunders Company. Philadelphia.

White, A., Handler, P., Smith, E., Hill, R., Lehman, I. *PRINCIPLES OF BIOCHEMISTRY*. Sixth Edition. 1978. McGraw-Hill Book Company. New York.

White, W. L., Erickson, M. M., Stevens, S. C. *CHEMISTRY FOR THE CLINICAL LABORATORY*. Fourth Edition. 1976. C. B. Mosby Company. St. Louis.

Chapter 9

Nuclear Medicine
(Wet Work)

RAYMOND L. METHOT
M.T. (ASCP), B.S., M.S.

OUTLINE

INTRODUCTION
RADIOCHEMISTRY
SAFETY RULES
    Biologicals
    Hygiene
    Radiation
    Documentation
RADIOCHEMISTRY
    Alpha Particles
    Beta Particles
    Gamma Rays
MATTER-RADIATION INTERACTIONS
    Photoelectric Effect
    Compton Effect
    Coherent Scattering
    Pair Production
    Photodisintegration
DECAY SCHEMES
    Alpha Particle Production
    Beta Particle Production
    Gamma Ray Production
UNITS OF MEASUREMENT
    Curie
    Decay Constant
    Half-Life
INSTRUMENTATION
INSTRUMENTS
    Film Badge
    Survey Meter
    Scintillation Counter

INTRODUCTION

The purpose of this chapter is to acquaint the student analyst with the prominent points of interest in radioisotope principles as they relate to the in-vitro- (wet-work) portion of radioimmunoassay. The radiochemistry section involves the safe handling of isotopes, particle and ray emissions, and interaction of radiation with matter. The instrumentation section is limited to the principles of the most widely used detector system in the clinical setting, the gamma counter. The radioimmuo-assay section deals with those principles most common to immuoassay namely; antibody interaction with antigen, the general testing procedures, pitfalls associated with various procedural steps, and the graphic expression of results. The last section outlines certain concepts in quality assurance as they pertain to the handling and control over the work spectrum.

Experience as a teacher can be very beneficial to a prepared mind; however, to help the student weather the occasional frustrations of the profession, one must adopt a good sense of humor which can best be expressed by briefly reviewing Murphy's experiences with the business world. He was so certain of his observations that he made them as immutable as laws. Let us examine closely what these observations are--Murphy's laws for implementation of planning and budgeting systems.

FIRST LAW: In any field of public or private endeavor, anything that can go wrong will go wrong.
Corollary 1:   Everything goes wrong at one time.
Corollary 2:   If there is a possibility of several things going wrong, the one that will go wrong is the one that will do the most damage.
Corollary 3:   Left to themselves, things always go from bad to worse.
Corollary 4:   Plans must be reproducible; they should fail in the same way.
Corollary 5:   Nature always sides with the hidden flaw.
Corollary 6:   If everything seems to go well, you have overlooked something.

SECOND LAW: It is usually impractical to worry beforehand about interference during system implementation; if you have none, someone will supply it for you.
Corollary 1:   Information necessitating a change in plans will be conveyed to you after, and only after, the plans are complete.
Corollary 2:   In listing alternatives, presenting one obvious right way versus one obvious wrong way, it is often wiser to choose the wrong way to expedite subsequent revisions.
Corollary 3:   The more innocuous a modification appears to be, the further its influence will extend and the more plans will have to be redrawn.

THIRD LAW: In any collection of performance and accounting data, the figures that are obviously correct and beyond all need of checking contain the errors.
Corollary 1:   Those you ask for help will not see the error.
Corollary 2:   Any nagging intruder who stops by with unsought advice will spot it immediately.

FOURTH LAW: If in any situation you find yourself doing an immense amount of work, the answer can be obtained by simple inspection.

SAFETY RULES

Having dealt with the lighter side, let us now buckle down to dealing with the safety precautions which will best protect the analyst from contact, aerosol or other hazards association with biologicals. These safety rules must be observed to insure some measure of protection. The rules can be categorized as follows: (1) biologicals; (2) hygiene; (3) radiation; (4) documentation.

BIOLOGICALS   It is vital that biologicals be preserved against deterioration, contamination or transmission of infectious diseases.

A. Refrigerate biologicals at 2 to 8 degrees centigrade.

B. Freeze serum or plasma at minus 20 degrees or lower if tests are not performed daily.

C. Dispose of waste biologicals through the sanitary sewage system or treat with 5% bleach or autoclave. For radioactive biologicals one must adhere to the individual state requirements for disposal and the permissable radiation levels for sewage disposal, if any.

HYGIENE   These rules deal with the analyst's safety.

A. Eating, smoking, drinking or the application of cosmetics in the laboratory environment is forbidden.

B. Where indicated, wear disposable rubber or plastic gloves.

C. Lab coats should remain in the work area and a "clean" coat should be worn outside the laboratory area.

D. Pipetting by mouth is to be avoided.

E. Operations which create aerosols should be controlled. Centrifuge serum tubes. Decant tubes with siphon set-ups utilizing a trap flash. The vacuum exhaust, from such devices, should be vented to the outside.

F. Film badges must be worn where required by state regulations.

G. Hand washing is essential after handling biologicals and isotopes.

RADIATION   Protection from exposure or cross contaminations is paramount to the analyst.

A. Decontaminate glassware with suitable detergent cleaners. Rinse with demineralized water.

B. Protect scintillator well with disposable plastic liners.

C. Cover work benches with plastic backed absorbent paper.

D. Dispose of solid waste in buckets containing disposable plastic liners which are properly labeled.

DOCUMENTATION   Obviously, records constitute prima facia evidence that work was performed.

A. A labeling system is important to identify tests and reagents.

B. Records of tests, quality control specimens, calibration, etc., must be preserved for the prescribed legal time limit based on accrediting agencies (usually 2 years).

C. Procedure manuals must be reviewed yearly and corrections duly noted.

D. Records of procedure validation should be preserved along with reference literature for the life of the procedure.

To the above list, everyone may wish to insert good standards of practice to provide better control over individual procedures, set limits, elaborate on criteria for unacceptable specimens, etc. Close scrutiny of each procedure is essential to eliminate misinterpretation of meaning; example, use of abbreviations must convey the same description to everyone. ASAP may mean "as soon as possible" to one person and "American Society of Apprehensive Pessimists" to another.

RADIOACTIVITY

Close observations and speculations by earlier scientists have lead to the discovery of a phenomenon that toppled the concept of immutability. Radioactivity proved to be a natural process by which atoms transmute or decay through emission of electromagnetic rays, and/or particles until a "stable state" is reached.

These emissions will be discussed briefly in the following paragraphs. More extensive information in nuclear physics is available by consulting the primary texts listed in the bibliography.

ALPHA PARTICLES   Alpha particles are helium nuclei having 4 atomic mass units (AMU) of 2 protons and 2 neutrons stripped of electrons with a positive charge of two. The particles are usually monoenergetic when extruded by a particular species of atomic nuclei at 1/10 the speed of light. The high energy particles may travel a distance of 8 centimeters in air, and 20-40 microns in water. Interaction with matter causes a great energy loss by inelastic collision with electrons leading to ionization. Loss of energy as the particle traverses matter, is called "linear energy transfer" (L.E.T.). Consider for a moment the make-up of matter—it is mostly space. If a proton were the size of a golf ball, its closest electron would be about 600 feet away.

The interaction of alpha particles with matter can be calculated in terms of ion pairs formed in the L.E.T. from alpha particles to the surrounding matter. As an example let us use the alpha particle ejected from 210-polonium which has an energy of 5.3 million electron volts (M.E.V.). To form 1 ion pair 32.5 electron volts are needed. Therefore approximately 163,000 ion pairs are formed.

$$\frac{5,300,000}{32.5} = \sim 163,000 \text{ ion pairs}$$

If the particles were to travel 38 millimeters in water, then approximately 4,400 ion pairs per mm. would be formed. Its ion density formation would be calculated as follows:

$$\frac{163,000}{38} = \sim 4,400 \text{ ion pairs per nm}$$

BETA PARTICLES (NEGATRONS)   The beta particle is an electron of nuclear origin which nearly approaches the speed of light. Its charge is minus 1 and is expressed as 1 electron mass units (EMU) or 5×10^{-4} AMU. A 3 M.E.V. particle can travel 13 meters in air with the formation of approximately 70 ion pairs per centimeter.

Elastic collision with matter leads to deflection of the beta particle, but collisions with orbital electrons leads to ionization and collisions with the nucleus causes the emission of X-rays equal to the electron volt unit of the particle.

POSITRONS   These are anti-particles to the electron having a positive charge and a weight of 1 E.M.U. Positron emissions occur in artificially produced isotopes in the process of changing a proton into a neutron.

GAMA RAYS   Like X-rays, gamma rays are electromagnetic radiations which travel with the speed of light. Gamma rays are nuclear in origin while X-rays originate from orbital electron transitions. Gamma rays appear to be cooling off energy in the isotopic transmutation process. They carry no charge, and at rest, have a mass of zero, but at 1 M.E.V. have an A.M.U. of 0.00107. These rays are very penetrating thus produce a low ion density. These may travel from a few centimeters to 100 meters in air depending on their energy content, but when in water, they may travel a few millimeters to several centimeters.

MATTER-RADIATION INTERACTIONS

There are two types of matter to consider when discussing interactions; the first being electrons, the other nuclei. Let us consider interactions with electrons first.

PHOTOELECTRIC EFFECT   The gamma photon may be absorbed by an orbiting electron producing secondary ionization in the form of beta particles, if all the energy is imported to the electron. This type of interaction occurs mostly with the innermost electron shells. The vacated electron-photon interaction allows an outer electron to fill in with consequent production of one or more characteristic X-ray. In doing so, the atom so ionized will attach to another atom forming an ion pair.

COMPTON EFFECT   Partial interaction between the electron and photon leads to a proportional decrease in the energy of the gamma photon and scattering of the more energetic electron which will lose its energy as it travels through matter. This high velocity electron is also referred to as a Compton electron. The gamma photon may undergo several other events before it has finally lost all of its energy.

COHERENT SCATTERING   Interactions of electrons with X or gamma rays may be elastic causing deflection of the X or gamma ray from its path with no loss of energy. Let us now consider the nuclear interactions with gamma photons.

PAIR PRODUCTION   A gamma ray of greater than 1.02 M.E.V. may interact with the nucleus with the splitting of the gamma photon into two particles, 1 electron and 1 positron hence the term pair production. The ejected negatron and positron would decay in a manner previously discussed.

PHOTODISINTEGRATION   The gamma photon, when entering the nucleus of an atom, may result in the ejection of a neutron, proton, or alpha particle.

DECAY SCHEMES

In perusing the literature, the student may be exposed to several ways of expressing the decay schemes for the radionuclides. Consider the following simply decay modes as an example of nuclear decay. Many radionuclides are far more complex.

The international symbols for expressing an element have been greatly simplified. The expression of an isotope may be represented by the letter X. The graphic representation can be explained as follows where:

A = mass number
Z = atomic number
V = valance
N = neutron number

$$\begin{matrix} A & \diagdown & V \\ & \times & \\ Z & \diagup & N \end{matrix}$$

$$\begin{matrix} 206 & +2 \\ & Pb \\ 82 & 124 \end{matrix}$$

ALPHA DECAY   As represented by the element polonium

$$_{84}^{210}\text{polonium}_{126} \qquad _{2}^{4}\alpha_{2} + _{82}^{206}\text{lead}_{124}$$

$$+ \quad \begin{array}{c} _{}^{210}\text{Po} \\ \hline \alpha \searrow \quad 100\% \\ 0.80 \ \lessgtr \quad 5.3 \text{ MEV} \\ \hline \text{Pb(stable)} \end{array}$$

BETA DECAY   As represented by the element phosphorus

$$_{15}^{32}\text{P}_{17} \qquad _{1}^{0}\text{e}_{1} + _{16}^{32}\text{S}_{16}$$

$$+ \quad \begin{array}{c} _{}^{32}\text{P} \\ \hline \\ \searrow 1.707 \text{ MEV} \\ _{}^{32}\text{S} \end{array}$$

GAMMA DECAY   As represented by the element iodine

$$_{53}^{125}\text{I}_{72} + _{1}^{0}\text{e}_{1} \qquad \gamma + _{52}^{125} + \text{e}_{73}$$

$$+ \quad \begin{array}{c} _{}^{125}\text{I} \\ \hline \text{EC} \swarrow \text{ (electron capture)} \\ \lessgtr \quad 0.035 \text{ MEV} \\ \hline _{}^{125}\text{Te} \end{array}$$

UNITS OF MEASUREMENTS

As with any discipline there are units of measurements to contend with. The original unit was the CURIE which represented the decay of 0.66 cubic meters of radon gas formed by 1 gram of radium per second. This amounted to 3.7×10^{10} decays per second (DPS). At present CURIE represents the unit of activity equal to a decay rate of 3.7×10^{10} DPS. Several metric prefixes may be affixed to the curie to represent fractional portions of the curie since in the clinical setting, one does not normally deal with such high concentrations, such being the milli $\frac{1}{1000}$, or micro 1×10^{-6} or pico 1×10^{-12}. The CURIE may not necessarily represent the counted events on the scintillation counter, since as an atom decays and the events are recorded by a scintillator, there are geometric and barrier factors to change the recorded events. Example: for every 100 atom decays of I-125, there are 144 events recorded by a scintillation counter.

When one speaks of decay, this brings to mind that a given point in time we will be left with fewer atoms than we originally started with. Several questions come to mind: (1) at what point in time? (2) what about activity?

Through experimental evidence it has been shown that different isotope species will decay at different rates. As of yet, there is no reasonable explanation why one atom species decays faster than another, therefore, the concept of the half life was coined. The half life can be defined as the length of time necessary for 1/2 of a particular number of atoms to decay. There is a wrinkle in this beautiful picture, i.e., atoms decay randomly, therefore the half life represents a statistical analysis of the decay. The bright side is that there exists a proportionality whereby a given number of atoms will decay within a given amount of time. Without this proportionality, radioactive decay events would be unreliably measured.

DECAY CONSTANT   This represents the fraction of total number of atoms present which decay per unit of time, or in equation (2) the number of atoms (N_t) remaining after a time (t) is equal to the number (No) at time (to) multiplied by $e^{-\lambda t}$, where e is the natural log base and λ is the decay constant.

$$(1) \quad -\frac{dN}{dt} = \lambda N \qquad or \qquad (2) \quad N_t = N_o e^{-\lambda t}$$

HALF LIFE   The half life can be shown to be related to the decay constant equation (3). One can substitute this expression for (λ) in the decay law to yield equation (4). To write the equation in terms of activity instead of numbers of atoms.

$$(3) \quad = \frac{0.693}{T^{\frac{1}{2}}} \qquad (4) \quad N_t = N_o e^{-\frac{0.693}{T^{\frac{1}{2}}}} \qquad (5) \quad A_t = A_o e^{-\frac{0.693}{T^{\frac{1}{2}}}}$$

INSTRUMENTATION

FILM BADGE   Earlier experimenters accidently discovered that photographic emulsions could be exposed by radiation emitted from mineral samples. This principle is put to use to monitor the exposure of laboratory personnel to radiation. Although its use is designed for individuals handling millicurie quantities of radioisotopes, some state nuclear regulatory agencies may require that analysts wear the film badges for all radiation work.

There are many variations of badges, from simple emulsions to complex shielded models for detection over the entire range of radiations. Shielding materials consist of varying thicknesses of aluminum, copper, and cadmium enclosed in a light tight case. The sensitivity may vary from a few millirads (unit of absorbed radiation) to 10,000 rads. This badge serves as a permanent record of an individual's exposure history on a monthly basis to insure that testing procedures do not result in overexposure or unnecessary exposure to radiation.

SURVEY METER   The commonly called Geiger counter was primarily designed to measure beta radiation and less so gamma radiation. In the laboratory the instrument is usually a battery operated, hand-held survey meter used to monitor the work and work benches. Certain technics of sampling along with the type of isotope element make this instrument less reliable. The "wipe test" which involves the use of a filter paper to wipe down a specified area at the work bench, refrigerator, centrifuge, etc., has a greater sensitivity to low M.E.V. isotopes such as I-125. The filter paper is then counted in the scintillation counter and the decision to decontaminate the bench or centrifuge is based on arbitrary standards set by the Nuclear Medicine Department.

Certain aspects of the meter should be reviewed before proceeding to another instrument type. The instrument consists of an ionization tube containing an inert gas such as argon and about 1% of a quenching gas such as chlorine. The tube is connected across a high voltage source which supplies the electrons to polarize the chamber followed by an amplifier and a meter or scaler to read the radiation level.

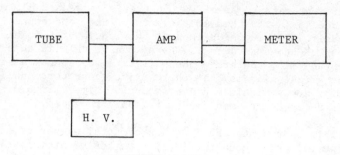

SURVEY METER

Ionizing radiation, penetrating into the chamber, causes the discharge of an electric pulse by the formation of an ion pair of gas molecules. The chlorine acts to avert a continuous discharge due to secondary ionization as it spreads throughout the tube.

Examine the voltage curve of a Geiger Mueller ionization tube and note that, in the presence of a radiation source, the detector will operate within a specified voltage range, i.e., at the plateau region. By varying the voltage applied to the

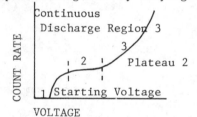

detector, the curve will show three major points: (1) the starting voltage where the applied voltage causes radiation counts to register on the meter; (2) the plateau which shows a flattened area of a uniform count rate even though the applied voltage is greatly increased; and (3) the continuous discharge region produced by electrons "boiling" off the cathode with excessive voltage. Even in the absence of radiation, the excess voltage will bridge the gap between the cathode of the detector and its anode resulting in the continued pulsing.

The counting efficiency of the survey meter is very low as compared to other instrument types designed to measure specific radiation sources--e.g., 1% efficiency for gamma rays.

SCINTILLATION COUNTER   As with any dynamic field of technology, the effect of auto-mation and computerization has revolutionized the shape, size and complexity of the scintillation counter. However, the basic principles still remain essentially the same. By concentrating on the basics, the student analyst will be able to decipher the more complex systems.

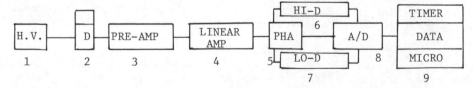

BLOCK DIAGRAM OF SCINTILLATION COUNTER

1. HIGH VOLTAGE (H.V.)   The variable high voltage supply sets up the electromotive force to allow the photomultiplier tube to amplify the weak signal produced by the light sensitive coating on the photomultiplier photocathode.

2. DETECTOR (D)   This is one of the most vital portions of the system and consists of three portions: (1) the crystal; (2) the photocathode; and (3) the dynodes.

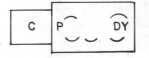

The crystal (c) is usually composed of a solid crystal of sodium iodide of different diameters (1 to 3 inches or greater) depending on the sensitivity of the instrument. There may also be an engineered impurity of thallium which acts as a quenching substance. A core may be drilled out to allow a glass tube to be placed into the center so that the crystal gives maximum radiation detection. The smaller crystals may be used flat against the radiation source. The entire crystal section is enclosed by a very thin, light, and tight aluminum can glued to the face of the photomultiplier tube adjacent to the photocathode.

The photocathode (p) within the glass case of the photomultiplier tube serves to connect light impulses from the crystal into electrical pulses.

The Dynodes (DY) amplify the electrical impulses of the photocathode a million or more times. The amplification will depend on the applied voltage.

PRE-AMPLIFIER   The very weak signal produced by the photomultiplier needs to be further amplified before it can be presented to the linear amplifier, this is the function of the pre-amp.

LINEAR AMPLIFIER   This section proportionately amplifies the signal pulse by the same ratio as the pulse presented to it by the pre-amp. The amplification can sometimes be controlled by an external "gain" control.

PULSE HEIGHT ANALYZER (PHA)   The pulses from the linear amplifier have the same proportional amplitude as the energy absorbed by the crystal. The counting of these pulses is accomplished by the PHA and, together with the low and high discriminator, serve to choose the energy spectrum of an isotope or focus on a peak energy source to enable the analyst to literally discriminate by rejection of all but a very narrow band of the desired spectrum. The narrow band is called a "window". By proper calibration, a prominent photopeak is selected and a section from 0.5% to 10% of the peak may be focused upon.

Examine the diagram of the PHA in action. The X axis shows the peak height in electron volts E.V., K.E.V., or M.E.V. The X axis shows vertical pulses entering the PHA over a period of time. The height of the pulses may be selected electronically by establishing cut off points through the high and low discriminator thus setting up a "window". All pulses falling within the window are counted, i.e., all those marked with "o" and "*"; however, those marked with "x" are ignored. The pulses may further be separated, if the instrument has 2 channels. Channel I will count the pulses marked with an "*", and channel II will count the pulses marked with "o".

PULSE HEIGHT ANALYZER

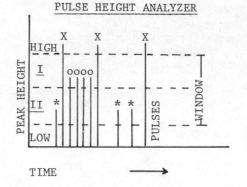

A/D CONVERTER   The function of this electronic circuitry is to convert an analog to a digital signal to facilitate its use by the microprocessor (computer) and data system.

TIMER   The timer section allows the analyst to preset any desired time for counting or to preset the number of pulses to be counted.

DATA REDUCTION   With the incorporation of microcomputers, the scintillator systems are now able to be hooked up directly to a central computer.   This facilitates the transfer of information and assumes better control over data validation.   The information may be sent in various ways such as: raw counts, net counts, plot curves, convert unknown sample results directly into unit values, etc.   The versatility of the computerized systems cannot be overstated.

COUNTING GEOMETRY   There are several other salient points that need mentioning to caution the student against making assumptions which could lead to statistical or careless errors.   The items may be grouped under the broad term of "counting geometry".

DISTANCE   The inverse square law states that the intensity of radiation from a point source varies inversely to the square of the distance from the source.

$$\frac{I_1}{I_2} = \frac{(R_1)^2}{(R_2)^2}$$

In counting practices, it is vital that the radiation source always be in the same position as seen by the terms $(R_1)^2$ and $(R_2)^2$ where distance can magnify an error, if changed.

RESOLVING TIME   This term relates to the ability of the instrument to count closely occuring radiation events, e.g., the typical scintillator may have a resolving time of 1 microsecond (10^{-6} seconds), while a Geiger tube may have a 200-300 microsecond (2×10^{-4} seconds) resolving time--an order of 2 magnitudes difference.

In simpler terms, it would be the ability of the instrument to recognize two or more radiation pulses that enter the detector almost simultaneously.   This also means that a detector cannot be inundated with very active sources without experiencing a loss in counts, e.g., millicurie quantities.

COUNTING EFFICIENCY   This function is multifaceted and takes in the detector size, radiation type, reproducibility, stability, thermal noise, etc.   Only a few functions will be discussed here.

DETECTOR SIZE   The larger the crystal the more photons will likely interact with it. While discussing the crystal and efficiency, it is a good time to review the interaction of matter with radiation, since it will affect efficiency directly.   The following may happen to a photon when entering the crystal environment: (1) there may be no interaction, i.e., the photon passes through the detector and is not counted; (2) the energy of the photon is completely absorbed and 1 pulse is counted; (3) a compton interaction with escape of the photon; (4) two compton interactions counted as one because of the closeness of the events; (5) pair production with both photons escaping detection; (6) pair production with 1 escaping photon; and (7) pair production with both photons absorbed and recorded as 1 photopeak.

RADIATION TYPE   Alpha particles require a different set up for counting than a crystal detector, i.e., a gas operated proportional counter or a liquid scintillation counter. The same applies to beta particles of low energy which cannot penetrate the casing of the scintillator crystal. Energetic beta particles may also require an anthracene crystal to improve efficiency rather than a sodium iodide crystal. The scintillator crystal is more sensitive to gamma and X-rays up to about 1.02 M.E.V. of energy.

CROSS OVER   Analysts using instruments to measure two isotopes in the same test system must guard against overlapping of energy ranges resulting in cross over radiation detection. Example I-131 and Cr-51 show a close photopeak at 0.36 M.E.V. (I-131) and 0.32 M.E.V. (Cr-51). The window could not be set narrow enough without losing sensitivity and count rate and still function well with both isotopes.

DECAY SCHEME   By reviewing the mode of decay of an isotope, the complexity of decay schemes can be appreciated. The scintillation counter could detect virtually 100% of I-125 decay but only 93% of cesium-137 and 77% or less of uranium-238 because I-125 produces photons which will interact fully with the detector while 77% of U-238 decays by gamma radiation and 23% by alpha particle radiation.

BACKGROUND RADIATION   Lastly, this topic is a fuzzy description given to radiation events, or what is counted as radiation events, which encompass such things as cosmic radiation, natural radiation in the construction materials, electronic noise, etc., or whatever contributes to count rates in the absence of a radiation source. Certain safeguards can be taken to shield the detector from stray radiation, but not from overt contamination by the analyst.

RADIOIMMUNOASSAY

INTRODUCTION

This section entitled radioimmunoassay is the result of evolutionary changes within the field of immunoassay as an attempt to measure the heretofore unmeasurable by coupling antigens and antibodies with radioactive tracers. The first assays involved the use of plasma protein as binders, such as thyroxine binding globulin and transcortin. By agreement the use of plasma protein as binders are known technically as "competitive binding assays", while the use of radiolabeled antigens are known as "radioimmunoassays" and the use of radiolabeled antibodies as "immunoradiometric assays".

The student analyst will be confronted with a host of "kits" which include all working reagents. This type of commercial packaging is meant to offer the "best" quality proven set-ups, however Murphy's Law inevitably catches up with the best. For this reason this section will treat only general principles of radioimmunoassay since in whatever laboratory a student interns the "way of doing things" has already been predetermined by validation studies. In the following section an "*" represents a radiolabeled substance.

There are general steps that are common to the reactions to be discussed: (a) mixing of reactants; (b) incubation to equilibrium; (c) separation; (d) counting; and (e) calculations.

COMPETITIVE BINDING ASSAY   Plasma proteins have been isolated elecyrophoretically and some fraction found to be carriers for certain hormones. Thyroxine binding globulin (TBG) was found to bind thyroxine, the hormone from the thyroid gland. In the circulation TBG facilitates the transport of thyroxine by resisting denaturation until the receptor site of the hormone is reached. By mixing radiolabeled thyroxine (T_4*), nonlabeled T_4 and TBG followed by incubation and absorption the ratio of <u>bound</u> T_4* and <u>free</u> T_4* can be measured. By varying the amount of T_4 (nonlabeled) in the test system, a standard curve can be plotted.

Refer to the following diagram for clarification. Each step will be discussed in greater detail later on.

$$T_4* + T_4 + TBG \rightleftharpoons \begin{matrix} T_4*TBG \\ T_4TBG \end{matrix}$$

Note that the amount of TBG is exactly saturated by T_4* and T_4. Since the system is in dynamic equilibrium the reaction is reversible so that a serum containing T_4 can compete for binding sites with T_4* by a certain ratio. The % T_4 bound to TBG decreases proportionately to the amount of serum T_4 under test.

The next step in the process is to absorb out the free T_4* and T_4 with a substance such as resin that can remove the unbound fractions. The resin is washed and counted so that the % uptake can be determined by comparing it to a standard curve.

RADIOIMMUNOASSAY   This testing procedure has been described as an isotope dilution technic. Specific binding reagent (antibody) is used at a limited concentration and need not be monospecific. Only antibodies which bind to the tracer are involved.

$$AN* + AN + Ig \rightleftharpoons \begin{matrix} AN*Ig \\ ANIg \end{matrix}$$

The above equation bears a semblance to the competitive binding assay; the difference being that the <u>Ig</u> (antibody) was produced in an animal to react with <u>AN</u> (antigen). This technic offers greater sensitivity over the competitive binding assay by increasing the affinity for the antigen.

IMMUNORADIOMETRIC ASSAY   The antibody is used essentially to prepare the labeled derivative whose molar concentration is proportional to, and ideally identical with, the molar concentration of antigen in the unknown.

There are variations of this tool. When <u>AN</u> (antigen), from serum or plasma, is added to a mixture of antibody chemically bound to plastic beads tubes and incubated, the <u>AN</u> will bind to the antibody. When labeled antibody is added to the mixture, it will bind to the antigen (AN) forming a "sandwich" of antibody-antigen-labeled antibody. The concentration of antigen is determined by the amount of labeled antibody present after proper washing.

$$AN + Ig + Ig* \rightleftharpoons (Ig- AN - Ig*)$$

The greater the amount of antigen, the greater the radiation count.

Before straying too far from basics, the explanation of the mechanisms will help you to appreciate the developments in radioimmunoassays. Like all subjects, certain definitions need standardization between the analyst and subject matter. The following list will help you to cope with the subject at hand.

1. Antigen: A substance of sufficient molecular weight which, when introduced
    (immunogen)   into the body of an animal, stimulates the production of antibody.

2. Antibody: Specific immunoglobulins produced in response to an antigen
                     challenge.

3. Affivity: The degree of complementary determinant sites existing between
                     specific antibody and antigens.

4. Avidity: The degree of association or dissociation (binding) between anti-
                     body and antigen.

5. Adjuvant: A substance which will help maintain an antigen challenge by am-
                     plifying antibody response or prolong the absorption of antigen
                     by a constant antigen challenge over a period of time.

6. Specificity: A biologic response particular to an inducer substance. Example,
                     growth and somatotropin.
                     The term is also used to mean the degree of highly selective re-
                     action between two substances or the ability to detect only the
                     compound to be measured or the degree of freedom from interference.

7. Sensitivity   The smallest amount of an antigen or antibody that can be distin-
                     guished from zero (no antigen or antibody).

8. Cross   The ability or a chemically related substance to interfere with
     reactivity: the target substance to be measured.

The term antigen, as defined above, is very broad and is comprised of several groups; here are some examples:

A. Non-peptide hormones: 17B estradiol, corticosterone
B. Peptide hormones: gH (somatotropin), ACTH (adrenocorticotropin), HC
                           (somatomammotropin)
C. Substances: digoxin, morphine, LSD, chorioembryonic antigen
D. Enzymes: C_1 esterase, acid phosphatase
E. Protein: IgE, Kappa and lambda chains of immunoglobulins

BASIC KINETICS   The law of mass action. The interaction between antigen can be presented as a mathematical formula.

(1) $AN + Ig \xrightleftharpoons[K_2]{K_1} ANIg$

This formula represents a literal description of what takes place. To convert this to terms which can be mathematically manipulated the concept of quantities must be added. The molar concentration of the reactants are such terms. The non-hormonal inserted in the following equation focus on quantitative relationships which exist in this reaction mixture.

(2) $(AN)(Ig) \xrightleftharpoons[K_2]{K_1} (ANIg)$

The formula can further be modified by combining the K_1 and K_2 into a single ratio expression of R $\left(\frac{K_1}{K_2}\right)$

(3) $R = \frac{K_1}{K_2} = \frac{(ANIg)}{(AN)(Ig)}$

Another term can represent the total molar concentration of the antibody IgO

(4) $IgO = (Ig) + (ANIg)$

Combining the above equations a further expression evolves

(5) $R(IgO) - (ANIg) = \frac{(ANIg)}{(AN)}$

If we now represent the bound antigen as $\underline{B}$ (bound) B = (ANIg). If the free antigen is represented by $\underline{F}$ (free) F = (AN) the formula begins to appear as a linear equation where y - mx + b

(6) $B/F = R(IgO) - B$

The above equation can be plotted on a graph where the y axis is the ratio of the B (bound) to F (free) antigen and the x axis is the quantity of total antigen.   R = the slope of the equation.

(7) $B/F = \text{ratio} \left(\frac{K_1}{K_2}\right) ((AN) + (ANIg) - (ANIg))$

There are many factors influencing this simple equation which are not treated mathematically such as electrostatic forces, excess antigen or excess antibody, the homogenous or heterogenous mixture of antigen, etc.   The valence of the antibody is taken into account in the expression Ig = molar concentration x valence, where the valence of the antibody is not 1.

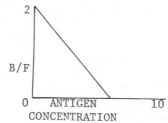

ANTIGEN PRODUCTION   To carry out the RIA, the substance to be identified (antigen) must somehow be purified so that it can be used to produce the necessary antibody. Also, the antigen is needed in the reaction to set up some form of competition with the antigen to be measured.   Next the antigen must be radiolabeled.   This process is more difficult than it sounds, because in the reaction mixture, there may be degraded antigen, pure antigen, mineral salts, and untreated isotope.   The characteristics that an antigen must possess are: (1) radiochemical purity whereby degraded antigen and free isotope may act as interfering agents; (2) immunoreactivity, meaning that the antigen must have an affinity for the antibody.   The degree of radiolabeling, chemical damage in the processing, and incubation damage caused by plasma components such as inactivators, serve to reduce the affinity.   The process is mainly trial and error until improvements in the procedure, to produce high quality antigens, become standardized; (3) the amount of radiolabeled antigen resulting from chemical manipulations that will show the greatest radioactivity.   The antigen with the greatest affinity for antibody may be the one which is least radioactive. However, some compromise must be reached to make the reaction detectable. The immunoreactivity of the labeled antigen must closely resemble that of the standard. It is not uncommon to find differences between labeled and unlabeled antigen; (4) sensitivity is the smallest quantity that can be detected. In RIA the common figure is about 10^{-8} moles per liter; (5) also, stability plays a vital role because in the process of radio-active decay, the labeled antigen will often lose some of its affinity. The trans-mutted element may have different chemical characteristics than the original element, e.g., I^{132} decay to xenon. The shelf life of the radiolabeled substance is a func-tion of the half-life of the radioactive tracer, liberation of free radiotracer and loss of immunoreactivity due to structural damage caused by the radiation itself. Storage is also problematical in that the substance is also a biological, and as such requires a stable temperature environment. Most peptide hormones will be well pre-served at $-20^{\circ}C$ or lower, but repeat thawing is to be avoided.

ANTIBODY PRODUCTION   As you may have realized from the previous discussion, the antibody is directly dependent upon the form the antigen is in when it is to be mea-sured, i.e., the form in serum samples may vary somewhat from that in purified test tube form. Every effort must be made to maintain the same reactivity otherwise what is proported to be measured is measured against a different yard stick. Be that as it may, let's review how antibodies are produced.

Milligram quantities of antigen are mixed with a "complete" adjuvant and injected subcutaneously, intracutaneously or intramuscularly, whichever route will yield the greatest amount of antibody. This is followed by "booster" injections of antigen mixed with "incomplete" adjuvant. The primary antibody response usually will pla-teau in 4-6 weeks. The secondary response, yielding of a 2-10 fold increase, may ac-company the booster injections. High avidity antibodies are produced by spacing the booster injections 3-6 months, since avidity has been shown to increase with time.

Rabbits, guinea pigs, goats and sheep or horses have all been tried with more or less success. Rabbits have been widely used. When larger volumes of antisera are necessary, goats and sheep are used. In RIA the volume of antisera for testing is not large. A good quality producer may necessitate a one to one million dilution of the antisera to make it usable. When dealing with commercial quantities of antisera, the problems become astronomical. There may be a great variability in the antisera between animal species as well as in the repeated use of the same animal. The history of antibody production of the animal is of vital importance as a control of consistency.

As you have probably learned by now, there may be several species of antibodies produced in the same animal such as IgM, IgG1$_{2,3,4}$. The radioimmunoassay must employ separation measures to remove those antibodies which may hinder the molar binding ratio in a reaction mixture. An IgM molecule may possess 5 binding sites as compared to 1 on the IgG molecule. It is also important that the reaction not use "helpers", such as complement, to force the reaction to equilibrium. These are some of the problems addressed in greater detail in textbooks of immunochemistry. Chemical agents may be added to remove all serum protein, except IgG, to increase specificity.

INCUBATION   This next step in RIA is an integral part of the reaction. It is the time and temperature required to reach equilibrium. An *, AN to be measured are al-lowed to compete for binding sites on Ig. The time required varies from a few hours to several days. The temperature required for equilibration will vary. The initial reaction $AN^* + AN + Ig \xrightarrow{K_1} AN^*Ig + ANIg$ is usually quite rapid, i.e., K_1 is terminated often within minutes. The ratio E (equilibrium) is really what is important to measure, therefore, the K_2 reaction must also be factored into the time reaction. Dissociation occurs more slowly than the K_1 (association) reaction. By lowering the incubation temperature, incubation damage produced by enzymes, oxidants, etc., can be reduced. The use of a minute quantity of serum in a larger reaction volume also benefits the non-specific effects.

Refer to the dissociation curve graph. Notice the effect due to incubation temperature. The E ratio is greatest at a lower temperature. Sensitivity and reproducibility is increased as the temperature is lowered.

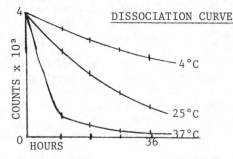

It has been theorized that conformational rearrangement of AN and Ig molecules increase the avidity by dissociation and reassociation. There may be a shift of Ig to more specific and avid antibody rearrangement.

SEPARATION AND COUNTING   The value of equilibration may be negated if in the end no simple method exists to separate the bound from the free antigen. Three principles are discussed here:

Precipitation: the bound antigen can be chemically precipitated with the immunoglobulin with organic acids such as trichloroacetic acid, the free antigen (AN*) can be poured off and the precipitate washed and counted. Three major problems exist with this technique: (1) the acid may not precipitate all of the bound antigen-antibody complex; (2) the antigen (AN*) may be eletrostatically bound to the coagulum resulting in elevated counts; and (3) the centrifugation force must be standardized to pack the coagulum to the bottom of the tube.

ABSORPTION   Initial success with this technique seemed promising. Lighter polypeptide hormones could be absorbed onto media such as charcoal, cellulose, resins, etc. Non specific absorption was found to be influenced by protein concentration, temperature, pH, ionic strength of diluent, etc. Any loss of absorber produced a false decrease in absorbed antigen (AN*).

DOUBLE ANTIBODY   A successful technique was discovered whereby the antibody in the initial reaction was precipitated by the addition of a second antibody B.

(1)   AN* + AN + Ig $\rightleftarrows$ AN*Ig / ANIg

(2)   AN*Ig / ANIg + IgB $\longrightarrow$ AN*IgIgB + ANIgIgB

The second antibody is produced by injecting another species of animal with the antibody of the first. Example: anti-rabbit antibody produced by injecting goats with rabbit antibody.

The separation phase is accomplished by centrifugation at high speed. An advantage is that the original antigen (AN), does not co-precipitate with the second antibody. The initial reaction (1) must not interfere with the second reaction (2). This method is best suited for high titer, and high avidity antibodies in the initial step.

Let us not overlook the disadvantages: (a) no precipitation will occur when the antibody concentration is 10^{-8} grams/liter or lower; (b) the incubation time may be prolonged overnight for adequate precision; (c) the reaction requires a large amount of the second antibody (relatively speaking); (d) the precipitate stability improves at lower temperature therefore centrifugation should be carried out in the cold.

COUNTING   Without automated systems, this phase may be the most tedious. Systems which are equipped with microprocessor can do all the counting, plot the necessary curves, choose the "best fit" curve, and express the unknowns directly in units of concentration.

Manual systems require at least a calculator. The analyst will count the background radiation, the total radiation count for each of duplicate tests which include 5-7 standards, 2-3 control specimens or more and duplicate unknown serums. After the completion of the reaction (incubation) separation, (centrifugation), the tubes will be counted again.

The method will usually specify if the supernatant or the precipitate will be counted. Whatever phase is employed, it must be standardized to minimize variations in technique. Each sample must be corrected for "background", unless the count rate is of such magnitude that it will not affect the outcome of the test.

Refer to dose rate curves. To measure the % antigen that is bound, one needs to know: (a) the total radiation count; and (b) the count rate of the precipitate. To measure the bound to free ratio, either the precipitate and the supernatant need to be measured or the total radiation and the precipitate. Subtracting the bound precipitate radiation from the total yield, the free antigen count is obtained. The ratio is then the bound radiation divided by the free radiation. Conversely, to calculate the % free antigen, the total radiation is equated to 100%, and the % bound is subtracted from 100% to yield the % free antigen by simple ratio and proportion.

DOSE RESPONSE CURVES   The method of expressing standard curves, from which to interpret unknown concentrations, may vary in character. The Y axis will present the data from the analysis versus the concentration of antigen on the X axis.

To plot the standards on the graph on the next page, you must reduce the count rate of each standard to the terms of the Y axis (such as % bound, the bound to free ratio or % free antigen) to suit the curve selected. The concentration of each standard is then plotted along the X axis. By plotting the Y value against the concentration on the X axis, a "best fit" curve is traced stringing together all the standard points. The resultant curve should resemble the pattern of one of the curves in the diagrams.

After reducing the calculations of the unknown to the terms of the appropriate Y axis (i.e., % bound B/F ratio, % free antigen, and determining the concentration plot along the X axis) you need only to follow the calculated value of the unknown on the Y axis until it intersects with the plotted standard curve. After this, drop to the X axis to read the concentration of the unknown.

COMMERCIAL KITS   Commercial kits, containing all the necessary reagents and standards

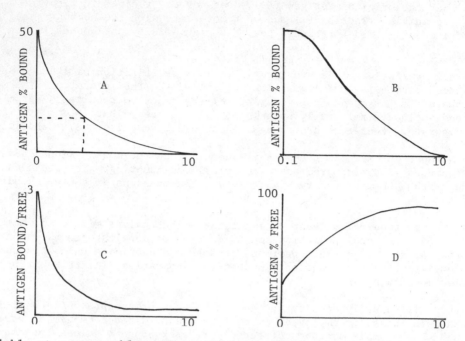

are available at a reasonable cost provided a sufficient number of tests are done. Certain key parts need to be addressed such as reproducibility. The package insert usually provides a guide to this parameter, but does not reflect your testing conditions. Also, always verify for reproducibility. Next, determine the usefullness of the procedure in-house and its clinical relevance. Compare with other products as to which technique you wish to use. Research the specificity claims through journals and peer evaluations. Carefully evaluate the reference values stated. Do not accept the normal values based on 10-20 or so "patients". Establish your own values by comparative testing and review the data pertaining to disease states.

Read and understand the precautions and limitations of the procedure by reviewing the sensitivity, precision, source of the standard, cross reactivity, etc. Carefully note the type of specimen required and whether the procedure can be used for analyzing other body fluids. In short, use constructive skepticism.

QUALITY ASSURANCE

INTRODUCTION

When speaking of scientific matters, it was always assumed that the end result was always the absolute truth. However, based upon the technology of the time, the word absolute may be shaded by degrees. This is where the emphasis or quality assurance comes in to support the degree of truth. It seems very legitimate to question the truth as to its "trustworthiness" or "believability", especially as it applies to physical matters. Time and again, the "truth" about the age of the earth, the origin of life, the length of a foot has been tampered with. It often came down to what you could make people believe. This is a very silly way to treat physical matters because the matter of "proof" is really what makes truth what it is, and on what standard the proof is based upon. Quality assurance seeks to control those variables which would make those truths less believable. In the course of your experience you will find that quality control is greatly emphasized where certain numbers can be

ascribed to certain outcomes and less credibility is given to areas of personal attitudes, equipment maintenance, and dynamic processes. No common set of values can be
ascribed to these, therefore, analysts tend to forget them.

PERSONNEL   It is difficult to measure the "trustworthiness" of an individual without
considering the entire spectrum of the person's make-up. You will find yourself in
the same dilemna of trying to "grade" an individual performance. Under today's laws
there are certain questions which an individual is not compelled to answer, therefore,
some aspect of personnel quality control cannot be defined. Some basic foundations
for determining quality are: (1) establish some form of pre-testing insurance that
a skilled person has the minimum knowledge and experience to do the work; and (2)
establish the work level until proven experience and knowledge leads to a higher level
of work. Monitoring a person's performance is a part of the control. External information is often vital, however, references are no substitute for good interviews.
Continuing education is at the other end of the spectrum. Analysts will find that
most of their life is spent studying comething or other. Some states have made education compulsory, but this may not always produce the desired results. You may have
heard of the saying: "You can lead a horse to water, but you can't make it drink",
well, you certainly could make it thirsty. In my experience there is no substitute
for personnel motivation!

SAMPLES   Three major factors can be identified. The important issue is that the
target substance to be measured remains unaltered or is altered as little as possible
so that the results will remain medically useful.

1. Collection: This can further be subdivided as to the type of specimen (serum,
                  urine, etc.) the site of collection (vein, heart,, kidney), the time
                  (AM, PM), the patient's position, sex, age (recumbent, etc.), in-
                  terfering drugs. Each of these parameters must be addressed and
                  specified in a procedure so as to assist the physician in interpret-
                  ing the final results. Example: (1) plasma renin collected in a
                  chilled container at $r^{o}C$; (2) collected above the right kidney in
                  the inferior vena cava while the female 75 year-old patient was
                  recumbent; (3) the specimen was collected at 8:00 AM following
                  (4) an injection apresoline HCL.

2. Handling: This includes the proper identification of the specimen, the trans-
                  portation, clotting, separation, aliquoting, the type of tube,
                  preparation in work set-up, and pipetting. Example: T_4 is known
                  to be retained by certain types of ceramic filters, plasticizers
                  may leak into the serum sample making it useless.

3. Storage: The idea behind storage is to help retain the original amount of the
                  target substance without undue alteration in amount of activity,
                  thereby rendering the information useless. For most RIA work, it is
                  recommended that the analysis be done as soon as possible, if not
                  yesterday. It may not always be feasible to perform a procedure for
                  one specimen, therefore the batching economics dictates that the
                  specimen be stored until tested. This is usually carried out at
                  minus $20^{o}C$ or lower. The length of storage will vary with each
                  analyte.

4. Procedure: The ultimate responsibility rests with the analyst. If the analyst
                  were to study a procedure and record where "things can go wrong"
                  it would undoubtedly span this chapter. It is not accidental that
                  a procedure is formulated the way it is. Quality control insists
                  that each step be carried out in a predictable manner so that the out-
                  come can be just as predictable.

There are many items to consider when relating to procedures: (a) understand the testing principle; (b) check the quality of the reagents; (c) check the pipetting precision; (d) check the incubation temperature and time; (e) verify the separation of fractions; (f) check the counting; (g) verify the calculations; (h) check the transcribing of the report; (i) post the reports on the proper charts; (j) note the precision of "in-run" duplicate and replicate determinations; and (k) interpret the results accurately.

Each of the above merits a paragraph of its own.

TESTING PRINCIPLE   How do you know if anything went wrong in the testing, if you do not understand how the procedure works? The answer rests with the educational process. As a teacher has a responsibility to the student, so to the student has a responsibility to seek to understand the subject matter.

REAGENT QUALITY   This may be more difficult or even beyond the control of the analyst since many testing kits are packaged and tested by the manufacturer. However, if reagents are made "in-house", it is vital that records of their performance be available for inspection to alert the analyst of any possible deterioration. Why do you take your drinking water for granted? Perhaps because there is someone overseeing its fittness for consumption. This is quality assurance.

PIPETTING   Pipetting is one of the greatest sources of error. When microliter quantities are at stake, it does not require excessive dehydration or carryover to disturb RIA tests. Consider for a moment a batch of pregnancy tests where the use of pipetting equipment resulted in excessive carryover of serum, the result: someone's test is "slightly positive". Well, no one is slightly pregnant!! All pipetting devices should be periodically checked for precision and cleanliness.

TEMPERATURE AND TIME   These parameters may already have been predetermined, but someone had to do it originally. It is not uncommon to see analysts anticipate timed reactions "hoping" that the variation will not affect the test results. The individual who calibrates stop-watches may be wasting time by doing so, if no one uses them properly. Water bath temperatures must be monitored or, if room temperature incubation is required, how much error will a draft introduce in the testing procedure? These are all minor, but serious questions. Would you want someone counting out your pay in front of an oscillating fan?

SEPARATION   The control of this function mainly re-emphasizes the need to standardize the centrifuge speed so that the proper "g" forces are applied to sediment a precipitate.

COUNTING   The equipment for counting is usually quite reliable provided the instrument has enough radiation to count. To yield a probable counting error of less than 1%, the statistical magic number quoted is usually 10,000 counts per minute. As the counts decrease to about 200 C.P.M., the probable error increases to about 6%. The analyst can determine what the probable error is for the instrument in use.

CALCULATION   Refer back to Murphy's third law. Semi-automated instruments have significantly reduced mathematical errors. Programmable calculators are available. There may still be that forgotten digit or excessive "rounding off" which creates more errors. Don't forget that the final answer reported encompasses the sum total of all the conscious or unconscious errors inherent or explicit in the procedure.

TRANSCRIBING   Needless to say, we all make clerical errors. After all, our art is analysis not transcribing. This may be the excuse given to justify neglect, but what if you sold your company for 10^6 dollars and you received a check for 10^{-6} dollars?

POSTING   You undoubtedly have heard about Mrs. Jones getting Mrs. Smith's operation? Remind me to tell you about it someday.

PRECISION   Statistical data can be manipulated by various formulas to reflect whatever terms we wish the results to be expressed in. Precision is such a mathematical reflection, it can take on the terms of coefficient of variation, standard deviation, percentile, average, etc., it is a measure of agreements between a series of test results. Precision can be measured with a "run-on" duplicate samples, between consecutive runs, etc. It is a means of measuring confidence or trustworthiness in the test results. As an example, if the cofidence in the test is 95% ± 5%, it simple means that the results reported can be relied upon of 90 to 100% of the stated value.

To assist in determining precision, one or two control samples are run with the tests and, after accumulating sufficient data say 20 sets, the formulas can be applied to reflect the true nature of the testing procedure. By producing such analyses day after day, or month after month, some degree of confidence can be established so that a certain degree of predictability can be achieved. On a day to day basis, it may not always be possible to monitor trends or lack of sensitivity, but precision by setting limits, can show if the test system is out of control. Example: 5-10% within assay duplicate and 8-15% between assay replication. One little note: the reaction system can have a high degree of precision, but lack accuracy. In other words, if the standardization is not correct, no matter how precise the test system is, the results cannot be believable.

CALIBRATION   Calibration is a process which assures performance on a continual basis and within predictable limits. Although it would be a blessing if analysts could be this way, it would not be a pleasant world to live in. We can rest assured that the analysts we have are of a certain "caliber".

Instrument and standard calibrations are essential for these are the basis against which all measurements are taken.

INSTRUMENT   The scintillator will usually require a constant check or background radiation. This guards against contamination and checks for reproducibility. A radioactive source such as Cesium-137 can be used. The latter will measure the day to day variation in counting. When the drift jeopardizes the validity of the results, it must be corrected. The scintillator also requires frequent checks of the peak energy setting, the window setting, the gain, etc. To be of value, all data pertaining to the instrument settings must be recorded in an easily scannable manner.

STANDARD   This is the most important calibrant. It should be referenced against an international standard of measurement so that everyone will interpret test results identically. It must be stable and homogenous. It must have the same reactivity as the substance to be measured.

MAINTENANCE   Quality assurance can be enhanced by preventive maintenance. Instrument failure is often a precipitous occurence, but if it can be averted by cleaning fans, filters, oiling necessary parts, cleaning electronic contact points, etc., the frequency or failure may be reduced significantly. There are two prevailing attitudes: (a) don't touch it if everything is going right, and (b) fix it before it goes wrong. Instrument experience frequently influences the analyst's attitudes. Obviously, the answer is to know the instrument and anticipate "down time" and also to develop and maintain alternate "back up" systems. With expensive systems, there are no back-ups --just anticipation.

DOCUMENTATION   There is no greater let down than to be told that you may have made a mistake. The only defense you may have is proper documentation of your work. Laboratory inspectors have for a motto: "If it is not documented, it was never done." Keep this in mind.

BIBLIOGRAPHY AND RECOMMENDED READINGS

Arena, V. *IONIZING RADIATION AND LIFE*. 1971. The C. V. Mosby Company.

Bruer, H., D. Hamel, and H. L. Krüskeper. *METHODS OF HORMONE ANALYSIS*. 1976. John Wiley and Sons Company.

Day, E. *ADVANCED IMMUNOCHEMISTRY*. 1972. The Williams and Wilkins Company

Freeman, L. and D. Blaufox. *RADIOIMMUNOASSAY*. 1975. Grune and Stratton.

Inhorn, S, *QUALITY ASSURANCE PRACTICES FOR HEALTH LABORATORIES*. American Public Health Association, Byrd Pre-Press Inc.

Odell, W. D. *PRINCIPLES OF COMPETITIVE PROTEIN-BINDING ASSAYS*. 1971. J. B. Lippincott Company.

Race, G. J. *LABORATORY MEDICINE*. 1980. Harper and Row Publishers.

Rose, N. and H. Friedman. *MANUAL OF CLINICAL IMMUNOLOGY*. 1976. American Society for Microbiology.

Spinks, J. W. T. and R. J. Woods. *AN INTRODUCTION TO RADIATION CHEMISTRY*. 2nd Ed. 1976. John Wiley and Sons Company.

THE LIGAND QUARTERLY. Vol. 2 N. 4. December 1979.

The American Association of Clinical Chemists, Inc. *CLINICAL RADIOASSAY PROCEDURES: A COMPENDIUM*. 1975. Academic Press.

Thorell, J., and S. Larson, *RADIOIMMUNOASSAY AND RELATED TECHNIQUES*. Methodology and Applications. 1978. The C. V. Mosby Company.

Weir, D, M. *HANDBOOK OF EXPERIMENTAL IMMUNOLOGY*. 1978. J. B. Lippincott Company.

Chapter 10

Urinalysis/Body Fluid Analysis

ALBERT E. PACKARD, BS, MT (ASCP)
Instructor of Biology
Natural Science Division
Notre Dame College
Manchester, New Hampshire

INTRODUCTION

The analysis of urine, and other body fluids, has traditionally been performed with mixed emotions. A well performed urinalysis may provide more information concerning the general condition of the body than any other single set of tests. Despite this well known fact, the analysis of urine is most often relegated to the "low-man-on-the-totum-pole", and most often is performed in the least well equipped, and often isolated laboratory. This is due, in part, to the analysis of urine as a "routine" procedure, and also in part to the poor esthetic reputation of urine.

The analyses of other body fluids are also shunned by many clinical laboratory practitioners. Speculation as to the reasons for this include: (1) these specimens are not seen frequently enough for the practitioner to feel comfortable with the analyses; (2) the lack of a large number of samples makes the quality control of the analyses difficult; and (3) there is a general lack of knowledge about these specimens with regard to their composition and normal vs. abnormal findings.

Hopefully, the "routineness" of urine analysis and the foreignness of other body fluids will be overcome, when the student of clinical laboratory science and the clinical laboratory practitioner come to believe in the value of body fluid analyses as important diagnostic tools.

The intent of this chapter is to provide the student and practitioner of clinical laboratory science with a concise review of the analysis of urine and other body fluids.

URINALYSIS/BODY FLUID ANALYSES

URINALYSES

Physical Tests   The physical examination of urine includes the evaluation of the color, appearance, odor, dissolved solids content, and, in some instances, the volume excreted.

COLOR   Normal, fresh urine has a color that ranges from clear and colorless or yellow to slightly amber, depending upon the concentration of the sample. The normal yellow to amber color is due to the presence of normal pigments known as urochromes. Dilute samples tend to be lighter in color, while concentrated samples tend to be darker.

Abnormal urine color may be almost any clor of the rainbow, depending on the source of the pigment. These abnormal colors include:

A. Various shades of orange which may be due to bile pigments, the food pigment in rhubarb, or a variety of medications;

B. Various shades of red to purple which may be due to hemoglobin, myoglobin, porphyrins, dyes, or a variety of medications;

C. Various shades of brown to black which may be due to hemoglobin, methemoglobin, porphyrins, melanin, homogentisic acid, the food pigment in rhubarb, phenolic drugs, dyes, or a variety of medications;

D. Various shades of yellow to green which may be due to riboflavin, bile pigments, dyes, and a variety of medications, and

E. Various shades of blue which may be due to dyes and a variety of medications.

A smokey color may also be seen. This is most commonly due to the presence of red blood cells.

The presence of these abnormal colors will often depend upon the pH of the urine or the amount of time that the sample has been standing.

APPEARANCE   Normal urine samples may be clear or cloudy. Cloudy or turbid urine samples are most commonly due to the presence of dietary urates or phosphates found in samples collected after meals. Abnormal cloudiness or turbidity may be due to the presence of white blood cells, red blood cells, bacteria, yeasts, or large amounts of lipids.

ODOR   Normal urine has a mildly aromatic odor that is generally not considered offensive. Other odors, although not considered clinically significant, may be detected. Certain foods such as asparagus or garlic may impart distinctive odors to the urine. The presence of acetone may give the urine a fruity odor. Bacterial decomposition of urea may give the urine a rather offensive ammoniacal odor. The presence of phenylketones may give the urine a "mousey" odor. Maple syrup urine disease will give the urine a maple syrup odor.

DISSOLVED SOLIDS CONTENT   Measurement of dissolved solids, or total solids, may be accomplished by one of the following methods:

A. *SPECIFIC GRAVITY:* The specific gravity of urine is measured by the use of a floatation device known as a urinometer. The urinometer is calibrated at $20^{\circ}C$ using distilled water for a reading of 1.000. The procedure calls for approximately 15-20 ml or more of urine. The urinometer is floated in the urine and readings taken from the scale on the urinometer at the surface of the urine. Since the urinometer is calibrated at $20^{\circ}C$, variations in room temperature must be taken into consideration. Each $3^{\circ}C$ above $20^{\circ}C$ readings must be corrected by adding 0.001 and each $3^{\circ}C$ below $20^{\circ}C$ readings must be corrected by subtracting 0.001. Corrections must also be made for the amount of glucose or protein present. For each gram of glucose per hundred ml of urine, 0.004 must be subtracted from the reading. For each 0.4 gm of protein per hundred ml, the reading must be corrected by subtracting 0.001. Normal urine has a specific gravity range from 1.010 to 1.025. Abnormal specific gravity is either increased, decreased, or fixed specific gravity.

Increased specific gravity, that is values over 1.025, may be due to excessive water loss, nephrosis, X-ray contrast media, diabetes, congestive heart failure, or liver disorders. Decreased specific gravity, that is, values below 1.010, may be due to renal disorders involving tubular damage, increased fluid intake, diabetes, or sickle cell disease. Fixed specific gravity, isothenuria, is usually associated with the inability of the kidney to concentrate urine. The inability to concentrate urine is usually due to severe damage of the renal tubules.

B. *REFRACTOMETRY:* Refractometry is the measurement of the refractive index of urine. The refractive index is the ratio of the velocity of light in the air to the velocity of light in solution. The refractive index and specific gravity are closely related in that they both increase with increasing amounts of dissolved solids. For the sake of simplicity in comparison of results, the refractive index obtained from the Goldberg refractometer is usually expressed in terms of specific gravity. This method is widely used because it is rapid, simple, and requires a very small volume of urine (only one drop). The refractometer, also known as the American Optical TS meter, may be obtained in models that are hand held, mounted on lighted bases, or mounted on lighted bases with automatic self rinsing capacity. Since the refractive index is usually expressed in terms of specific gravity, normal and abnormal values may be found in the text discussing specific gravity.

C. *OSMOLALITY:* Osmolality is probably the most accurate way to determine the amount of dissolved material in a urine sample. Osmolality is usually determined with the use of an osmometer which measures the osmolality by determining the freezing point depression or vapor pressure of the urine sample. Osmolality is expressed in terms of milliosmoles. A one molal solution, or 1000 mOsm per kilogram, depresses the freezing point of water by $1.86^{o}C$. Osmolality measures the colligative properties of a solution which depends on the number of particles present in the solution. Normal urine has an osmolality range of 5000 to 800 mOsm per kilogram of water. An osmolality of 800 mOsm is approximately equivalent to a specific gravity of 1.025. Increased osmolality may be seen in water retention, cirrhosis of the liver, congestive heart failure and high protein diets. Decreased osmolality may be seen in diabetes, increased water loss, hypokalemia and hypercalcemia.

D. *FALLING DROP:* The falling drop method is based on the urine falling a specific distance through an immiscible fluid. The time required for the drop to fall a specific distance is inversely related to the specific gravity. This method is utilized in the Ames Company automated urinalysis instrument CLINILAB®. Results are expressed in terms of specific gravity.

E. *VOLUME:* The normal volume of urine excreted in a 24 hour period ranges from 600 to 2,000 mls with the day volume being two to three times the night volume. Volumes in excess of 2,000 mls per 24 hours are termed polyuria, while volumes of less than 500 ml per 24 hours are termed oliguria, and a complete stoppage of urine formation is termed anuria. Increased urine volumes may be due to diabetes, excessive water intake, renal failure or some adrenal disorders. Decreased urine volumes may be due to dehydration, nephrosis, acute glomerulonephritis, or renal obstruction.

Chemical Tests   The chemical tests employed in the analysis of urine include: pH, glucose, proteins, ketones, hemoglobin, myoglobin, bilirubin and urobilinogen, enzymes, phenylketones, calcium, porphyrins, nonprotein nitrogenous compounds, and special chemistry tests.

pH   Normal freshly excreted urine has a pH that generally falls between 5.5 and 6.5. However, urine pH may be found to be anywhere from 5.0 to 9.0. The pH of urine is one of the tests commonly performed in "routine" urinalysis. Methods of determining urine pH vary depending on the desired level of accuracy. These methods include: litmus paper tests, dipstick tests, nitrazine indicator papers, and pH meter determinations.

LITMUS PAPER TESTS   The litmus paper test is useful as a screening test to determine the acidity or alkalinity of a urine sample. The major drawback to this procedure is simply that there is no differentiation in relation to the degree of acidity or alkalinity.

DIPSTICK TESTS   The dipstick test for urine pH is probably the most widely used method since it is simple and provides some differentiation of the degree of acidity or alkalinity. Also, this test is relatively inexpensive, and is usually one portion of a multiphasic screening dipstick. The test employs two indicators impregnated onto filter paper strips attached to a paper or plastic holder. The two indicators, methyl red and bromthymol blue, provide color changes that indicate pH values ranging from 5.0 to 9.0. The color produced on the strip is visually compared to a color chart that is provided with the strips.

NITRAZINE INDICATOR PAPERS   Nitrazine indicator papers are used in much the same manner as the dipstick tests, providing a color change that spans from a pH of 4.0 to a pH of 8.0. As in the case of the dipstick tests, the nitrazine papers are simple, provide some differentiation of the degree of acidity or alkalinity, and are relatively inexpensive. Unless the purpose of examination is strictly to monitor urine pH, it appears that testing for urine pH with nitrazine papers would be un- necessary since most "routine" urinalysis performed today employs some form of mul- tiphasic screening, and most of these methods employ dipsticks with a pH strip.

pH METERS   pH meters provide the most accurate means of measuring urine pH. How- ever, unless this accuracy is necessary, the use of pH meters for the determination of urine pH, is impractical. Acid pH is associated with normal freshly voided urine samples, high protein diet, acidosis, diabetes, and certain medications. Night urine is usually more acid than day urine, and since clinically important crystals and casts are destroyed or dissolved by alkaline media, the first morning specimen is usually the specimen of choice for urinalysis. Alkaline pH is associated with the post-prandial alkaline tide, which occurs approximately one hour after meals, urine specimens that have been left standing, bacterial decomposition of urea releasing ammonia, some medicines, and more specifically some antibiotics.

GLUCOSE   Glucose is one of the "threshold" substances found in the urine. Threshold substances are those substances which are selectively reabsorbed by the renal tubules up to a certain level or threshold. Normally, the kidney will reabsorb glucose at levels of 160 mg/dl $\pm$ 20 mg/dl. Therefore, glucose will appear in the urine in ap- preciable levels in only two instances: (1) when the renal threshold has been ex-- ceeded, that is, the blood levels are over the threshold limit as in diabetes melli- tus, or, (2) when the renal threshold is lower than normal, a condition referred to as renal glycosuria. A "routine" urinalysis almost always includes a screening test for glucose. The methods employed are generally of two types; those that are testing for the presence of reducing substances, or those that are specific for glucose. These methods include: the Benedict's test and the dipstick tests utilizing glucose oxidase.

THE BENEDICT'S TEST   Benedict's test is based on the principle that reducing sub- stances will reduce copper ions in a hot alkaline solution. This procedure, and its modification, known as the Clinitest Tablets®, is a semiquantitative method. This procedure, particularly its modification, is easy to perform. This is utilized as a screening procedure, and is utilized by many diabetics to monitor and regulate their insulin intake. The major drawback to this procedure is that it is not specific for glucose. Any reducing substance present in the urine will result in a positive re- action. Some of the more common reducing substances that will give a positive reac- tion include: galactose, fructose, lactose, pentoses, homogentisic acid, high levels of creatinine and uric acid, ascorbic acid, certain antibiotics and formaldehyde. There is one advantage of this non-specificity in that it allows the detection of galactosemia in infants. The reaction for this procedure is:

$$\text{Cupric ions} + \text{Reducing} \xrightarrow[\substack{\text{alkaline} \\ \text{medium}}]{\text{heat}} \text{Cuprous ions} + \text{Oxidized}$$

Cupric ions	+ Reducing	Cuprous ions	+ Oxidized
(Blue)	Substance	(Orange)	Reducing
			Substance

ENZYMATIC TESTS   Most of the dipstick tests available for the detection of glucose in urine, utilize an enzymatic procedure that is specific for glucose. Two forms of this procedure are available: (1) a glucose oxidase method with o-tolidine as a chromogen, and (2) a glucose oxidase method with an iodine complex as a chromogen. The test is based on the principle that glucose oxidase catalyzes the oxidation of glucose to gluconic acid and hydrogen peroxide. The hydrogen peroxide with the enzyme peroxidase results in the oxidation of the chromogen which results in a color change of the chromogen. The distinct advantage of utilizing the enzymatic procedure for the determination of the presence of glucose is that is is specific for glucose, and that normal constituents of urine do not result in false positive results. False positive results obtained with this procedure are usually due to the presence of some contaminant in or on the glassware or collection containers such as hydrogen peroxide or bleach, both of which may be found commonly in many homes. False negative results are more frequently encountered. The procedure that utilizes o-tolidine as the chromogen receptor will yield false negative results in the presence of large amounts of ketones in the urine, as well as with large amounts of strong reducing substances such as ascorbic acid, which compete with the chromogen for the oxygen released in the reaction. The procedure that utilizes the iodine complex as the chromogen receptor does not result in false negative results in the presence of large amounts of ketones, but does result in false negatives in the presence of large amounts of strong reducing substances. The reactions for these procedures are as follows:

1. Glucose + Oxygen $\xrightarrow{\text{glucose oxidase}}$ Gluconic acid + Hydrogen peroxide

Hydrogen peroxide + o-tolidine (Chromogen) $\xrightarrow{\text{peroxidase}}$ Oxidized o-tolidine + H_2O

2. Glucose + Oxygen $\xrightarrow{\text{glucose oxidase}}$ Gluconic acid + Hydrogen peroxide

Hydrogen peroxide + Iodine comples (Chromogen) $\xrightarrow{\text{peroxidase}}$ Oxidized Iodine Complex + H_2O

PROTEINS   The measurement of proteins in urine is probably the most sensitive indicator of renal damage. Normally, protein in the urine does not exceed 20–25 mg/dl. Levels above 25 mg/dl may indicate some form of renal tubular damage. Elevated or abnormal urine protein levels are referred to as proteinuria. Proteinuria exists in several forms, ranging from proteinuria due to renal damage, proteinuria due to pre-renal disorders, and benign proteinuria due to orthostatic or transitory proteinuria. Renal causes of proteinuria include acute and chronic glomerulonephritis, nephrosclerosis, nephrotic syndrome, polycystic kidney disease, renal tubular disorders, and renal damage associated with systemic lupus erythematosus. Pre-renal causes of proteinuria include cardiac disorders, convulsive disorders, febrile disorders, liver disorders, and hematologic disorders. Benign proteinuria is that type of proteinuria that is not associated with disease and includes proteinuria resulting from: excessive exercise, prolonged exposure to heat or cold, emotional stress, and ingestion of large amounts of protein. Orthostatic proteinuria is that type of proteinuria that is associated with a postural defect resulting in disappearance of the proteinuria when the patient lies down. There are several methods that are available for the determination of proteinuria, including:

A. *PROTEIN ERROR OF INDICATORS:* This method is used for a rapid, colorimetric, screeming of urine samples for proteinuria. The dipstick methods utilize this principle. This method is based on the principle that in the presence of protein, some acid-base indicators will change color without a change in pH. The dipstick methods utilize tetrabromphenol blue, which is yellow at a pH of 3 and blue at a pH of 5. The filter paper strip is impregnated with tetrabromphenol blue and a buffer to maintain the pH at 3. In the presence of protein, the color of the strip will change from yellow to green to blue, depending on the amount of protein present in the sample. False positive values occur in urine samples that are highly alkaline and actually produce a pH change.

B. *SULFOSALICYLIC ACID METHOD:* This method is one of the semi-quantitative methods. This method is based on the principle that most urine proteins are coagulated in dilute solutions of sulfosalicylic acid, and this forms a turbid solution which can be interpreted visually. Visual interpretation may be standardized, to some degree, by using a set of Kingsbury standards for comparison. False positive results may be obtained if the urine contains tolbutamide metabolites, mucin, high concentrations of uric acid, penicillin, or some X-ray contrast media. False negative results may be obtained with highly buffered alkaline urines.

C. *HEAT AND ACETIC ACID METHOD:* This method is another of the semi-quantitative methods. The principle of this method is that proteins are coagulated by heat resulting in the formation of a turbid solution which can be interpreted visually. The acetic acid is utilized to prevent turbidity that may result from the presence of phosphates or mucin. False positive results may be obtained if the urine contains tolbutamide metabolites, large quantities of penicillin, or some X-ray contrast media. False negative results may be obtained with highly buffered alkaline urines.

D. *ESBACH'S METHOD:* This method is a quantitative method. This method is based on the principle that proteins are precipitated with picric acid, and that the amount of precipitate produced may be measured in standardized tubes. This method is usually used for determining the total amount of protein excreted in a 24 hour period.

KETONES   Acetone, diacetic acid, and beta-hydroxybutyric acid are collectively known as ketone bodies. Ketone bodies are not normally found in the urine, but may be found whenever there is increased fat metabolism. Increased fat metabolism occurs whenever there is a decrease in carbohydrate metabolism such as in diabetes, starvation, severe diarrhea and vomiting, and low carbohydrate diets. The ketone bodies are formed from the accumulation and condensation of excess acetyl-Co A in the liver. The condensation of acetyl-CoA results in the formation of acetoacetic acid, some of which is reduced to beta-hydroxybutyric acid, and some of which is decarboxylated to form acetone. The simplified relationship of these compounds is as follows:

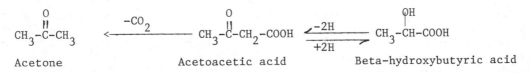

Acetone   Acetoacetic acid   Beta-hydroxybutyric acid

Excess concentrations of ketone bodies in the blood results in their excretion into the urine. It is possible to detect the presence of acetone and acetoacetic acid in the urine, however, there is no direct test available to determine the presence of beta-hydroxybutyric acid. Several methods are available for the detection of ketone bodies in the urine, including:

A. *ACETEST® METHOD:* The principle of this test is that sodium nitroprusside reacts with acetone and acetoacetic acid to form a colored complex. It does not react with beta-hydroxybutyric acid. The color produced by this reaction is purple, and ranges from lavender, to deep purple depending upon the amount of ketones present. False positive results may be obtained when the urine contains phthalein compounds, melanogens, cystine, or large amounts of phenylketones.

B. *DIPSTICK METHODS:* The dipstick methods utilize reagents similar to those used in the Acetest® method. The principle and results are similar to those of the Acetest® method.

C. *GERHARDT'S TEST:* Gerhardt's test is used to detect the presence of acetoacetic acid in urine. This method is based on the principle that acetoacetic acid will react with a 10% ferric chloride to produce a red complex. False positive results may be obtained when the urine contains salicylates, phenothiazides, or phenols. These false positive tests may be differentiated from reactions with diacetic acid by boiling the solution. If, after boiling, the color disappears the test was positive for acetoacetic acid, whereas, if the color persists after boiling, the reaction was due to some interfering substance.

D. *ROTHERA'S TEST:* This method is used to detect the presence of acetone and aceto-acetic acid. The test is based on the principle that acetone and acetoacetic acid will react with sodium nitroprusside to form a red-purple colored complex. False positive reactions will occur if the patient has received phthalien dyes.

E. *HART'S TEST:* Hart's test detects the presence of beta-hydroxybutyric acid. As was mentioned earlier, there is no direct test available for detecting beta-hydroxybutyric acid. This test measures the presence of beta-hydroxybutyric acid indirectly by first boiling the urine to remove any acetone or acetoacetic acid that may be present. After the urine has been boiled, hydrogen peroxide is added to the sample to reduce any beta-hydroxybutyric acid that is present. After reducing the sample, a nitroprusside test is performed to detect the presence of acetoacetic acid.

HEMOGLOBIN AND MYOGLOBIN Both hemoglobin and myoglobin are threshold substances. Hemoglobin has a renal threshold level of 100-140 mg/dl, while myoglobin has a renal threshold of approximately 20 mg/dl. Since free hemoglobin in the plasma is bound by haptoglobin, hemoglobinuria is usually found when the serum haptoglobin levels fall. The causes of hemoglobinuria include: incompatible blood transfusions, hemolytic anemias, burns, paroxysmal cold hemoglobinuria and paroxysmal nocturnal hemoglobin-uria. The causes of myoglobinuria include: crushing injuries, severe muscle damage due to exercise, electrical shock, and progressive muscle diseases. Hemoglobin and myoglobin are discussed together because the testing procedures used for the determination of hemoglobin in urine will result in positive tests in the presence of hemo-globin, myoglobin, and red blood cells. Methods of determining these substances include the following:

A. *BENZIDINE TEST:* This test is based on the principle that benzidine is oxidized by the oxygen released from hydrogen peroxide which is decomposed by the peroxidase activity of hemoglobin or myoblobin, and charged to its blue colored form. This is a very sensitive test. Care should be taken when using this method since benzidine has been found to be a potential carcinogen. When the microscopic examination is performed, the presence or absence of red blood cells may be established. If no red blood cells are found, and the benzidine test is positive, further testing will be necessary to determine whether the positive results are due to the presence of hemoglobin, myoglobin, or some other substance.

B. *ORTHOTOLIDINE METHOD:* This method is utilized in the dipstick procedures for the detection of hemoglobinuria, hematuria, or myoglobinuria. The test is based on the following principle. Hydrogen peroxide is decomposed by the peroxidase activity of hemoglobin and myoglobin. The oxygen which is released then oxidizes orthotolidine to its blue colored form. As in the benzidine method, microscopic examination for red blood cells must be performed. If no red blood cells are found, further testing will be necessary to determine the source of the positive results.

C. *AMMONIUM SULFATE TEST:* This test is used to determine the presence of myoglobin in the urine. This test is based on the principle that myoglobin is soluble in 80% ammonium sulfate while hemoglobin is not. Therefore, hemoglobin will preci- pitate in the 80% ammonium sulfate solution. Since substances such as porphyrins, dyes, and homogentisic acid will also produce a red color in urine, the sample should be tested for the presence of protein before continuing with the ammonium sulfate test. If the ammonium sulfate test is positive, confirmation of the pre- sence of myoglobin may be accomplished by testing the sample with a saturated solution of ammonium sulfate which should precipitate myoglobin.

BILIRUBIN TEST   Bilirubin is a bile pigment which, when found in the urine, is a sign of liver disease. The detection of bilirubin in the urine may indicate one of several liver diseases including: obstructive jaundice, and hepatocellular damage. Screening for bilirubin is of value because urine bilirubin levels are often elevated before other signs or symptoms of disease are found. Bilirubin in urine may be detected by several methods, including:

A. *PRESUMPTIVE OR SHAKE TEST:* This test is based on the finding of a yellow foam on the urine after it has been shaken. This is only a presumptive test and re- quires confirmation with tests that are specific for bilirubin.

B. *GMELIN TEST:* This test is based on the principle that bile pigments will be oxidized by nitric acid to provide a rainbow of colors at the interface of the reaction. The colors produced range from brown to red, purple, violet, blue, green and yellow.

C. *HARRISON TEST:* This test is based on the principle that bile pigments may be ex- tracted from urine onto barium chloride and oxidized by ferric chloride in trich- loroacetic acid to yield blue, green or yellow colored complexes. False positive results may be obtained if the urine contains salicylates.

D. *FREE AND FREE'S ICTOTEST:* This test is based on the principle that diazo salts will form colored complexes with bilirubin. This method is very sensitive and easily performed. A blue or purple color is a positive test, while the presence of salicylates, urobilin, or indican will produce an orange to red color.

E. *DIPSTICK METHOD:* This method is based on the same principle as the Ictotest, and utilizes a diazotized 2, 4-dichloroanaline as the active reagent. Bilrubin in the urine will react with the diazotized 2, 4-dichloroanaline to produce a brown colored compound. False positive results may be obtained if the urine contains large amounts of chlorpromazine or phenazopyridine.

UROBILINOGEN   Urobilinogen is another of the bile pigments. Normal urine contains very small amounts of urobilinogen. Urobilinogen levels are significant if they are either elevated or decreased. Increases in urobilinogen are associated with a vari- ety of disorders, including: hepatitis, portal cirrhosis, hemolytic anemias, malaria, and infectious mononucleosis. Decreased levels are associated with biliary obstruc- tion and antibiotic therapy. It has been shown that urobilinogen is excreted at the highest rate between the hours of 2:00 PM and 4:00 PM. Samples of urine to be tested for urobilinogen should be collected over that two hour period, preferably in a brown bottle, and tested as soon as possible. Urobilinogen may be detected by a variety of tests, including:

A.   *DIPSTICK METHOD:* This method is only useful in detecting elevated levels of urobilinogen. This method employs paradimethylaminobenzaldehyde which will react with urobilinogen to form yellow to brown colored complexes. Positive reactions are also obtained when the urine contains porphobilinogen or para-aminosalicylic acid.

B.   *EHRLICH'S TEST:* This method may be performed as a qualitative procedure or as a quantitative procedure. The method is based on the principle that urobilinogen will react with Ehrlich's aldehyde reagent to produce a cherry red color. Ehrlich's aldehyde reagent is utilized in other testing procedures for urobilinogen and is composed of concentrated hydrochloric acid, para-dimethylaminobenzaldehyde and distilled water. False reactions are obtained with other substances that produce red colors, including phenazopyridium, indole, and porphobilinogen.

C.   *WATSON-SCHWARTZ TEST:* This test is a qualitative test for both urobilinogen and porphobilinogen. This test is based on the principle that both urobilinogen and porphobilinogen will react with Ehrlich's aldehyde reagent and that the urobilinogen complex is soluble in chloroform, while the porphobilinogen complex is soluble in both chloroform and n-butanol. In this procedure, a pink pigment that is extractable with chloroform is due to the presence of urobilinogen; a pink pigment that is extractable with chloroform and then with n-butanol is due to the presence of porphobilinogen; and a pink pigment that is extractable with n-butanol but not with chloroform is due to the presence of some other substance.

Other Chemical Tests   There are a variety of other chemical tests which may be performed on urine samples. These tests include the analysis of aminoacidurias, catecholamines, carbohydrates, electrolytes, mucopolysaccharides, and phenolic acids. Since some of these groups of compounds overlap, these tests will be listed alphabetically by the condition or by the particular chemical tested for in the urine.

ALCAPTONURIA   Alcaptonuria is an inborn error of metabolism in which the patient is unable to oxidize homogentisic acid. This inability to oxidize homogentisic acid results in increased amounts of homogentisic acid being excreted in the urine. Several presumptive tests for alcaptonuria include: alkalinization of the urines to produce a brown to black color; Benedict's test, which will produce a green to black color with a black precipitate; the ferric chloride test which will produce a green color followed by a black precipitate and the Fishberg method which produces a blackening or developing of photographic paper when alkalinized urine containing homogentisic acid is dropped on it. The presumptive test should be confirmed by chromatographic procedures.

AMYLASE   Amylase is normally found in the urine of healthy individuals. The clinical value of urinary amylase levels is significant in acute pancreatitis and renal insufficiency. Elevated levels of urinary amylase may be observed in acute pancreatitis, while the rate of excretion of amylase may be of value in the diagnosis of renal insufficiency. The procedures available for the measurement of urinary amylase activity are the same as those used in the serum determination of this enzyme.

CALCIUM   Urinary calcium determinations are useful in the diagnosis of a variety of diseases. Elevated urine calcium levels may be found in hyperparathyroidism, bone tumors, hypervitaminosis D, hyperthyroidism, and Cushing's syndrome. Decreased urine calcium levels may be found in hypoparathyroidism, vitamin D deficiency, sprue celiac disease, and decreased calcium intake. Determinations of urine calcium may be accomplished by a semiquatitative method or a quantitative method. The semiquantitative method is known as the Sulkowitch test. The Sulkowitch test is based on the formation of calcium oxalate, which will precipitate, when the urine calcium reacts with ammonium oxalate. This procedure is only a screening test, but may be useful as a screening mechanism for hypoparathyroid patients for the regulation of their medication, and as an emergency method for the determination of hypercalcemia.

CATECHOLAMINES   The determination of urinary catecholamines is of value in the assessment of adrenomedullary function, specifically in the diagnosis of pheochromocytoma and neuroblastoma. The determination of total catecholamines is rapidly being replaced by specific tests for the metabolites of the catecholamines which provide more accurate information. Elevated levels of catecholamines will be found in patients with pheochromocytomas and neuroblastomas, but, may also be found in patients with widespread burns, muscular dystrophy, myasthenia gravis, and patients taking tetracyclines or methyldopa.

CHLORIDE   Urinary excretion of chloride varies considerably from one individual to the next. Normally, urine levels of chloride will decrease with a concurrent decrease in the serum chloride level. The estimation of urine chloride levels may be of use in the diagnosis of Addison's disease, since urinary chloride levels will still be considerable despite the fact that the serum levels have fallen below 100 mg/dl at which normal patients show very low levels of urinary chloride.

CREATININE   The estimation of urinary creatinine by itself is of little clinical value. However, the estimation of urinary creatinine along with that of plasma or serum creatinine levels is useful as a tool for the determination of the glomerular filtration rate. Creatinine determinations have advantages over some of the other clearance tests in that creatinine tests are not affected by a high protein diet, and creatinine is cleared at a high rate without appreciable reabsorbtion.

CYSTINE   The presence of cystine in the urine is associated with two conditions known as cystinosis and cystinuria. Cystinosis is due to the inability of the kidney to reabsorb substances such as glucose and amino acids. Cystinuria is not an inborn error of metabolism as in other aminoacidurias, but, is due to the inability of the kidney to absorb cystine, arginine, and ornithine. Increases of urinary cystine are often detected by the presence of cystine crystals in the urine sediment. The finding of these crystals must be confirmed by chemical methods. A qualitative test for cystine utlizes sodium nitroprusside which reacts with cystine to produce a magenta color. Since other compounds, including acetone, acetoacetic acid, melanogens, and salicylates will produce colored complexes with sodium nitroprusside, confirmation of the presence of cystine must be made by chromatographic methods.

HOMOVANILIC ACID   Urinary levels of homovanilic acid (HVA) are normally rather low, that is, below 15 mg/24 hours. HVA is a metabolite of the catecholamines and is found elevated in patients with neuroblastomas. HVA assay is particularly useful in distinguishing between neuroblastomas, which will produce elevated levels of HVA, from pheochromocytomas which will not produce elevated levels of HVA.

17-HYDROXYCORTICOSTEROIDS   The estimation of urinary 17-hydroxycorticosteroids is one of several hormone analyses that may be performed to assess adrenocortical disorders. The Porter-Silber reaction is the most widely used method for the determination of these hormones. For more extensive coverage of these compounds the reader is referred to clinical chemistry texts and texts on endocrine function.

5-HYDROXYINDOLACETIC ACID   The urinary estimation of serotonin, as its metabolite 5-hydroxyindolacetic acid (5-HIAA), is useful in the diagnosis of carcinoid tumors or argentaffinomas. Decreased levels of 5-HIAA may be obtained if the urine contains methyldopa or phenothiazines. Falsely elevated levels of 5-HIAA may be encountered with the metabolites of various drugs, such as phenacetin, and with the ingestion of certain foods that are high in serotonin, such as bananas, pineapples, and avocados.

INDICAN   Indole, normally produced by bacteria in the intestinal tract, is excreted in the urine in the form of potassium indoxyl phosphate which is better known as indican. Most of the indole produced by the bacteria is eliminated in the feces. Urinary elevations of indican are usually related to putrifactive disorders of the intestines, such as intestinal infarctions, gastric cancer, and gangrene. The Obermayer test will detect increased levels of indican in the urine. The Obermayer test utilizes a ferric chloride in hydrochloric acid reagent which will produce a faint blue color in normal urine samples, and deep violet-blue color when the urine contains elevated levels of indican.

17-KETOSTEROIDS   The 17-ketosteroids are a group of hormones that may be assayed in the assessment of adrenocortical disorders. As in the discussion on 17-hydroxycorticosteroids, the reader is referred to clinical chemistry texts and endocrinology texts for further, more extensive discussion of these compounds.

MELANIN   Melanin, a normal skin pigment, and its precursors known as melanogens, will only be present in the urine, in quantities sufficient to detect, in disorders such as malignant melanoma. There are two screening procedures that are used for the detection of melanin and melanogens, a ferric chloride test and the Thormählen test. The ferric chloride procedure utilizes a 10% ferric chloride reagent which will produce a gray-black precipitate if melanin or melanogens are present in abnormal quantities. The Thormählen test is also known as the nitroprusside test. Elevated levels of melanin in the urine will produce a blue-black color in strongly alkaline solutions of urine after acidification of the urine with glacial acetic acid.

MUCOPOLYSACCHARIDES   The mucopolysaccharides, dermatan sulfate, heparan sulfate, and keratan sulfate, are found in abnormal amounts in the urine in patients with genetic disorders such as Hurler's syndrome, Hunter's syndrome, Sanfilippo syndrome and Morquio syndrome. A screening procedure utilizing toluidine blue to form metachromatic complexes with the mucopolysaccharides will yield positive results with urine samples that contain elevated quantities of mucopolysaccharides.

PENTOSES   Urine levels of pentoses may be elevated after the ingestion of fruits high in pentoses, and in a rare disorder known as essential pentosuria. Pentoses will yield positive results with the reducing tests that are used in urinalysis, but not with the enzymatic tests. Definitive identification of the presence of specific pentoses may be accomplished with chromatographic procedures.

PHENYLKETONURIA   Phenylketonuria is an inborn error of metabolism which results in the excretion of increased amounts of phenylpyruvic acid in the urine. The build up of phenylketones is the result of inability to metabolize phenylalanine to tyrosine. If this disorder is detected early enough, before the age of four months, the disorder and its complications may be treated and prevented. Screening tests are available for the detection of increased urine levels of phenylpyruvic acid. These screening tests include: the diaper test or ferric chloride test, and the dipstick method. The diaper test or ferric chloride test is based on the principle that ferric ions will react with phenylpyruvic acid to form green to gray colored complexes. The diaper test is performed by adding ferric chloride directly to a baby's urine soaked diaper. The test is considered positive if a gray-green or olive green color appears on the diaper within three minutes. The ferric chloride test may also be performed on urine directly, with the same criteria for a positive test as that of the diaper test. The dipstick method is based on essentially the same principle as the ferric chloride test. Again, ferric ions in the test strip will react with phenylpyruvic acid to produce blue, gray, or green complexes. Positive results with either of these methods requires confirmation by blood analysis. This is normally accomplished by the Guthrie bacterial-inhibition test.

PHOSPHOROUS   Phosphorous may be excreted in the feces and the urine. Approximately 60% of the phosphorous excreted is excreted in the urine. The amount excreted by the kidney depends, for the most part, on the dietary intake of phosphorous. Increased phosphorous excretion in the urine may be due to primary hyperparathyroidism, while decreased excretion may be due to hypoparathyroidism. Testing procedures are the same as those used to determine the serum or plasma levels of phosphorous.

PORPHYRINS   The determination of urinary porphyrins is of value in the diagnosis of the various porphyrias. Porphyrins are tetrapyrolle structures that are intermediate to the formation of hemoglobin and cytochromes. Excess urine porphyrins may be detected by screening mechanisms such as the Watson-Schwartz test or the fluorescence tests. The Watson-Schwartz test employs Ehrlichs reagent. This has been previously discussed in the testing procedures for urobilinogen. The fluorescense tests will be positive in the presence of urinary porphyrins that have been adsorbed to an anion exchange resin, acidified, and then subjected to ultraviolet light at 380 nm.

SUGARS (OTHER THAN GLUCOSE)   Various mono- and disaccharides appear in the urine of patients with rare metabolic disorders. These sugars include: galactose, lactose, fructose, and sucrose. Each of these sugars, with the exception of sucrose, will yield positive results with the reducing tests that are normally used in urinalysis. Confirmation and identification of the specific sugar must be accomplished through chromatographic procedures.

VANILMANDILIC ACID   Vanilmandilic acid (VMA) levels will be elevated in the urine of patients with pheochromocytomas and neuroblastomas. For more detailed discussion of VMA, the reader is referred to texts on clinical chemistry and endocrinology.

MICROSCOPIC EXAMINATION OF URINE   The microscopic examination of urine is one of the most vital aspects of the "routine" urinalysis. The task of the clinical laboratory scientist, in the microscopic examination of urine, is to be able to distinguish between those items found in the urine sediment that are in fact significant, and those items that are artifactual. Among the significant items found in the urine sediment are: casts, cells, crystals, and microorganisms. Since the clinical significance of some of these items is based on the actual numbers present in the sediment, it is necessary to establish some form of standard procedure for quantitation. Unfortunately, there is no standard procedure for quantitating items found in the urine sediment. One method that has been suggested could, if accepted universally, provide a means of relating microscopic analysis of urine between clinical laboratories. This method calls for the centrifugation of a fixed volume of urine, ten to twelve ml, decantation of the supernatant urine, which is saved for chemical analysis, and the reconstitution of the sediment to one ml with the supernatant. Utilization of such a method would provide the physician with a more reliable day-to-day comparison of the formed elements that are excreted in the urine, and provide a mechanism for interlaboratory comparison.

CASTS   Casts are delicate cylindrical structures that are formed in the renal tubules. Three conditions for the formation of casts are essential; an acid pH, the proper solute concentration, and the Tamm-Horsfall mucoprotein. The matrix of the cast is composed of the Tamm-Horsfall mucoprotein in which organized structures, such as cells, may become encased. Casts are soluble in alkaline urines, therefore it is necessary to examine a freshly voided sample that has an acid pH. Casts are most commonly classified by their inclusions.

A. *HYALINE CASTS:* Hyaline casts are the most commonly found casts. The hyaline cast is essentially the coagulated mucoprotein without any inclusion bodies. The Tamm-Horsfall matrix has a refractive index that is close to that of glass which may make them difficult to see. Hyaline casts arc best detected when viewed under low power with reduced lighting.

B. *CELLULAR CASTS:* Cellular casts consist of the coagulated Tamm-Horsfall mucoprotein with cells encased. These casts are classified according to the type of cell encased in the matrix. The cellular casts include: red blood cell casts, white blood cell casts, and renal tubular epithelial cell casts. Red blood cell casts are indicative of damage to the glomeruli or the renal tubules which allow red cells to escape into the lumen of the nephron. Red blood cell casts are most commonly associated with diseases such as acute glomerulonephritis and systemic lupus erythematosus. White blood cell casts are most commonly associated with renal infection and may be found in patients that have pyelonephritis and lupus erythematosus. Renal tubular epithelial casts are associated with damage to the renal tubules resulting in the cuboidal epithelial cells of the tubules being deposited in the lumen of the tubules. Renal tubular epithelial casts are most commonly associated with acute and chronic glomerulonephritis.

C. *GRANULAR CASTS:* Granular casts are formed as the result the degeneration of cellular elements that were once contained in these casts. As the cells degenerate, the cast takes on a coarsely granular appearance with the casts then being referred to as coarsely granular casts. Further degeneration results in a finely granular appearance with the casts being referred to as finely granular casts. The granular casts are most commonly associated with acute and chronic renal disorders.

D. *WAXY CASTS:* Waxy casts are highly refractile, brittle casts with squared ends and prominent cracks. Waxy casts are formed as the result of further degeneration of the once cellular casts. Waxy casts are rarely found, and are associated with chronic, long-term, renal disorders. A variety of the waxy casts, known as the broad casts (because of their wide diameter) are most often associated with renal failure and are sometimes called renal failure casts.

E. *HEMOGLOBIN CASTS:* Hemoglobin casts are formed from the hemoglobin present following intravascular hemolysis.

F. *FATTY CASTS:* Fatty casts are casts which contain lipids. These casts, like the waxy casts, are associated with chronic renal disorders. The lipids contained in these casts are anisotropic and are best demonstrated by the use of polarized light microscopy.

Proper identification of casts with standard light microscopy is difficult. Ideally, interference phase contrast microscopy would be used since this provides excellent three dimensional images of the casts and makes identification and differentiation of casts much easier. However, since interference phase microscopes are expensive, and since the urinalysis laboratory is usually the poorest equipped laboratory, it is unlikely that many clinical laboratories will afford this luxury.

CELLS   Various cellular elements may be found in the urine sediment. These cells include red blood cells, white blood cells, and epithelial cells.

A. *RED BLOOD CELLS:* Red blood cells in urine indicate some form of damage to the elements of the urinary tract. They will appear as round, refractive structures and, depending on the tonicity of the urine sample, may be crenated, biconcave, or spherical. It is important to differentiate red blood cells from other urine sediment elements such as yeasts and oil droplets. This differentiation may be accomplished by adding dilute acetic acid under the cover glass and re-examining the sediment. If the structures observed were red blood cells, they will have disintegrated, whereas yeasts, oil droplets and crystals will not have disintegrated.

B. *WHITE BLOOD CELLS:* Few white blood cells may normally be found in urine sediments. However, an increased number of white blood cells may indicate some form of infectious process in the urinary tract. The most common type of white blood cell observed is the polymorphonuclear neutrophil, which, in hypotonic solutions, may display Brownian movement giving the cells a "glittering" appearance. These cells are often referred to as glitter cells.

C. *EPITHELIAL CELLS:* Squamous epithelial cells may normally be found in urine sediments. The source of these cells is most frequently the urinary bladder. The presence of large numbers of these cells is of no clinical significance, however, large numbers of these cells may obscure the view of other significant elements in the sediment. Renal tubular epithelial cells are cuboidal cells which, when released into the urine, tend to become round, and are easily mistaken for white blood cells. Staining the urine sediment may aid in the differentiation of renal tubular epithelial cells from white blood cells by providing a better view of the large prominent nucleus of the cuboidal epithelial cell.

CRYSTALS   A wide variety of crystals, both normal and abnormal, may be found in the urine sediment. These crystals, for the most part, may be separated into two major groups; those found in acid urines, and those found in alkaline urines. Normal crystals that may be found in urine sediments include: amorphous urates, uric acid, calcium oxalate, calcium phosphates, and occasionally calcium sulfates. The abnormal crystals are only found in acid urines, and these include: cholesterol, cystine, leucine, and tyrosine. The normal crystals that may be found in alkaline urine sediments include: ammomium magnesium phosphates (triple phosphates), amorphous phosphates, calcium phosphates, calcium cabonates, ammonium biurates, and calcium oxalates.

Amorphous urate crystals are red crystals that when present in large amounts, tend to give the urine a pink color. Large amounts of amorphous urates are of no clinical significance, however, large quantities of these crystals may obscure the view of other significant elements in the sediment. Amorphous urates may be removed by heating or treatment with alkali. Uric acid crystals may normally be found in the urine sediment. Uric acid crystals may appear in a variety of shapes, however, most generally are found in the shape of whetstones, six sided plates, and in rosettes. These crystals are most frequently yellow in color, but may be colorless. Occasionally, these crystals may be found in the form of pseudocasts. Calcium oxalate crystals are the only crystals that are normally found in acid, neutral, or alkaline urine. These crystals are most commonly seen as refractive double envelope forms, however, they may be found as oval forms. Calcium phosphate crystals may be found in acid urines, although they are more frequently found in alkaline urines. The normal crystals of alkaline urines also exhibit a variety of shapes. The ammonium magnesium phosphate or triple phosphate crystals are colorless crystals that may be found in the shapes of coffin lids or hip roofs. Amorphous phosphates appear as white, small, amorphously shaped crystals which are of no clinical value. They may appear abundantly after meals. These crystals are insoluble when the urine is heated, but are soluble when acetic acid is added. Calcium phosphates are also found in alkaline urines, and appear as colorless, slender, prisms or needles. These crystals are also insoluble when the urine is heated, but soluble in acetic acid. Calcium carbonate crystals appear as small dumbbell shaped crystals that are soluble, with effervescence, in acetic acid, Ammonium biurate crystals appear as yellow to brown crystals with characteristic thorn apple appearance. The crystals are soluble when the urine is heated.

The abnormal crystals, when found in the urine sediment, are of greatest significance. Although they are rarely encountered, it is of utmost importance that they be recognized, and, in all cases, chemically confirmed. Cholesterol crystals are found as colorless, flat plates with notched corners. These crystals may be found in acid urines, and occasionally in neutral urines. Cystine crystals are found in both primary and secondary cystinuria. These crystals are found as colorless, transparent, hexagonal plates. These crystals are only found in acid urine samples and will readily dissolve as the urine becomes alkaline. Tyrosine crystals appear as colorless to yellow, fine needles or sheaves of these needles. As in the case of the cystine crystals, these crystals will dissolve in alkaline urines. Leucine crystals are also rarely encountered. They appear as spheres with radial striations that are yellow to brown in color. These too will dissolve in alkaline urines. As mentioned earlier, all findings of abnormal crystals must be confirmed with chemical tests. The chemical tests for these crystals are as follows: (1) cholesterol crystals may be confirmed by their solubility characteristics; (2) cystine crystals may be confirmed with the nitroprusside reaction; (3) tyrosine crystals may be confirmed with Mörner reagent; and (4) leucine crystals may be confirmed with the Salkowski test.

In addition to the crystals mentioned, it is also possible to encounter crystals from the sulfa drugs. These crystals are considered to be abnormal crystals and must be chemically confirmed by applying diazo reagent.

MICROORGANISMS   A variety of microorganisms may be encountered in urine sediment, either as pathogenic agents or as contaminants. These organisms range from bacteria to yeasts, or from flagellates to ova of larger parasites. The presence of bacteria may be due to actual infection or to contamination of the urine. In either case, a "clean-catch" urine specimen should be obtained for culture and possible susceptibility tests. Yeasts may also be found in the urine. The usual cause of yeast in the urine is due to vaginal contamination, and the organism most frequently encountered is *Candida albicans*, the causative agent of monilia. Another fairly frequent vaginal contaminant is a parasite known as *Trichomonas vaginalis*. Trichomonads are easily recognized by their swift jerky movement in urine sediment. The ova of two other parasites are sometimes encountered in urine sediment. The ova of *Enterobius vermicularis*, the common pin worm, may be found in the urine as the result of fecal contamination, and the ova of *Schistosoma haematobium* may also be found since the eggs of *Schistosoma haematobium* are deposited in the wall of the urinary bladder and occasionally erupt into the bladder.

Other Urine Sediment Findings   S   In addition, components other than cells, casts, crystals, and microorganisms may be encountered in urine sediment. Among the items often encountered are spermatozoa, mucus, powder crystals, pollen grains, starch granules, hair fibers, and cloth fibers. It is absolutely essential for the clinical laboratory scientist to be able to differentiate between these contaminants and clinically significant organized sediment. Spermatozoa may normally be found in the urine sediment of male patients, but in female patients, the finding of spermatozoa is a direct indication of vaginal contamination of the urine specimen.   Mucus, cotton, and wool fibers must be distinguished from the more symmetrical casts that are found in urine sediment. Pollen granules and starch granules must be carefully distinguished from parasites and abnormal crystals respectively.

ANALYSIS OF CEREBROSPINAL FLUID (CSF)

The analysis of cerebrospinal fluid (CSF) is of great importance in the assessment of central nervous system disorders, particularly those of an inflammatory nature. The complete analysis of CSF includes physical examination, chemical examination, microscopic examination, and microbiological examination of the fluid.

Physical Tests   The physical analysis of CSF includes the assessment of the color, appearance, measurement of dissolved solids, and clot formation.

COLOR   Normal CSF is crystal clear and colorless. Abnormally clolored CSF is usually the result of the presence of blood or xanthochromia. Red or pink CSF may be due to the presence of blood in the fluid. Blood in the CSF may be the result of a bloody tap, or a subarachnoid hemorrhage. It is important to distinguish between these two causes. Methods for distinguishing between a bloody tap, and a subarachnoid hemmorrhage may include: (1) the amount of blood in each tube of CSF, which in the case of a bloody tap, will decrease in each consecutive tube while blood from a subarachnoid hemorrhage will remain fairly uniform in all of the tubes; (2) the formation of clots in the CSF which in the case of a bloody tap, will appear when the CSF is incubated at 37°C while no clot formation will take place if the blood is due to a subarachnoid hemorrhage; and (3) repeating the tap at a higher location, which in the case of a bloody tap, will often produce a clear fluid, while in the case of a subarachnoid hemorrhage the fluid will be similar to the first tap. Xanthochromia is a yellowish discoloration of the CSF which may be due to bilirubinemia, subarachnoid hemorrhage, or intracerebral hemorrhage. The presence of xanthochromia may be semiquantified using a 1+ to 4+ range depending on the amount of discoloration, a 1+ value being given to a pale yellow CSF, a 4+ value to an orange colored CSF. Xanthochromia is due to either the disintegration of blood or the presence of bilirubin.

APPEARANCE   Normal CSF is clear. A cloudy or turbid CSF is usually the result of the presence of cellular elements such as white blood cells, bacteria, or yeast. Microscopic and microbiologic examinations will be necessary to determine the cause of the turbidity.

MEASUREMENT OF DISSOLVED SOLIDS   The measurement of dissolved solids in CSF may or may not be a routine practice depending on the individual laboratory performing the CSF analysis. If this measurement is performed, it is mot frequently determined as specific gravity. The normal specific gravity of CSF is 1.006 to 1.008. Elevations of CSF specific gravity may be due to the presence of increased amounts of glucose or proteins in the fluid.

Chemical Tests   Chemical analysis of the CSF includes the measurement of protein, glucose, electrolytes, and enzymes.

PROTEIN   The normal CSF protein level falls in a generally accepted range of 20-50 mg/dl of fluid. This 20-50 mg/dl range is for adults. To date, there is no generally accepted "normal" range for children. Elevations of CSF protein may be due to: brain lesions, meningoencephalitis, intracerebral hemorrhage, Guillain-Barré syndrome, tuberculosis meningitis, tumors, and degenerative disorders. Methods for the determination of CSF protein vary from quantitative methods such as the sulfosalicylic turbidimetric procedures and the modified biuret procedure, to electrophoretic procedures which determine levels of specific proteins. Other testing procedures for proteins, including the Pandy test, the Nonne-Apelt test, and the colloidal gold test are now considered antiquated especially in light of the availability of electrophoretic procedures.

GLUCOSE   The normal level of CSF glucose is approximately 70% that of the serum glucose level, with a normal range of approximately 50-90 mg/dl.   Increases in CSF glucose correspond to increased serum glucose levels.   There is a time lag of 1 to 3 hours between the rise in serum glucose and the corresponding rise in the CSF glucose. Decreased CSF glucose levels may be obtained in a variety of disorders, including: hypoglycemia, bacterial and fungal meningitis, subarachnoid hemorrhage, sarcoidosis, leukemias, and toxoplasmosis.   Methods used to determine glucose in CSF are the same as those used for serum glucose determinations.

ELECTROLYTES   The determination of levels of certain electrolytes may be of considerable value in the diagnosis and confirmation of tuberculous meningitis.   These electrolytes include calcium, magnesium, and chloride.

CALCIUM   CSF calcium levels are normally approximately 2.3 mEq/L.   In tuberculous meningitis, the CSF calcium levels will be elevated.   The methods used for determining CSF calcium levels are the same as those used for serum calcium levels.

MAGNESIUM   CSF magnesium levels are normally approximately 2.2 mEq/L.   In tuberculous meningitis the CSF magnesium level will be decreased.   The methods for determining CSF magnesium levels are the same as those used for serum magnesium levels.

CHLORIDE   CSF chloride levels are a reflection of the serum chloride levels and consequently determinations of serum and CSF chloride should be performed simultaneously.   CSF chloride levels are normally higher than serum chloride levels, having a normal range of approximately 115-130 mEq/L.   In tuberculous meningitis, and other bacterially caused meningitis, both the CSF and serum chlorides will be decreased. The methods used for the determination of CSF chloride levels are the same as those used for serum chloride levels.

ENZYMES   The estimation of CSF enzyme levels may or may not be a part of a "routine" CSF analysis, depending on the particular laboratory.   There is some disagreement concerning these determinations, nevertheless, the determination of CSF levels of aspartate transferase, lactate dehydrogenase, and phosphohexose isomerase will be discussed.

ASPARTATE TRANSFERASE   Aspartate transferase (also known as glutamic oxalacetic transaminase (GOT)) levels in CSF have a normal range of 0-19 units.   Elevations of aspartate transferase in CSF have been associated with cerebral infractions, meningitis, and subarachnoid hemorrhage.

LACTATE DEHYDROGENASE (LDH)   Lactate dehydrogenase levels in CSF are normally approximately one-tenth of the serum levels.   Elevations of CSF lactate dehydrogenase have been associated with bacterial meningitis and cerebrovascular accidents.

PHOSPHOHEXOSE ISOMERASE (PHI)   Phosphohexose isomerase levels in CSF are normally very low, having a range of approximately 0-4 Bodansky units.   Elevations of CSF phosphohexose isomerase are associated with brain tumors and infections of the central nervous system.

Microscopic Examination   The microscopic examination of CSF is of significance in the assessment of meningitis.   The microscopic examination of CSF should include enumerative procedures for red blood cells and white blood cells, gram stain and acid-fast stain for bacteria, and an India ink preparation.

RED BLOOD CELLS   The microscopic examination of the CSF sediment should include a determination of the number and condition of red blood cells.   The enumerative procedures for the determination of the number of red blood cells in the CSF may be found in most hematology texts. In addition to the number of red blood cells present, the condition of these cells may be significant, consequently, it should be noted whether these cells are fresh or crenated.

WHITE BLOOD CELLS   The determination of the number and type of white blood cells present in the CSF is of greater importance in the diagnosis of meningitis. Red blood cell determination is secondary to this determination. The enumerative procedures for the enumeration of white blood cells present in the CSF may be found in most hematology tests. Increased white blood cell counts must be confirmed by determination of the type of white blood cells present. The type of white blood cells present may be determined by performing a differential white blood cell count. The procedure for performing differential white blood cell counts may be found in most hematology texts. Normally, the CSF contains only 0-5 cells per cubic millimeter, and most of these will be lymphocytes. Elevations of the total white blood cell count may be found in meningitis, syphilis, and Guillain-Barré syndrome.

BACTERIA   In all cases of suspected meningitis, the CSF sediment should be examined for the presence of bacteria. The examination of the CSF for bacteria should include a gram stain and an acid fast stain. In all cases, the sediment should be cultured on appropriate media and under appropriate conditions. The procedures for staining and culturing CSF may be found in most medical microbiology texts.

FUNGI   The sediment of the CSF should also be examined for the presence of *Cryptococcus neoformans*. This is best accomplished with India ink. The procedure for this preparation may be found in most medical microbiology texts.

ANALYSIS OF SYNOVIAL FLUID

The analysis of synovial fluid is of importance whenever there is excessive accumulation of the fluid in a joint. The analysis of synovial fluid should include physical tests, chemical tests, and microscopic examination.

Physical Tests   The physical analysis of synovial fluid should include determinations of the color, appearance, viscosity and clot formation.

COLOR   Normal synovial fluid is pale yellow in color, however, this is of little value since patients with various forms of arthritis will also have a pale yellow fluid. Abnormal synovial fluid colors may be a deeper yellow due to xanthochromia, or brown due to previous hemorrhage.

APPEARANCE   Normal synovial fluid is clear. Abnormal synovial fluids may be turbid, milky, or bloody. Turbid fluids may be due to the presence of increased numbers of white blood cells. Milky fluids may be due to lymphatic drainage into the joint while bloody fluids may be due to traumatic taps or hemophilia. In the case of bloody fluids, it is important to differentiate between a traumatic tap and frank bleeding in the joint. If the blood present is due to a traumatic tap, there may be uneven distribution or streaking of the blood in the syringe, with the blood clotting within 10-15 minutes. If the blood present is due to frank bleeding in the joint, particularly in the case of hemophilia, there will be a more even distribution of the blood in the syringe and the blood will not clot.

VISCOSITY   Normal synovial fluid is a rather viscous fluid. The viscosity is a reflection of the hyaluronic acid content of the synovial fluid. If the fluid drips like water, it has a low viscosity. Decreased viscosity is associated with effusions due to inflammatory processes.

MUCIN CLOT FORMATION   The mucin clot test, also known as the Ropes' test, is a measure of hyaluronic acid. The test is based on the principle that mucin will form a clot or ropy mass when added to acetic acid. The consistency of the clot is graded as good, fair, poor, or very poor. Normal synovial fluid will form a good clot, that is, one that is compact and will not break up when the container is agitated. The softer and more friable the clot, the poorer the grade.

CLOTTING OF THE SYNOVIAL FLUID   Normal synovial fluid does not contain fibrinogen or other clotting factors, therefore, it does not clot. Inflammatory processes allow fibrinogen and other clotting factors to enter the synovial fluid. When the cotting factors are present, and the fluid is left to stand, a clot will form. The rapidity of clot formation, and the volume of fluid involved in the clot, are directly proportional to the extent of the inflammation.

Chemical Tests   The chemical tests used in the analysis of synovial fluid include tests for protein, glucose, and enzymes.

PROTEIN   Normal synovial fluid has approximately 2.0 gm/dl of protein. Increased synovial fluid protein is associated with inflammatory processes. The tests employed for the total protein in synovial fluid are the same as those used to determine serum total protein. If there is a need to determine specific proteins, electrophoretic procedures may be used. The procedure for synovial fluid electrophoresis is the same as that used for serum protein electrophoresis with the exception that the hyaluronic acid must first be removed. Removal of the hyaluronic acid may be accomplished by treating the sample with hyaluronidase or by refrigerating the sample for 2-3 days.

GLUCOSE   The normal glucose level of synovial fluid is approximately 10 mg/dl lower than that of the serum. Differences of this ratio are apparent in patients with arthritis. Patients with severe inflammatory arthritis tend to have synovial fluid glucose levels anywhere from 25-50 mg/dl lower than the serum glucose. Patients with non-inflammatory arthritis tend to have synovial fluid glucose levels that are anywhere from 10-20 mg/dl lower than the serum glucose. The methods used for synovial fluid glucose determinations are the same as those used for serum glucose determinations.

ENZYMES   Synovial fluids may also be tested for the levels of acid phosphatase, alkaline phosphatase, and lactate dehydrogenase.

ACID PHOSPHATASE   The acid phosphatase levels of synovial fluid have been shown to be elevated in patients with rheumatoid arthritis, while they are normal in patients with bacterial arthritis.

ALKALINE PHOSPHATASE   The synovial fluid levels of alkaline phosphatase have been shown to be lower than the serum alkaline phosphatase levels.

LACTATE DEHYDROGENASE   Normal synovial fluid levels of lactate dehydrogenase will be found in normal patients and patients with degenerative joint disorders. Elevated synovial fluid lactate dehydrogenase activity will be found in patients with rheumatoid arthritis, and gout.

Microscopic Examination   Microscopic examination of synovial fluid should be performed to detect the presence of various cellular elements, crystals, and microorganisms.

CELLS   The cellular elements that may be found in synovial fluid include white blood cells, red blood cells, LE cells, RA cells, and Reiter cells.

A. *WHITE BLOOD CELLS:* The white blood cell count in normal synovial fluid is generally under 200 cells per cubic millimeter. Elevated white blood cell counts in synovial fluid may be found in a variety of disorders, including septic conditions, gout, rheumatoid arthritis, lupus erythematosus, rheumatic fever, and scleroderma. As in the case of other fluids, a differential white blood cell count is necessary to determine exactly what types of white blood cells are present. Normally, the majority of white blood cells in synovial fluid are lymphocytes and monocytes. There is one draw back to using the normal counting procedures, namely that the usual diluting fluid for white blood cell counts is acetic acid, which will precipitate the hyaluronic acid and make the enumeration of the cells extremely difficult, if not impossible. When counting white blood cells in synovial fluid it is necessary to use a red cell lysing agent that will not precipitate hyaluronic acid.

B. *RED BLOOD CELLS:*The actual enumeration of red blood cells in synovial fluid may be purely academic, since red blood cells are not normally found in synovial fluid. The presence of red cells is important to determine whether they are present as the result of a traumatic tap or as the result of frank bleeding into the joint cavity, as in the case of a hemophilic patient with a hemarthrosis.

C. *LE CELLS:* The presence of LE cells in synovial fluid may indicate that the patient has either lupus erythematosus or rheumatoid arthritis. At least 30% of the patients that have rheumatoid arthritis exhibit the presence of the antinuclear antibody in their synovial fluid. All of the patients that have systemic lupus erythematosus will have antinuclear antibody in their synovial fluid.

D. *RA CELLS:* RA cells, also known as ragocytes, are actually neutrophils containing an inclusion body. Approximately 95% of the patients suffering from rheumatoid arthritis will exhibit RA cells in their synovial fluid. The presence of RA cells in the synovial fluid is not diagnostic, since these cells may also be found in patients with disorders that are associated with increased quantities of granulocytic cells in the synovial fluid.

E. *REITER CELLS:* Reiter cells may also be found in synovial fluid. Reiter cells are actually large phagocytic cells that have ingested neutrophils. Reiter cells are non-specific cells and may be found in the synovial fluid of patients with a variety of conditions.

CRYSTALS   Monosodium urate crystals, calcium pyrophosphate dihydrate crystals, and cholesterol crystals are of greatest importance in synovial fluids.

A. *MONOSODIUM URATE CRYSTALS:* The presence of monosodium urate crystals in synovial fluid is associated with gout. In acute gout cases, these crystals are most frequently found in phagocytes, while they are often found extracellularly in cases of chronic gouty arthritis. These crystals must be distinguished from the calcium pyrophosphate dihydrate crystals. The differentiation may be accomplished using polarized light microscopy.

B. *CALCIUM PYROPHOSPHATE DIHYDRATE CRYSTALS:* Calcium pyrophosphate dihydrate crystals may be found in the synovial fluid of patients with "chondrocalcinosis", also known as pseudogout. The clinical importance of these crystals lies in the ability of the examiner to distinguish between these crystals and monosodium urates. This differential identification is important because patients with chondrocalcinosis have symptoms that mimic gout.

C. *CHOLESTEROL CRYSTALS:* Cholesterol crystals in the synovial fluid are associated with chronic inflammation of the joint. These crystals appear as plates and are not often confused with either momosodium urates or calcium pyrophosphate dehydrate crystals.

MICROORGANISMS   Synovial fluids should always be examined for the presence of microorganisms. To accomplish this, synovial fluid sediments should be gram stained and acid fast stained. In all cases the sediment should be cultured on appropriate media so as to detect aerobic, anaerobic, and acid fast organisms.

ANALYSIS OF SEROUS FLUIDS

The serous fluids, pleural fluid, pericardial fluid, and peritoneal fluid, are ultrafiltrates of the plasma. The serous fluid effusions are usually classified as either transudates or exudates. Differentiation between transudates and exudates is best accomplished by determining the protein level of the fluids. Transudates usually have total protein levels below 3 gm/dl while exudates usually have total protein levels above 3 gm/dl. The examination of serous fluids should include physical examination of the fluid, chemical examination of the fluid, microscopic examination of the fluid, microbiological examination of the fluid; also Papanicolaou smears are made to detect malignant cells.

Pleural Fluid   Pleural fluid analysis is indicated whenever there is an abnormal accumulation of pleural fluid.

Physical Examination   The physical examination of pleural fluid should include: assessment of the color, appearance, volume, clot formation, and specific gravity of the fluid.

COLOR   Normal pleural fluid is pale yellow or straw colored. Abnormal pleural fluids may be red, yellow, or white. Red pleural fluid is usually due to the presence of red blood cells. Yellow pleural fluid may be due to xanthochromia, however, this is often difficult to assess since the normal fluid is pale yellow. White pleural fluid is usually due to fats.

APPEARANCE   Normal pleural fluid is clear and transparent. Abnormal fluids may be turbid, bloody, milky or creamy in appearance. Turbid pleural fluid is usually due to the presence of increased numbers of white blood cells in the fluid. Bloody fluid may be due to pulmonary infarcts, tumors, or trauma. Milky fluid may be due to the presence of cholesterol in the fluid, while creamy fluid may be due to damage to the thoracic duct.

VOLUME   The normal volume of pleural fluid is one to ten milliliters. Abnormal volumes are associated with increased capillary permeability, hypoproteinemia, increased hydrostatic pressure or decreased lymphatic drainage.

CLOT FORMATION   Normal pleural fluid does not clot. Clot formation in the pleural fluid indicates the presence of fibrinogen in the fluid and can be associated with damage to the capillary walls.

SPECIFIC GRAVITY   Normal pleural fluids have a specific gravity approximately 1.015. Transudates may have specific gravity values that range from 1.010 to 1.020, while exudates may have higher specific gravity values. The increased specific gravity of exudates is associated with the increased protein level.

Chemical Examination   The chemical examination of pleural fluid should include determination of total protein, glucose, and enzymes.

TOTAL PROTEIN   The determination of pleural fluid total protein is valuable in determining whether the effusion is a transudative or exudative effusion. The normal pleural fluid total protein is approximately 1-2 gm/dl. Pleural fluid total proteins above 3.0 gm/dl are suggestive of exudative effusions. Methods of determining the total protein include the Rivalta test, which is a screening test, quantitative total protein determinations, and electrophoretic procedures. The Rivalta test employs an acetic acid solution which is added to the pleural fluid. The mixture is observed for cloudiness or precipitation. Normal fluids do not get cloudy. Transudates may produce some cloudiness, and exudates may produce heavy cloudiness and precipitation. Quantitative procedures are the same as those used for serum total protein determinations. Specific protein concentrations may be determined by performing electrophoretic procedures on the fluid.

GLUCOSE   Normal pleural fluid glucose levels are essentially the same as the serum glucose levels. Changes in the blood glucose levels will be reflected in the pleural fluid one to three hours later. Decreases in the pleural fluid glucose of as much as 40 mg/dl are associated with bacterial infections and malignancies. The methods used for the pleural fluid glucose determinations are the same as those used for serum glucose determinations.

LACTATE DEHYDROGENASE   Normal pleural fluid lactate dehydrogenase levels are essentially the same as those of the serum. Elevated pleural fluid lactate dehydrogenase levels are associated with malignancies and inflammations. If the fluid is bloody, these determinations may be of little value because enzyme from the hemolized red cells will also result in elevations of the lactate dehydrogenase activity.

AMYLASE   Normal pleural fluid amylase levels are essentially the same as those of the serum. Elevations of the pleural fluid amylase activity may be found in patients with acute pancreatitis. These patients will not only have higher pleural fluid amylase than serum amylase levels, but the higher pleural fluid amylase levels will remain higher for a longer period of time.

Microscopic Examination   The microscopic examination of pleural fluid should be performed to determine the number and type of cells present, and observation for the presence of crystals.

CELLS   Pleural fluid sediment should be examined for the presence of white blood cells, red blood cells, mesothelial cells and malignant cells.

WHITE BLOOD CELLS   Enumerative procedures for white blood cells should be performed whenever inflammatory processes are suspected or whenever the pleural fluid is turbid. Elevated white blood cell counts (over 1,000 white cells per cubic millimeter) are suggestive of inflammatory processes. A differential white blood cell count should be performed to determine the percentages of specific types of white blood cells.

RED BLOOD CELLS   Red blood cells are not normally found in pleural fluid. The presence of red blood cells indicates either trauma or malignant processes.

RA CELLS   RA cells are occasionally found in pleural fluid, but they are generally considered to be non-specific.

CRYSTALS   Chylous and pseudochylous fluids should be examined for the presence of cholesterol crystals. Cholesterol crystals are flat, plates with one corner notched.

Pericardial Fluid   The analysis of pericardial fluid should be performed whenever there is an abnormal accumulation of pericardial fluid.

Physical Examination   The physical analysis of pericardial fluid should be essentially the same as that of pleural fluid.

COLOR   Normal pericardial fluid is pale yellow. Abnormal pericardial fluids may be found in patients with hemorrhagic and pseudochylous effusions. Hemorrhagic fluids will produce a pink to red color and may be due to trauma or hemorrhagic effusion. Pseudochylous fluids will appear white and are associated with inflammatory disorders.

APPEARANCE   Pericardial fluid is normally clear and transparent. Abnormal fluids may be cloudy or turbid, bloody or milky. Cloudy or turbid fluids are associated with inflammatory disorders, bacterial infections and chronic effusions. Bloody fluids are associated with trauma and hemorrhagic disorders such as, hemorrhagic pericarditis and leaking aortic aneurysms. Milky fluids may be due to chronic pericarditis.

VOLUME   The normal volume of pericardial fluid is approximately 20-50 milliliters.

Chemical Examination   The chemical examination of pericardial fluid is essentially the same as for pleural fluid, except for the enzyme analyses.

PROTEIN   As in the case of pleural fluid, total protein analysis will assist in the determination of whether the effusion is transudative or exudative. The methods of determination are the same as those used for pleural fluids.

GLUCOSE   The pericardial fluid measurement of glucose content may be useful in the diagnosis of bacterial pericarditis. In bacterial pericarditis, the glucose level will be lowered.

Microscopic Examination   The microscopic examination of pericardial fluid is usually performed strictly for the determination of the number and types of white blood cells that may be present. Enumerative procedures and differential white blood cell counts should be performed as in the case of pleural fluids.

MICROBIOLOGICAL EXAMINATION   All pericardial fluids should be stained and cultured for the presence of bacterial and fungi.

Peritoneal Fluid   Peritoneal fluid is, like pleural fluid and pericardial fluid, an ultrafiltrate of the blood. Peritoneal fluid should be analyzed whenever there is an abnormal accumulation of peritoneal fluid, or when intra-abdominal hemorrhage is suspected.

Physical Examination   The physical examination of peritoneal fluid is similar to that of   pleural or pericardial fluid.

COLOR   Normal peritoneal fluid is pale yellow. Abnormal peritoneal fluids may be pink to   red, due to the presence of red blood cells, green, due to the presence of bile, or white, due to the presence of fats.

APPEARANCE   Normal peritoneal fluid is clear and transparent. Abnormal peritoneal fluids may be bloody, due to trauma, turbid, due to bacterial infection, or milky, due to chylous ascites.

VOLUME   Normally, there is under 100 milliliters of peritoneal fluid. Abnormal volumes are associated with a variety of disorders including, nephrotic syndrome, cirrhosis, peritonitis, duodenal ulcers, or perforated intestines.

Chemical Examination   Peritoneal fluid, like pleural fluid and pericardial fluid, is classified as either a transudate or exudate. The chemical analysis of peritoneal fluid includes measurement of total protein, enzymes, ammonia, creatinine and urea nitrogen.

TOTAL PROTEIN   The determination of peritoneal fluid total protein is valuable in the differentiation between transudative and exudative effusions. The methods for determining the total protein levels are the same as those used for pleural and pericardial fluids.

AMYLASE   Elevated levels of peritoneal fluid amylase activity are associated with pancreatitis and bowel necrosis.

LACTATE DEHYDROGENASE   Elevated lactate dehydrogenase activity in peritoneal fluid is associated with peritonitis, malignancies, and hemorrhagic effusions.

ALKALINE PHOSPHATASE   The estimation of alkaline phosphatase activity in peritoneal fluid may be of diagnostic value in the determination of a rupture of the small intestine.

AMMONIA   Elevated ammonia levels in peritoneal fluid may be found in patients with intestinal perforation or necrosis.

CREATININE AND UREA NITROGEN   The estimation of creatinine and urea nitrogen in peritoneal fluid is of differential diagnostic value in patients suspected of having ruptured urinary bladders. These determinations are also useful when a puncture of the urinary bladder is questioned to determine whether the fluid being analysed is in fact peritoneal fluid and not urine.

Microscopic Examination   As in the cases of pleural fluid and pericardial fluid, the peritoneal fluid should be examined for the presence and type of white blood cells, for red blood cells, and for tumor cells. In addition, microbiologic procedures should be performed to diagnose or rule out bacteriologic infection of the peritoneum.

ANALYSIS OF AMNIOTIC FLUID

   The analysis of amniotic fluid was originally employed for the detection of erythroblastosis fetalis (hemolytic disease of the newborn). Since then, amniocentesis has played a major role in several other aspects of the estimation of fetal maturity and development. Chemical analysis of amniotic fluid is now available for the determination of fetal death in utero, and fetal lung maturity. Karyotyping is now available for the detection of genetic disorders and family counceling. This section will briefly review the chemical analysis of amniotic fluid. For further information with regard to karyotyping for genetic defects the reader is referred to texts on cytogenetics.

TESTS FOR ERYHTROBLASTOSIS FETALIS   The tests most frequently used for the detection of erythroblastosis fetalis are the spectrophotometric analysis of the amniotic fluid and a quantitative determination of the level of bilirubin in the amniotic fluid.

SPECTROPHOTOMETRIC ANALYSIS   This test is based on the principle that increased levels of bilirubin will produce a distinguishable deviation from the normal curve produced by normal amniotic fluid. The specimen is filtered and read, spectrophoto-metrically, at a number of wavelengths ranging from 350 nanometers to 700 nanometers. Normal amniotic fluid will produce an almost straight line through each of the points on the graph. Amniotic fluids with elevated bilirubin levels will produce a curve that has a distinguishable "hump" at 450 nanometers. The difference in absorbance between the reading at 450 nanometers in the specimen, and the projected reading constitutes a value known as the Δ450. This value may then be plotted on one or more of the charts, such as the Lily graph, and an estimate of fetal damage and fetal sur-vival may be made.

Quantitative analysis of the level of bilirubin in amniotic fluid may be assessed by methods that are employed in the determination of serum bilirubin levels.

ENZYMES   Two enzymes, lactate dehydrogenase and creatine kinase, may be of diagnos-tic value in questions of fetal death.

LACTATE DEHYDROGENASE   Elevated levels of lactate dehydrogenase activity in amniotic fluid may be due to damage to the placenta, or fetal death.

CREATINE KINASE   Elevated creatine kinase levels, unlike lactate dehydrogenase, does not reflect damage to the placenta. Elevated creatine kinase levels in amniotic fluid are usually associated with fetal death in utero.

CREATININE   The estimation of amniotic fluid creatinine may be of use in the assess-ment of fetal maturity. Amniotic fluid levels of creatinine in premature infants is usually 1.0 mg/dl or less, while higher levels of 1.5 mg/dl or higher are usually indicate fetal maturity.

LECITHIN/SPHINGOMYELIN RATIO   The ratio of the phospholipids lecithin and sphingomy-elin is useful in the assessment of fetal lung maturity and is of value in the diag-nosis of respiratory distress syndrome. The measurement of the phospholipids is accomplished by thin-layer chromatographic procedures. L/S ratios of less than 1.5 respiratory distress syndrome is almost certain, while L/S ratios of approximately 1.5 indicate that there will be some degree of respiratory distress syndrome, and L/S ratios of 2.0 or greater indicate fetal lung maturity and respiratory distress syndrome should not occur.

ANALYSIS OF SEMINAL FLUID

The analysis of seminal fluid is of diagnostic value in the determination of male infertility. The examination should include at least a physical examination and a microscopic examination.

Physical Examination   The physical examination of seminal fluid should include assessments of the amount, appearance, vicosity, liquifaction, and ph.

AMOUNT   The average volume of seminal fluid is between 2.0 and 5.0 milliliters. Increased volumes are usually associated with sterility.

APPEARANCE   Freshly ejaculated seminal fluid is thick, white to gray-white, and opaque.

VISCOSITY   Normal seminal fluid, which is freshly ejaculated, is a very viscous coagulum. The coagulum generally liquifies within 10-20 minutes, and is considered abnormal if it does not.

pH   Normal seminal fluid has a pH of approximately 7.4.

Microscopic Examination   The microscopic examination of seminal fluid should include determinations of the number of sperm, the motility of the sperm, and an assessment of the morphology of the sperm.

NUMBER   Normal seminal fluid has a range of approximately 60 to 150 million spermatozoa per milliliter of seminal fluid. Sperm counts of less than 20 million per milliliter are associated with infertility.

MOTILITY   Motility of the spermatozoa in the seminal fluid decreases with time. Normal values for motility change with each passing hour. Normal values for motility are: greater than 70% for the first four hours, greater than 50% for the next three hours, and greater than 35% for the next three hours

MORPHOLOGY   Normal sperm morphology may exhibit slight variations in the shape of the sperm. At least 80-85% of the sperm should have normal morphology. Abnormal spermatozoa may exhibit changes in the shape and size of the head, may have cytoplasmic appendages, or may be double forms. Adequate estimates of sperm morphology should be performed on stained specimens which are examined under oil immersion. At least 200 spermatozoa should be observed, recording the percentages of normal and abnormal forms found.

BIBLIOGRAPHY AND RECOMMENDED READINGS

Bauer, J. D., Ackermann, P. G. and G. Toro. *BRAY'S CLINICAL LABORATORY METHODS.* Eighth Edition. 1974. The C. V. Mosby Company. St. Louis.

Frankel, S., Reitman, S. and A. C. Sonnenwirth (Editors). *GRADWOHL'S CLINICAL LABORATORY METHODS AND DIAGNOSIS.* Volume II. Seventh Edition. 1970. The C. V. Mosby Company. St. Louis.

Freeman, J. A. and M. F. Beeler. *LABORATORY MEDICINE-CLINICAL MICROSCOPY.* 1974. Lea & Febiger. Philadelphia.

Henry, J. B. (Editor). *TODD-SANFORD-DAVIDSOHN CLINICAL DIAGNOSIS AND MANAGEMENT BY LABORATORY METHODS.* Sixteenth Edition. 1979. W. B. Saunders Company. Philadelphia.

HENRY, R. J., Winkelman, J. W. and D. C. Cannon (Editors). *CLINICAL CHEMISTRY PRINCIPLES AND TECHNICS.* Second Edition. 1974. Harper and Row Publishers. Hagerstown, Maryland.

Race, G. J. and M. G. White. *BASIC URINALYSIS.* 1978. Harper and Row Publishers, Hagerstown, Maryland.

Raphael, S. S. (Senior Author). *LYNCH'S MEDICAL LABORATORY TECHNOLOGY.* Volume I. Third Edition. 1976. W. B. Saunders. Philadelphia.

Tietz, N. W. (Editor). *FUNDAMENTALS OF CLINICAL CHEMISTRY.* Second Edition. 1976. W. B. Saunders. Philadelphia.

Chapter 11

Quality Control/Management in the Clinical Laboratory

SHIRLEY H. BRIEN, BA, MT (ASCP)
Chief Technologist, Catholic Medical Center
Manchester, New Hampshire
Assistant to Regional Inspector for the College
of American Pathologists' Inspection and
Accreditation Department
Skokie, Illinois

OUTLINE

INTRODUCTION

The purpose of this chapter on quality control is twofold. The first reason is not to confuse and complicate life for the young laboratorians, but rather to make them understand exactly why they are doing what they are, and by incorporating this knowledge into their workday, reduce frustration on the part of their supervisors who might valiantly be trying to guide these young persons as they begin their journey in the world of clinical medicine.

The second reason for this synopsis on quality control, is to help the young supervisors who may not have too many years of bench experience before being in a management roll and with it the responsibility (very often without authority) of providing the patient and the physician with a laboratory that produces reliable data.

The young supervisors must also be ready to face the myriads of accrediting agencies such as Joint Commission, College of American Pathologists, State Licensing Agencies, Center for Disease Control, and the Occupational Safety and Health Act of 1970. These agencies require statistical data as well as documentation of just about every action that takes place within the confines of the laboratory. When inspectors say "show me", if the supervisors or bench technologists cannot produce--automatically this assumes a negative action on the part of the laboratory. Perhaps my years of experience can help to uncomplicate a complicated process. You might be tempted to say that ignorance is bliss, but not in this case--ignorance is guilt!

QUALITY CONTROL/MANAGEMENT IN THE CLINICAL LABORATORY

NEED FOR QUALITY

Anyone who is going out to buy an article of clothing, furniture, food or any item he or she may want, will shop with one thought in mind--translated into words that thought is, "quality". Everyone wants to buy something that will last, look good and perform in the manner for which it was intended. The idea of quality is not new; I'm certain that cavemen worked diligently at making their caves the best and their weapons to outshine their neighbor's. And so on throughout civilization was the word quality always on the tongues of our ancestors. Quality was always something that people took pride in doing, so controlling quality was never really a problem. Then came the industrial age and with it mass production as well as "piece work". The more items an individual produced the more money he made--so what happened to "quality"? It lost its flavor. So emerged industrial quality control to help produce better quality items and still try to keep up production as well as good salaries for personnel. Major task? I would have to say so, but as a result the first "quality control" programs were put into action in industry during the middle 1920's.

BRIEF HISTORY OF CLINICAL LABORATORY AND QUALITY CONTROL

If one glances briefly at the history of clinical laboratories, one knows that in the 1920's they were just starting to develop as a part of the hospital setting. Most hospital administrators gave the physician in charge of the laboratory (who most likely was not a pathologist) a small room in the darkest corner of the basement and said, "Bless you, go and multiply." And that is precisely what the physician did-- he multiplied and multiplied and multiplied until today, only 50 years later, the laboratory is probably the largest ancillary department in the hospital, revenue

producing and quite vital to the financial survival of every medical institution.
With this growth, emerged the profession of Medical Technology and more physicians
turned their gaze to pathology as their specialty.

Like industry, the larger our laboratories grew and the more mechanized they became, the greater became the problem of quality. Nothing of great importance took
place in the area of "quality control" until 1950 when Levy and Jennings brought forth
the idea of using sera of known values and plotting daily results on a wall chart.
This was the beginning of quality control in laboratory medicine. As I said, that was
just the beginning and for years it was the only item in quality control programs.

Today, with laboratories being the complex unities that they are, our attention
must now turn to quality control but not merely in the light of a Levy-Jennings' chart
but to a concept of total quality control. This may sound like an impossible task,
but if the program is well organized it can be the best source of management the supervisor could have.

As overused as the expression might sound, the only reason for the existence of
quality control is "for better patient care". The quality of work produced by a
laboratory is dependent on many factors, but the most important factor is that all
members of the clinical team must want quality. To want it, they have to be motivated.
This means that the primary motivator must be the pathologist himself. His enthusi-
asm must be felt throughout the laboratory. He must be ready and willing to spur his
staff to produce quality work. This means he himself must be versed in all aspects
of quality control and impart his knowledge to his employees.

In many instances however, the entire responsibility for quality control will
rest on the shoulders of the laboratory supervisor or chief technologist, whatever
title best fits the situation. Most of us are called just about everything and anything and then some. If the responsibility is solely yours as a young supervisor,
"cry first", then plunge into the task at hand and know that once you begin, it's an
ongoing process that never ends.

SETTING UP A TOTAL QUALITY CONTROL PROGRAM

The following text will attempt to set up, as uncomplicatedly as possible, a
quality control program that might fit or could be tailored to fit your situations.
We will base ourselves on major points that should constitute your program. As you
read through these pages there might be perhaps 5 or 6 more points that you feel are
more important than the ones mentioned. This only proves that a quality control program is very specific to each setting. It also means that once a quality control
program has been set up, you cannot sit back and keep doing the same things year after
year. The points which are important to you today, in your own laboratory, might not
fit the situation tomorrow because of new tests, new facilities, new physicians, new
evaluating and certifying agencies. Your program must be a changing one and the
technologists must be motivated to accept change if the program is to fulfill the
need and dimensions for which it was intended. Remember that the most important asset
to a quality control program is common sense, but more realistically speaking it is
safe to say that "educated common sense" is the best choice of words.

Many of the factors that play an important part in quality control occur away from
the laboratory and as such are sometimes hard to control. However, a good interde-
partmental as well as intradepartmental communication system can control these factors as much as possible.

Let us now list the areas that are important in setting up a quality control program; one that will satisfy all concerned that the laboratory is really a patient-

focused laboratory and simultaneously is satisfying all the agencies that are forever making demands on clinical areas. To be able to produce quality work, the following are some points that will be discussed as important in setting up a total quality control program.

1. Manual describing the laboratory's quality control program
2. Physical restraints
3. Personnel needs
4. Nonlaboratory dependent sources affecting quality
5. Specimen collection--preparation
6. Procedure manual
7. Water analysis
8. Instrument maintenance
9. Purchasing of quality supplies and inventory
10. Error detection--normal and abnormal controls
11. External survey programs
12. Quality evaluation
13. Continuing education program
14. Method evaluation and selection
15. Supervision

These are only a few of the areas to be looked at but are adequate to start a total concept of quality control in your setting or probably cause you to add a few points here and there.

Many people have the wrong idea of what a Quality Control Program is, and will therefore have a tendency to make it quite complicated where in reality it can be set up with ease. The secret behind its success is that the laboratory personnel not look upon the program as unnecessary paper work. A point to remember is that quality control is a "friend" willing to help you if you let it. It will prevent you from making errors and will defend you when your neck is in a noose. But, to be able to do this, you must make certain that quality control remains healthy and that means daily, weekly, monthly and yearly check-ups. If anything is physically wrong, it must be dealt with. Then and only then will the program repay you one hundredfold.

Let's begin our journey up the mountain of "statistics" by focusing our energies on the Department of Chemistry. The bulk of our quality control process takes place in this section of the laboratory. Whatever we discuss pertaining to the chemistry area can be modified and adapted, in part, to other sections. It is not the intention at this time to go indepth through all the divisions of pathology, but to leave some processes to your inventiveness.

Quality Control Manual

The most appropriate way to start your trek is by defining exactly what your Quality Program is going to comprise. This can be done by means of a manual. A brief outline of the items in your manual could be as follows:

1. Program description (total or per section)
2. Goals
3. Objectives
4. Specific quality control procedures for each section
5. Acceptable performance defined
6. Guidelines on course of action to take when out-of-control situations occur
7. Means by which the action is taken
8. Definition of terms used in quality control.

The following terms are but a few that you will need if a decent quality control program is to exist in your laboratory. At this point, it would be appropriate to define them:

1. Quality: all of the features of a service that will permit it to satisfy the need for which it was intended.

2. Quality Assurance: simply put, it is all activities the laboratory will engage in to ensure that all data generated by the clinical setting is correct. This means that there is an ongoing evaluation of the quality control program.

3. Quality Control: in laboratory medicine this term refers mostly to repeated measurement of the same specimen. From these measurements laboratory personnel can determine the mean, standard deviation and coefficient of variation and by using a Levy-Jennings chart plot these determinations daily to show upper and lower levels of "control".

4. Precision: merely reproductibility.

5. Accuracy: how close a test result comes to the true value.

6. Reliability: the ability of a method to maintain both accuracy and precision even after months of usage.

   Reliability of a method is a very important aspect of quality control. My reasons for saying this are simply that most laboratories will definitely acquire new technologists, change of reagents or probably even keep the same reagents, but they will be used on a different instrument. This could all happen within a short period of time and if the method in question retains its precision and accuracy in spite of this, it is now said to be quite reliable and worthy of keeping as part of your procedures.

7. Control: used to check on performance of laboratory. Control samples will monitor the precision (reproducibility) of a technique. The control sample must be close in texture to the specimen being analyzed. Controls therefore have the same base, that is, serum or urine and as such reduce interference from outside sources.

8. Standard: the term used most frequently in our clinical settings these days is "calibrator." A calibrator is used to establish the accuracy of a method. A laboratory depends totally on calibrators for assigning values when analyses are performed--in other words, they are used to set up curves, etc.

   There are two types of calibrators:

   A. Primary calibrators--pure substance in solution.

   B. Secondary calibrator--also called reference sera. These are pools of sera with chemicals added to reach the level desired. It should always be checked against a primary standard. The reason for secondary calibrators is that some authorities feel that the presence of sera in the calibrator permits a closer texture to the real samples. This point is still controversial and probably will be for some time to come.

9. Standard Deviation: important as a decision making tool is quality control. It measured the distribution of values to the average value of a group or series of measurements.

± 1 Std Deviation = 67% of the group of values
± 2 Std Deviation = 95% of the group of values
± 3 Std Deviation = 99.7% of the group of values

The above figures are represented by what we call a normal distribution curve or Gaussian curve (See Figure 1)

FIGURE 1*

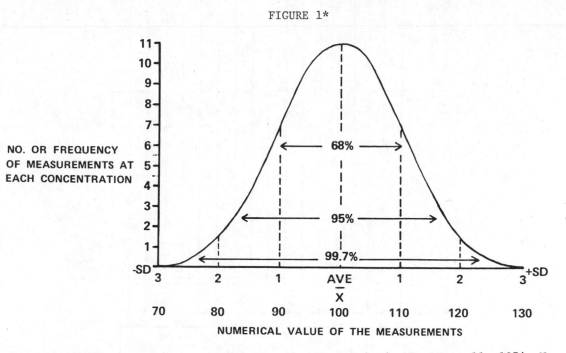

NO. OR FREQUENCY OF MEASUREMENTS AT EACH CONCENTRATION

NUMERICAL VALUE OF THE MEASUREMENTS

*Permission for reproduction given by Bradley E. Copeland, MD, April 11, 1974, New England Deaconess Hospital, at the ASCP Training Institute in Clinical Chemistry, Merrimack College, Andover, MA.

To calculate standard deviations for specific prodedures, one must have a series of 20 or more test results and apply these results to Figure 2.

10. Coefficient of Variation--the standard deviation expressed as % of the mean

$$CV = \frac{SD}{Mean} \times 100$$

Federal regulations allow ±1 SD to equal the following CV's:

5% CV for all quantitative determinations
10% CV for enzymatic determinations
3% CV for electrolyte determinations

This means that according to the Gaussian normal distribution curve, 1-68% of all control data for quantitative analysis such as glucose creatine etc., should fall within ± 5% of the mean.

FIGURE 2

MONTHLY QUALITY CONTROL REPORT

Procedure		1. Average $\bar{X}$ =	Evaluation:
Date		2. Std. Dev. =	
Pool #		# out of control	

Procedure for Calculating Average and Standard Deviation:

1. Record control analyses in column one.
2. Add column one.
3. Calculate average - line A.
4. Calculate and record in column two individual differences from average.
5. Square each individual difference, and record in column three.
6. Add column three.
7. Calculate standard deviation (SD) - line B.
8. Control limits: ± 3 x SD = 3 x _____ = _____

Average: (3)			Diff. from Average:	Squared diff. from Average:
1				
2				
3				
4				
5				
6				
7				
8				
9				
10				
11				
12				
13				
14				
15				
16				
17				

FIGURE 2 (continued)

MONTHLY QUALITY CONTROL REPORT

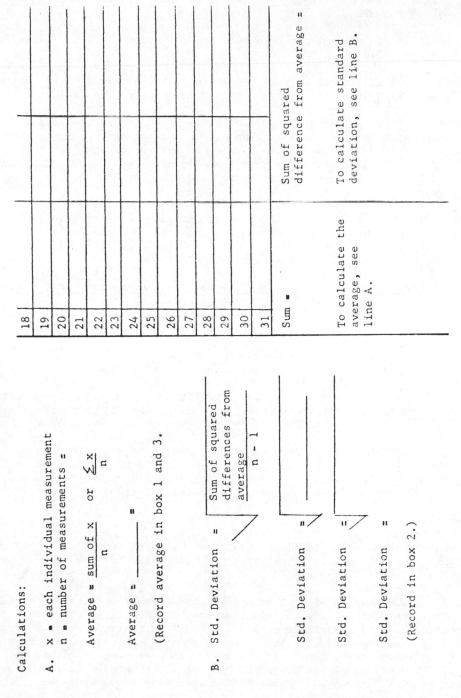

Calculations:

A. x = each individual measurement
    n = number of measurements =

Average = $\frac{\text{sum of x}}{\text{n}}$ or $\frac{\sum x}{n}$

Average = _____ =

(Record average in box 1 and 3.)

B. Std. Deviation = $\sqrt{\dfrac{\text{Sum of squared differences from average}}{\text{n} - 1}}$

Std. Deviation = $\sqrt{}$

Std. Deviation = $\sqrt{}$

Std. Deviation =

(Record in box 2.)

18	
19	
20	
21	
22	
23	
24	
25	
26	
27	
28	
29	
30	
31	
Sum =	

To calculate the average, see line A.

Sum of squared difference from average =

To calculate standard deviation, see line B.

Permission for reproduction given by Bradley E. Copeland, MD, New England Deaconess Hospital, April 11, 1974, at the ASCP Training Institute in Clinical Chemistry, Merrimack College, Andover, MA.

2-68% of all control data for enzymatic determinations should fall within $\pm$ 10% of the mean.

3-68% of all control data for electrolyte determination should fall within $\pm$ 3% of the mean.

11. Constituent: the substance in the sera to be analyzed, for example, cholesteral or sodium.

12. Mean: the arithmetic average of several results. In quality control, usually 20 determinations are necessary to derive a decent mean value.

13. Quality Control Charts (Levy-Jennings): graph paper with days on the horizontal axis and the concentration of the constituent in appropriate units on the vertical axis. Charts have a mid horizontal line for mean value and one parallel line above and below the mid line for $\pm$ 1 SD values and another parallel line above and below the $\pm$ 1 SD line for $\pm$ 2 SD values. Some laboratories may elect to go to $\pm$ 3 SD (Figure 3).

14. Tonk's Formula: used to calculate acceptable limits of error. This is not the most ideal way to determine acceptability, but it's a guide.

Acceptable limit of error in percentage:

$$\frac{1/4 \text{ upper limit of normal range - lower limit of normal range x 100}}{\text{mean of normal range}}$$

or 10% whichever is smaller. This formula can be used to check limits on the control charts.

15. Trend: gradual change in values either upward or downward on a Levy-Jenning chart. Downward may indicate breakdown of reagent--standard is becoming too concentrated or perhaps instrument problem. Upward trend means breakdown of standard, dirty instrument, etc. Both give clues to the technologist that investigation is needed.

16. Shift: abrupt change in values either upward or downward on a Levy-Jenning chart. This could be due to a bad lot of reagents or standards. This problem could be avoided if old lots of reagents and standards are checked against new lots before being put into use (Figure 4).

Physical Restraints

It is hard enough under ideal physical conditions to establish a quality control program, but if your physical situation is not adequate the task will probably be very difficult, but not impossible.

Administration must be willing to support the cost of quality in the laboratory. There is no doubt that it is going to be expensive. Sometimes there is a tendency to compromise definite essentials such as: amount of controls, number of personnel, and salaries. Consequently, the quality of personnel suffers, equipment of inferior quality is purchased or perhaps there is a lack of proper equipment to do the job correctly. This will definitely hinder the laboratory and the quality of work produced and one will find oneself compromising with objectives and goals.

There is no easy answer if you have this problem. Obviously cost containment is

FIGURE 3

MONTH ─────────

YEAR ─────────

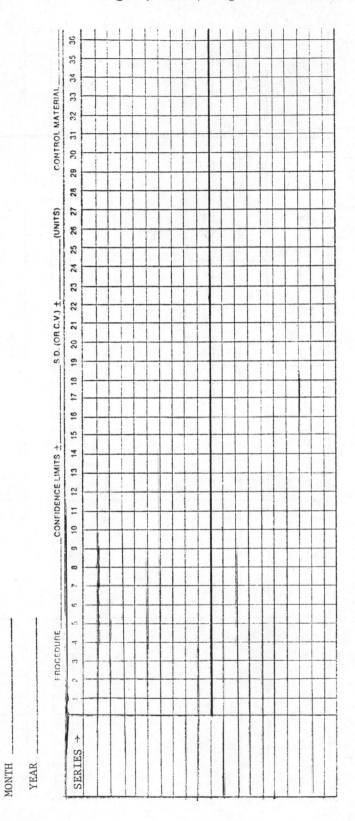

FIGURE 4

REAGENT QUALITY CONTROL: CHEMISTRY

REAGENT	OLD LOT # –	OLD STD. VALUE	OLD CONT. VALUE	NEW LOT #	NEW STD. VALUE	NEW CONT. VALUE

very important to administration, but if it is such that the quality of work is affected, then I feel that restrictions in the amount of work and services should be the items held back and not producing poor quality in the laboratory. To be practical about the situation, we all know that there will always be financial constraints on the laboratory. A sincere effort on the part of administration and the laboratory director must be made so that a fairly reasonable balance will exist between quality and cost. In other words, basically what I'm saying is that quality at any cost is not reasonable and that the middle line or being slightly a bit on the plus side of the line must exist to have a good quality control program in a laboratory.

Personnel Needs

It is ideal to have all the necessary equipment, controls and reagents in the laboratory, but if the number and/or number of reliable technologists is low, the quality of work will reflect the existing condition, without a doubt. Again, cost containment is the reason for this problem. At times the people who determine quantity, quality, and distribution of laboratory personnel have nothing directly to do with the laboratory and have no knowledge whatsoever about the activities of the clinical laboratory. In spite of technical deficiencies, it seems they have the supreme power to decide what type personnel you have, what will happen to them, and how you will use them. A perfect example of such a situation is having an outside agency come and spend time in your laboratory to determine if you are making use of time correctly. This is not objectionable if done by an agency that deals strictly with clinical laboratories and as such will have developed techniques of measuring that are both geared to the laboratory and to the hospital setting. But as I sit here writing these lines I can feel my blood pressure rising because I know that all of you out there, as well as myself, have been involved in a situation where the evaluator has dealt strictly with industry prior to setting foot in your laboratory and as such all of his/her analogies were based on a production line. After lowering your productivity by bothering your technologists for 3 months, a report is sent to administration, that of course, must be implemented because "the experts" have spoken.

Situations like this can really do a number on the quality of work in a laboratory because it demoralizes the staff in many ways. Most of all, I think it makes the staff feel they're just a number in the crowd and no one really cares about their situation. Instead of bettering the situation usually it is only aggravated. This opinion is a personal one based on my own experience. I'm certain there are many good agencies that could render a service to the laboratory director. Before the agency comes, the laboratory director should have some input into the planning and the choice of the agency that is to come.

A quality situation cannot exist in your laboratory unless you have the following situations: (1) the skill mix must be balanced and adequate; (2) section supervisors must be away from bench work to be able to supervise; (3) there must be evening, night and week-end supervisors; (4) as productivity increases more technical help must be acquired; (5) if the laboratory is large enough, a quality control manager should be available; and (6) staff salary must be comparable if not better than the hospital in your area.

If you remember at the beginning of this chapter, we said that the first factor that had to exist in a good quality control program was that "the technologists had to want quality". To want quality they must themselves be first well qualified--and to obtain well qualified people the salary must be well qualified.

The needs of the personnel in your laboratory are not to be ignored. The technologists, technicians, secretaries, housekeepers, all these people will play a vital role in your quality control program, and their needs must be met if they are to meet yours.

Non Laboratory-Dependent Sources Affecting Quality of Work (Nursing Manual)   ; MANUAL)

There are many areas other than the laboratory per se that affect the internal quality of the work produced. These areas we will mention only briefly mainly because there is no set rule as to what to do and what not to do. Perhaps you are not experiencing problems in these areas, but in my years of personal experience, as well as in communicating with other laboratory supervisors, the succeeding areas are a definite source of concern and should be controlled as much as possible.

It is probably quite safe to say that the entire process of what laboratory quality represents depends solely on the initiator of the request, namely the physician. The manner in which his requests are stated on the chart could result in either serious misunderstanding or the smooth flowing of the many processes that will follow after his initial step. The instant the laboratory is notified, a system is set into action.

However as all of us know, to deal with new physicians, at times, can be a bit frustating. In spite of this it is vital when a new physician arrives on the scene, that he be introduced to the Pathologist and laboratory supervisor and that reliable communication take place between those involved. The laboratory should know what the physician expects of the laboratory and the physician should be made aware what services are available to him and when.

Once this initial introduction has taken place, Nursing Service is the next group of people who can help the laboratory immensely by being the next step in the long chain of processes that take place before a reliable result reaches the physician. To help ease the process, communication by means of a Laboratory Procedure Manual is one way to help smooth out any rough spots and prevents the laboratory office from receiving unnecessary phone calls. To permit the manual to function as expected, periodic in-service programs with nursing service, and the continuous giving of corrected information to people who stray from the expected process will work. The following outline is the one from our own Nursing Service Laboratory Procedure Manual.

I. General Remarks

   Here we explain how the laboratory functions.

II. Working Hours

III. Definitions

   A. Stat
   B. Routine
   C. Today, etc., etc.

IV. Requisition

   How to complete

V. Routine Laboratory Tests

   A. Preparation
   B. Normal Values
   C. Requisition slip to use

VI. Profiles

     Each defined

VII. Special Procedures

    A. Histology
    B. Hematology
    C. Blood Bank
    D. Urinalysis
    E. Stool Specimens
    F. Chemistry
    G. Microbiology

Figure 5 is section IV of our manual while Figure 6 is an example of section V. Figure 7 and Figure 8 are parts of section VII. These are just examples of what best suits our needs--yours might be entirely different.

Specimen Collection and Preparation

Remember, a test result will only be as good as the manner in which the sample was obtained. To insure that quality exists from the beginning, a manual of some kind is needed that will contain all the details to guide the technologist, technician, phlebotomist, nurse, physician, whoever will be the first contact with the sample to be examined. This manual can be incorporated into the Nursing Service Laboratory Procedure Manual or may be a manual of its own.

As a manual standing by itself, it should first fit your situation--I sound like I am repeating the same thing over and over again, but believe me an inspector knows if the manual you have at the bench is one that was put out just for the inspection and was copied from someone else's manual, or if it really fits your actual situation.

The following outline again is just a guide as to what the manual should contain. I will not add descriptions after each heading; that is where you fit in.

The manual should be divided perhaps into four sections:

A. Blood Specimens
B. Urine Specimens
C. Body Fluids
D. Send-outs to Reference Labs

A few sub-titles for each heading could probably be as follows:

A. Blood Specimens

    1. How to do a proper venipuncture
    2. How to do a proper finger or ear stick
    3. How to draw blood from newborns for (a) hematology, (b) chemistry, or
        any other item needed in your clinical setting
    4. Transport of specimens
    5. Storage of specimens
    6. Proper anticoagulant to use
    7. Proper preservation
    8. Drug interference
    9. Identification of specimen

    10. Patient preparation
    11. Instructions for timing of specimens
    12. Interfering substances such as bile or lipidemia
    13. Type sample needed: plasma, serum, etc.
    14. Specific instructions for a specific test
    15. Any other item or items specific to your needs

B. Urine Specimens

    1. Patient identification
    2. Preservatives
    3. Clearly defined instructions for obtaining urines in the following manner:

        a. voided
        b. clean-catch
        c. catherized

    4. Type specimen needed for specific test Ex. - culture - clean catch
    5. Patient preparation
    6. Storage of specimens
    7. Specimen identification
    8. Any other detailed item or items specific to your clinical setting

C. Body Fluids

    1. Preservatives relative to specific fluids and for specific analyses
    2. Preparations for specific fluids for specific analyses
    3. Proper containers for different fluids
    4. Time allowed for specimen arrival at laboratory after collection
    5. Details in identification

        a. time
        b. name
        c. fluid

    6. Manner of reporting. Figure 9 is the report sheet used at Catholic Medical Center

D. Send-Outs

    1. Name of reference laboratory with telephone number
    2. List of routine send-outs with proper amount of sample needed for each analysis
    3. Details on obtaining their service. Ex. - courier - describe process
    4. Any other information pertinent to your institution

At this time, let me stress once again how important the first encounter with the sample to be analyzed should be. It must be carried out with extreme care and concern. The need for a manual with as much information as possible will not only assure the quality of the analyses but will increase the productivity and the efficiency of the laboratory. With all the necessary information between two covers, the technologists will not have to search or perhaps ask several people for the "whereabouts" and the "howabouts" therefore increasing other people's efficiency. Another point which is not to be ignored, is that it will certainly make your life much easier when inspectors come around and ask for your "Sample Collection and Preparation Manual".

FIGURE 5

IV REQUISITIONS

Requisitions must be completely filled and include the following:

1. Patient's complete name
2. Complete address
3. Room Number
4. Date of Birth
5. Physician's name
6. Diagnosis
7. Date ordered
8. Tests requested
9. Charge number
10. Nurse initials

CHEMISTRY - requisitions for routine work must be in the laboratory by 6:30 A.M.

HEMATOLOGY - requisitions for routine work must be in the laboratory by 6:30 A.M.

URINALYSIS - routine urines must be in the laboratory by 7:00 A.M.

BLOOD BANK - Laboratory should be notified of Pre-Op crossmatch as soon as they are received from the doctor. Screening for antibodies is done early - thus preventing postponement of surgery should an unusual situation arise.

All other requisitions for blood except emergency cases are to be in the lab by 7:00 AM. Late requisitions may result in blood not being ready for the requested time.

BACTERIOLOGY - requisition must accompany specimen. Source of material is a must and the antibiotic treatment patient might be receiving. Time of specimen collection must also be specified.

TISSUES - These include paps, surgicals, bone marrows and any specimen requiring a pathological examination.

Requisitions must accompany all specimens sent to the tissue laboratory. They must indicate SOURCE OF SPECIMEN and DIAGNOSIS.

PAP requisitions must also list LMP and PREVIOUS MEDICATION.

All specimens received in histology that require inciniration must be accompanied by a signed permit for proper disposition. These permits can be obtained in the Medical Records Department.

FIGURE 6

TEST	PREPARATION	NORMAL VALUE	REQUISITION SLIP	PROFILE NORMAL
ASTO TITRE	1.0 ML SERUM	LESS THAN 200 TODD UNITS	SEROLOGY	
BARBITUATES	1.0 ML SERUM	NEGATIVE	MISCELLANEOUS	
BILIRUBIN – TOTAL – DIRECT	1.0 ML SERUM 1.0 ML SERUM	0-1.5 mg% 0-1.5 mg%	CHEMISTRY II CHEMISTRY II	0.2 – 1.2 mg%
BLEEDING TIME (IVY)		1 – 6 MIN.	COAGULATION	
BLOOD CULTURE ANAEROBIC & AEROBIC SEE BACTERIOLOGY PROCEDURE		NO GROWTH	BACTERIOLOGY	
BLOOD GROUP & RH	SERUM & BLOOD ONE RED TOP TUBE		BLOOD BANK	
BLOOD SUGAR FASTING RANDOM 2 HR PP	0.5 ML FAST. SERUM 0.5 ML RANDOM SERUM 0.5 ML SERUM AFTER LOADED MEAL OR DRINK	70 – 115 mg% LESS THAN 130 mg%	CHEMISTRY I CHEMISTRY I CHEMISTRY I	72 – 128 mg%
BONE MARROW	NOTIFY LABORATORY	INTERPRETED BY PATHOLOGIST	MISCELLANEOUS	
BUN	0.5 ML SERUM	5 – 25 mg%	CHEMISTRY I	5 – 26 mg%
C3 (B.A GLOBULIN)	1.0 SERUM	55 – 120 mg%	SPECIAL CHEMISTRY	
CALCIUM	1.0 ML SERUM	8.5 – 11.0 mg/dl	CHEMISTRY I	8.5 – 10.5 mg/dl
CEA (CARCINOEMBRYONIC ANTIGEN)	2 EDTA TUBES (SEND TO LEARY)	LESS THAN 5.0 ng/ml IN 98-99% OF NON-SMOKERS	MISCELLANEOUS	
CBC(INCLUDES WBC, DIFF.1 EDTA TUBE REC, HCT, HGB,			HEMATOLOGY SEE HEMATOLOGY REQ.	

PROCEDURES FOR COLLECTION, PREPARATION AND HANDLING OF MICROBIOLOGICAL SPECIMENS

GENERAL INSTRUCTIONS

1. Basic Principles

   As it defines the diagnosis and nature of disease, the microbiological investigation determines the mode and treatment as well as outlook for the patient affected. In the practice of medicine, specimen collection must be a crucial first step upon which rests the validity of each succeeding step.

   The results of laboratory tests can be no better than the specimen on which they were obtained. Thus, if the specimen is inadequate or rendered unsuitable by drying, exposure to heat or cold, contamination or improper collection, any results obtained may be grossly misleading to the clinician.

   In obtaining and submitting the diagnostic specimens, basic principles should be observed. Principles applicable to specimens submitted for isolation and identification of the etiologic agent include:
   a. Select the appropriate specimen.
   b. Obtain the specimens as early in the illness as possible.
   c. Identify the specimen completely.
   d. Request the specific test (S) desired and indicate etiologic agent suspected.
   e. Protect viability of organisms during transit.
   f. Sterile equipment must be used in the collection of any specimen and specimens deposited in a sterile container.
   g. The specimen must be collected from the actual site of the disease and not contaminated with bacteria from nearby areas.
   h. Adequate amounts of material should be collected; if swabs are used in specimen collection, two or more should be used if possible.
   i. No preservatives or antiseptics should be added to specimen, and specimens should be collected before the patient receives chemotherapy, if possible. If antibiotics are already being used, it should be noted on the requisition form.
   j. Requisition form should always include the following Information:
      1. Patient name
      2. Patient/ age/sex
      3. Room number
      4. Source/site of specimen
      5. Date/time of specimen collection
      6. Name of physician
      7. Examinations requested, one request per requisition form.
      8. Processing priority, stat or routine
      9. Clinical diagnosis
      10. Current antibiotic therapy.
      11. Charge number
      12. Specimens for urine culture must indicate "midstream" "clean catch" or catheterized" urine.

FIGURE 7

GENERAL INSTRUCTIONS
1. Basic Principles (cont.)
    K. A single specimen with multiple examination requests
        should be accompanied by a SEPARATE requisition form
        for each examination requested.
    L. Specimens will, in general, be rejected by the laboratory
        for the following reasons:
        1. Specimens delivered in non-sterile containers, with
        the exception of stool specimens submitted for enteric
        pathogen examinations.
        2. Specimens which are submitted in containers that
        are leaking, grossly soiled or contaminated externally,
        or which otherwise constitute a distinct biological
        hazard to laboratory personnel.
        3. Specimens submitted on dry swabs.
        4. Specimens submitted in containers that are unlabeled,
        on which the patient's name is not clearly discernable.
        5. Specimens submitted as sputum which clearly consist
        of saliva.
        6. Specimens obviously exposed to extreme temperatures
        of heat or cold.
    M. The specimens should be delivered directly to Bacteriology
        Laboratory as soon as possible. All STAT specs. are
        to be personally delivered to the laboratory: Do not
        leave them without notifying laboratory personnel.
        Never store specimens in refrigerator.

2. Specimens

    A. THROAT/TONSILS: Specimens should be collected using
        dual swabs, by using gently pressure over the infected area.
        Do not allow the swabs to dry. If a delay in delivery to
        the lab is anticipated, deposit swabs tips in transport medium
        available in Bacteriology Lab. Do not allow swabs to come
        incontact with the tongue or normal secretions of the mouth.
        Requisition slip should indicate if a routine culture or
        only a "Strep Screen" is desired.
    B. NASAL, SINUS AND NASOPHARYNX: Use a single swab on a bent
        wire or flexible plastic base, tilt head back, pass swab
        directly back to posterior wall, rotate swab and carefully
        remove. Sinus samples will be collected by clinician. Naso-
        pharyngeal swabs with media are available from the Microbiology
        Department.
    C. EAR: Excreta are collected from the external auditory canal
             after the outer ear has been wiped with 70% ethanol.
             Middle ear or mastoid samples are collected by clinician.
             Deposit swab in transport medium and send directly to the
             laboratory.
    D. EYE: Specimens will be collected by the clinican. Deposit
        swabs in transport media and transport directly to lab.
    E. TEETH/GUMS, ETC.: If abscesses are present, use pressure
        over infected area with sterile swab and collect specimen
        with second sterile swab. If Vincent's Angina is suspected,
        swab the inflamed peridontal area. Notify lab of suspected
        infection. Deposit swabs in Stuart's Transport medium and
        send directly to lab.

FIGURE 8   PROCEDURES FOR COLLECTION
PREPARATION AND HANDLING OF MICRO-BIOLOGICAL SPECIMENS

FIGURE 9

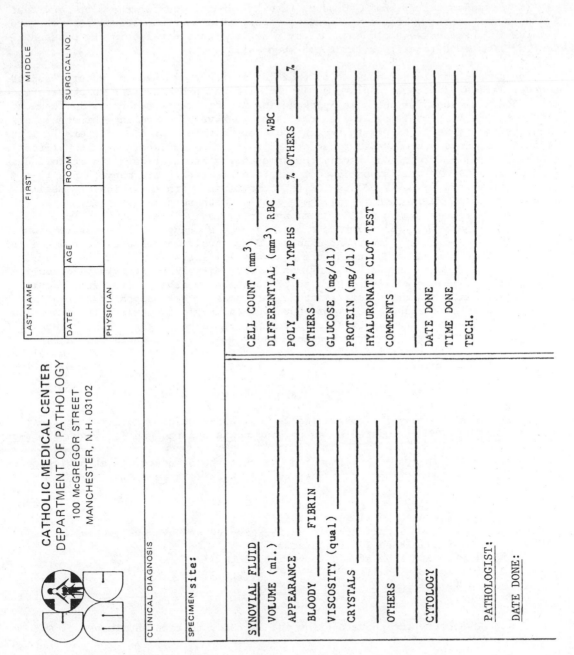

Procedure Manual

The Standard Operational Procedure Manual (SOPM) is one of the most important items at the bench. Laboratory Personnel could not function without it. The procedures in the manual should be so clearly defined that new laboratory personnel should be able to function without too much assistance.

The manual should not consist of package inserts from the manufacturer's kits. However, it is advisable to place an insert with the procedure for quick references, if needed. Reasons for not using package inserts are many, but probably the most important one is closely related to the story we have been telling throughout all of these pages. That is simply that each and every clinical setting differs from the next, therefore a procedure that was set up in a research laboratory in California certainly will not function exactly the same at the bench at Catholic Medical Center, Manchester, NH. As one is working out a procedure, there are many things that might be done a certain way only because of the conditions in that particular setting. The purpose of the SOPM is to have all these little idiosyncracies written. Also, as changes occur these are so noted, dated and initialed. This is a very important function of the SOPM. For example, there might be a change in temperature from 37°C to 40°C. This is a very important change and it should be so noted, dated and initialed so that all personnel doing the analysis will be aware of it. Another important reason not to use package inserts is that every laboratory should run its own normal values. These will vary because of location, weather, diet, etc. Normal values for California might differ enough for those in New Hampshire so that it should be so noted after running a study of about 40 healthy individuals. The mean should be calculated and the standard deviation determined. Values higher than the mean $\pm$ 4 SD and lower than the mean $\pm$ 4 SD are eliminated. The standard deviations are then recalculated with the remaining values. The process goes on until no values fall outside the $\pm$ 4 SD range. Then:

$$\text{Normal range} = \bar{x} - 2\ SD \text{ to } \bar{x} + 2\ SD$$

The SOPM is probably the most valuable tool and should be reviewed at least yearly, however the SOPM is updated on an ongoing basis and as such is always up-to-date.

The following is just a brief outline of what the Standard Operational Procedure Manual should contain. The more contained, the better it is.

1. Test Principle
2. Patient Preparation (if applicable)
3. Reagents (give location--this helps week-end and evening people)
4. Specimen Collection and Preparation
5. Procedure (don't be afraid to go into detail)
6. Calculation of Results
7. Normal Values
8. References

If one adheres to the above outline one is ready to face any inspector with an SOPM in hand.

Water Analysis

Water or dirty glassware are probably the two largest culprits responsible for poor laboratory results. A quality control program should include a glassware check procedure as well as a water quality control procedure.

Mr. Raymond Methot, BA, MS, MT (ASCP) who is our Maintenance and Safety Coordinator at Catholic Medical Center has put together the following quality checks which serve our needs quite well. Parts of it are CAP guidelines as well as some of our own. They may not suit your situation at all, but could give you ideas on how to set up your program. Figures 10 through 13 describe our program fully.

The glassware check is totally in the hands of our laboratory housekeeping section. They take great pride in their work and are constantly checking the glassware.

Instrument Maintenance

Laboratory results are only as good as equipment that is functioning properly. If a laboratory is going to give 24 hour service, downtime of instruments must be at a minimum. If preventive maintenance is not done on instrumentation, costly repairs will result as well as loss of laboratory service.

It matters not the size of the hospital, there definitely has to be a preventive maintenance program. Some hospitals have fairly elaborate systems while others keep it quite simple and practical.

Basically, we try to keep ours as simple as possible and involve or teach several people to avoid calling in technologists on shift.

A simple way might be the folllwing steps:

1. It is important to have a Service Contract with a reliable agency. This agency will come and do the preventive maintenance 2, 3 or 4 times a year, whichever best fits your needs. We have our PM 3 times per year. This is truly a necessity. You will find your downtime automatically reduced by about 50% after the first year that you're on a program.

2. It is important to do a daily check (every morning) of all instruments in the laboratory. (See Figure 14). This walk-through the laboratory assures that all instruments are functioning as expected. If an instrument should not be operational there is an Instrument Repair List used in conjunction with the Instrument Review Check List and the technologist would follow the directions on the Repair List.

3. Each instrument should have a separate function sheet for the daily, weekly and periodic checks for that particular instrument. Figures 15 through 19 are just a few examples of what these sheets can look like. As you can see they are not sophisticated, but are well accepted by inspectors and are easy for the technologists to use.

Most of our function sheets have been prepared by Raymond Methot guided with each Section Supervisor's input.

It is very important that the people who are doing the work be involved because they know what would make life easier for themselves.

People must be assigned specific duties. This is a very important point if the instrumentation part of the quality control program is to run smoothly. Every technologist must know what is expected of him/her.

This portion of quality can be quite elaborate, or as we do it, quite simply but clearly. Remember, documentation is the key word.

WATER

FIGURE 10

I. GENERAL

A. Pure water should be produced only at the rate needed, handled as little as possible, and used after minimum storage.
B. The water used and the processing systems must be checked frequently, regularly, and results of checks documented.

II. SAMPLING

A. The water specimens collected must be representative of that being used for test analysis. Collect specimens at the effluent site of the water processing system, at any storage site, and at any separate utilization point. Choose the points of any sampling carefully and keep a written description of their location.
B. The samples must represent the conditions existing at the point taken.
1. Collect specimens in polyethylene bottles as appropriately given for each testing method. The bottles must be processed and stored as follows:
a. Clean with soap and water.
b. Clean with Micro Cleaning solution.
c. Rinse out residula cleaning solution with reagent water.
d. Rinse thoroughly with reagent water.
e. Dry by draining.
f. Stopper and cover the bottle tops and necks with metal foil or parafilm dust covers.
2. Rinse the collection bottle at least three times with the water to be tested.
3. Fill the collection bottle quickly, allowing the water to run down the side and avoid frothing, to prevent changes in the carbon dioxide content.
4. Avoid excessive contact with air by filling the collection bottle to overflowing and then stoppering quickly and tightly.
5. The time interval between collection and sample analysis must be as short as possible.
6. The directions for collecting specimens for cultures is given in the methods section.

III. FREQUENCY

A. The testing must be accomplished frequently enough to insure a constant supply of reagent grade water that meets the requirements and specifications.
B. Source water-affluent to the water processing system. Check at least monthly to detect any changes in source water. The interval of time may be varied depending upon the local water situation.
C. Effluent water-direct discharge from the water processing system. Check that the effluent water meets all the specifications and requirements before using:
1. After cleaning or servicing the distillation apparatus.
2. After back-flushing, regenerating, or installing a new ion-enchange resin.
3. With each distinct batch of water processed in a distinctly discontinuous separate batch system.
4. At least once weekly with a continuous operation.
D. Stored water-should be kept at a minimum. Check the stored water for all specifications and requirements cannot be net for the procedures used, then stored water cannot be used and the water must be processed freshly as required.

E. Bench water—separate utilization points in the laboratory where separate containers of water are used for individual test analysis.

    1. This water should be obtained daily from the effluent of the water processing system. If this is a continual system, the once weekly effluent check will suffice.

    2. If obtained at different intervals or is obtained from a tested batch system, then this bench water must be tested at least weekly for the minimum specifications.

IV. REAGENTS

A. All reagents used must be free of interfering impurities and meet the specifications as outlined in Designation E-200 and the ACS reagents.

B. Blank tests and controls should be made where possible as outlined in the methods section.

C. Water being tested must be kept out of the reagents used for testing. Therefore, reagent grade water must be prepared or obtained separately.

V. REPORTING RESULTS

A. Keep accurate records.

    1. Performance of water processing system. Rate of effluent production or output.

    2. Dates of maintenance, servicing and changes.

    3. Keep graphs or charts of all specifications and requirements so that relative changes as well as absolute values can be compared. Report appropriate units. Adhere to the metric system and report in a weight/volume relationship of mg/liter rather than ppm.

VI. SPECIFICATIONS

Specification	Water Grade		
	Type I	Type II	Type III
Specific conductance, micromhos, maximum	0.1	2	5
Specific resistance, megohms, minimum	10	0.5	0.2
Silicate, mg/L, maximum	0.01	0.01	0.01
Heavy metals, mg/L, maximum	0.01	0.01	0.01
Permanganate reduction	Pass Test	Pass Test	Pass Test

The following requirements are also monitored to maintain acceptable standards for all water used as well as evaluate and maintain the water processing system.

Requirement	Level
Ammonia	Less than 0.1 mg/L
Carbon dioxide	Less than 3 mg/L
Culture	Interpretation
Hardness	Negative
pH	6.0-7.0
Sodium	Less than 0.1 mg/L *(0.4 meg/L)* *5-8-80*

SD

VII. REQUIREMENTS

A. Type I Reagent Water

    1. Used in methods intended to give maximum accuracy and precision.

    2. Atomic absorption spectrometry.

　　　　3.　Flame photometry.
　　　　4.　Enzymology.
　　　　5.　Blood gas and pH determinations.
　　　　6.　Reference buffer solutions.
　B.　Type II Reagent Water
　　　　Used for general laboratory testing. Chemical methods not specifically stated or proven to require Type I water may include most of the
procedures listed under Type I water depending upon the methodology,
the reagents used, and the sensitibity. The only group of procedures
determined to specifically require Type I water are those performed by
atomic absorptometry. Should include most hematological, serological, and
microbiological procedures.
　　　　All reagents not otherwise specified.
　C.　Type III Reagent Water
　　　　1.　Used for general alboratory testing.
　　　　2.　Satisfactory for most qualitative analysis procedures.
　　　　3.　Most urinalysis, parasitology and histological procedures.
　　　　4.　Rinsing glassware.
　D.　Reagent Water free of dissolved gas (Carbon dioxide free)
　　　　Used for those procedures where the normal limit of dissolved gases
(ammonia, carbon dioxide and oxygen) is excessive and affects the analysis.
The preparation directions are given in the methods section. Unless
otherwise specified, freshly boiled or adequately treated Type II water is
adequate.
Certain NBS and reference buffers.
Prothrombin times.

VIII.　TESTING

　A.　Substances reducing permanganate
　　　　1.　Sampling—Collect 500 ml of the water to be tested in a micro washed
　　　　　　stoppered bottle of chemically cleaned Pyrex glass. Perform the
　　　　　　analysis immediately.
　　　　2.　Method—The consumption of potassium permanganate by organic impurities
　　　　　　if judged by the disappearance of the permanganate color.
　　　　3.　Apparatus—None.
　　　　4.　Reagents
　　　　　　a.　Potassium permanganate, 0.1 N. Fisher chemicals # SO-P-288
　　　　　　b.　Sulfuric acid, concentrated. A.R. grade reagent.
　　　　5.　Standardization—None.
　　　　6.　Procedure
　　　　　　a.　Add 40 ul. of the potassium permanganate solution to a mixture
　　　　　　　　of 500 ml of the water and 1 ml of sulfuric acid.
　　　　　　b.　Stopper the bottle and mix well.
　　　　　　c.　Allow to stand for one hour at room temperature.
　　　　7.　Interpretation
　　　　　　a.　Consider the reagent water as having passed the test if the per-
　　　　　　　　manganate color does not disappear completely after standing for
　　　　　　　　one hour at room temperature.
　　　　　　b.　Ion-exchange materials may add organic contaminants to the water.

WATER (cont.)   FIGURE 10 (continued)

IX. TESTING: SODIUM
   A. Sampling- Obtain sufficient volume for flame photometric analysis in an
       acid-washed, chemically resistant glass or polyethylene bottle.
   B. METHOD_ Flame photometry.
   C. Apparatus- Flame photometer used routinely in the clinical laboratory.
   D. Reagents- Use the same standards and reagents as used with the clinical
       flame photometer. These standards and reagents must be prepared with Type I
       water. The ASTM specifies in addition the sodium or potassium content shall
       not exceed 0.01 mg/liter, or one percent of the maximum concentration in the
       range to be covered, whichever is greater.
   E. Procedure
       1. Open the Propane Shut-off Valve located at the top of the fuel cylinder,
           all the way open.
       2. Turn ON/OFF Switch to ON position. The Flame On Indicator Light should
           come on.
       3. Place a lithium blank solution or distilled water on the sample stand,
           raise the stand and aspirate for at least five minutes before calibrating.
       4. Change the lithium solution and aspirate a fresh lithium diluent.
       5. Set the needle on the Lithium Response meter at the center of the
           reference triangle with the Lithium Set Control.
       6. Set both the sodium and Potassium Digital Concentration Displays to
           0000 with their respective Zero Controls.
       7. Aspirate an appropriate working standard (140 Na/ 5 K). Dilute Two
           HUNDRED TIMES with the lithium diluent. 50 microliters of standard in
           10 ml of lithium diluent.
       8. Set both the Sodium and Potassium Digital Concentration Displays to the
           corresponding values of this standard with the respective Balance
           Controls.
       9. Replace the standard with an unknown sample correctly diluted with
           the lithium diluent and aspirate. (The dilution is made as for the
           standards). A direct read out is recorded.
       10. All samples, standards, and controls should be done in duplicate and
           should chekc within 1 mEq/L.
       11. After completing your determinations, aspirate lithium diluent or dis-
           tilled water through the unit for a few minutes.
       12. Turn the PROPANE Shut-off Valve at the top of the fuel cylinder clock-
           wise (closed). Do not overtighten this valve. When the Flame On Indi-
           cator Light goes out, the solenoid will shut off all gas supplies.
       13. Allow the Automatic safety Relief Valve at the bottom of the Air Filter
           to purge condensed water vapor from the compressed air supply.
       14. When dry, place the ON/OFF Switch to it's Off position.
   F. Interpretation- The acceptable limit of 0.1 mg/ liter is based upon the
       dilution and sensitivity of the flame photometer used. Each laboratory may
       have to establish their own limits on this basis. The one percent of the
       maximum concentration in the range to be covered is a good guideline for
       setting the upper limit. This calculation must include the dilution factor
       and represent the actual concentration measured, not the normal serum con-
       centration.
            An increase in sodium concentration may be the first sign of deficiency
       in the cation exchange resin. Also, it is a good indicator of the status of
       the distillation apparatus.

WATER (CONT.)

FIGURE 10 (continued)

B. Ammonia Nitrogen: 19mm cuvette
  1. Principle: Any substance containing an amino radical will react with the directly proportional to the concentration of ammonia nitrogen.
  2. Sampling: 8 ml water- test immediately.
  3. Reagents: Ammonium chloride 1000 mgN/ liter standard. Dissolve 3.819 gm. NH$_4$Cl resin treated water. Dilute to 1 liter. Intermediate standard 10.0 mgN/ liter. Dilute 1.0 ml ofstock standard (1.0 mg/ml) to 100 ml with resin treated water. Workingstandard 0.5mg N/liter. Dilute 5 ml of intermediate standard to 100 ml with resin treatedwater.
  Resin treated water: Use sterile water for irrigation 1000 mlvolume. Add 2 vials (10 gm) prep. resin to the bottle and mix thoroughly. Allow resin to settle before use. Store at room temperature. (Resin obtained from Hyland BloodAmmonia Test Kit).
  Phenol reagent: Chemistry II Refridgerator. 0.5% W/V sodium nitro-ferri-cyanide in phenol. Store at 4-8°C. Stable 6 months in brown bottle.
  Alkali hypochlorite reagent: Chemistry II refrigerator. 1.5% W/V sodium hypochlorite in 17.9% (W/V) NaOH. Store at 4-8°C. Stable 6 months in brown bottle.
  4. Procedure:
    a. Label the following series of 10 ml (15x100) new vacutainer tubes for each blank, standardand test.
    b. Add the indicated volumes of each reagent.

	0.50 mg/L N standard	Resin treated	water	Test water	Phenol reagent	Alkali hypochlorite
Reagent Blank	----	8 ml.		--	1 ml.	1 ml.
Standard I 0.125 mg/L N	2 ml.	6 ml.		--	1 ml.	1 ml.
Standard II 0.25 mg/1 N	4 ml.	4 ml.		--	1 ml.	1 ml.
Test water	--	--		8 ml.	1 ml.	1 ml-

    c. Mixwell and keep capped.
    d. Incubate at 37°C in a water bath for 15 min.
    e. Read absorbance in the spectrophotometer at 630 nm. in a19mm cuvette against the reagent blank.
    f. Calculations: Plot the standards on a regular graph paperopposite their absorbances. Read the concentration of the test water opposite their absorbances.
    g. The mg ammonia (NH$_3$)/ dl= mg N/dl x 1.2.
  5. Interpretation:
    a. Values greater than 0.1mg NH$_3$/ liter indicates eithercontamination or a breakdown of the ion exchange resin.
    b. A raised ammonia level is one of the first indications ofpoor quality water froma cation resin. Water must be checked from a new column immediately as high ammonia levels are found if the new column has not been adequately preconditioned.

  6. References:
  Hyland Blood Ammonia test Kit (at end). Also Henry R.J. Clinical Chemistry: Principle and Technics

FIGURE 11

CATHOLIC MEDICAL CENTER LABORATORY

WATER ANALYSIS   TECH.   DA   MO   YR

ACCEPTABLE VALUES	DISTILLED WATER	DEMINERALIZED	STAT LAB
SODIUM $<$ 0.4 mEq/L			
AMMONIA $<$ 0.1 mg/L			
KMNO$_4$ TO PASS TEST			
CONDUCTANCE $<$ 2.0umhos			
RESISTANCE $>$ 0.5 megohms	———————		———————
pH 6-7.0			

NOTE: THE SOURCE WATER FOR THE DEMINERALIZER IS FROM CENTRAL
SUPPLY DISTILLED WATER SYSTEM.

THE SOURCE WATER FOR THE DISTILLED WATER SUPPLY IS FROM
THE DISTILLER LOCATED IN CENTRAL SUPPLY. IT IS PUMPED IN
THRU A PLASTIC PIPING SUSTEM.

THE STAT LAB DEMINERALIZED WATER IS A STAND ALONE SYSTEM
CONNECTED DIRECTLY TO THE TAP.(CITY WATER SUPPLY).

COLLECTION:

1) ALLOW WATER TO FLOW FREELY FOR 5 SECONDS BEFORE COLLECTING.

2) FILL THE APPROPRIATELY LABELLED FLASKS TO THE BRIM.

3) THERE IS ENOUGH HEAD SPACE ABOVE THE 500 ml. MARK TO DO
ALL THE TESTING.

4) THE RESISTANCE READING OF THE DEMINERALIZED WATER IS TO BE
TAKEN OFF THE METER IMMEDIATELY AFTER SAMPLING. THE SAMPLING
STATION FOR DEMINERALIZED WATER IS AT THE METER OUTLET IN
THE GLASSWARE ROOM.

5) FOLLOW THE PROTOCOL OUTLINED IN THE WATER TESTING MANUAL
LOCATED AT THE SMAII REAGENT PREPARATION BENCH.

6) REPORT ANY UNACCEPTABLE VALUE TO THE RESPONSIBLE SUPERVISOR.

FIGURE 12

GLASSWARE DETERGENT CHECK

PRINCIPLE

The importance of using chemically clean glassware in the clinical laboratory cannot be overemphasized. This procedure is recommended as a method of testing glassware for proper removal of detergent during the cleaning process.

PROCEDURE

1. One randomly chosen piece of glassware is taken from each load, preferably a narrow necked flask, Erlenmeyer flask, or some other piece of glassware that is difficult to rinse adequately. (Also use a flask or tube containing detergent to see a positive reaction.)
2. Add 20 ml of deionized water to the pieces of glassware being tested and swirl the water within it.
3. Add 2 drops of BSP (Bromsulphthalein) solution to the water and mix.

INTERPRETATION

The appearance of a purple color in the water indicates the solution is alkaline, which may be attributed to residual detergent in the glassware. If the batch of glassware tests positive for the BSP test, it should be rewashed. Record the positive or negative reactions on the daily work sheet along with your initials.

REAGENTS

BSP solution: BSP ampules, 5% BSP solution (Hynson, Westcott and Dunnings, Inc. Baltimore, MD).

REFERENCE

Laboratory Medicine, May 1977, page 133.

_SB_ LAB SUPERVISOR

_RB_ LAB DIRECTOR

5-31-77

Rev. 10-17-78 SB

Rev. 8-21-79 SB

Rev. 8-27-80 SB

FIGURE 13

DAILY GLASSWARE BSP DYE QUALITY CHECK

DATE	TUBE	FLK	TECH	DATE	TUBE	FLK	TECH	DATE	TUBE	FLK	TECH	DATE	TUBE	FLK	TECH	DATE	TUBE	FLK

FIGURE 15

TECHNICON
BLOOD GAS - MAINTENANCE PROGRAM

MONTH ___ TO ___ YEAR

	1	2	3	4	5	6	7	8	9	10	11	12	13	14	15	16	17	18	19	20	21	22	23	24	25	26	27	28	29	30
DAILY ROUTINES																														
CHECK GASES																														
EXERCISE #12																														
#13																														
#14																														
#15																														
#16																														
#17																														
ASPIRATE 0.2% NAOCl																														
EMPTY WASTE BOTTLE																														
FILL BUFFER & SALINE																														
WEEKLY ROUTINES																														
ROTATE ELECTRODES																														
CHANGE MEMBRANES																														
#1 KCl																														
#1 pCO_2																														
#1 pO_2																														
#1 pH																														
#2KCl																														
#2 pCO_2																														
#2 pO_2																														
#2 pH																														
CLEAN pH ELECTRODE #1																														
CLEAN pH ELECTRODE #2																														
PREPARE 0.2% NaOCl																														
CLEAN STYLUS WITH WIRE																														
BAROMETRIC PRESSURE 7																														
REFRIDGE TEMPERATURE																														
HI																														
LO																														
GLASS THERMOMETER																														
TECH. SIGNATURE																														

FIGURE 14

INSTRUMENT REVIEW
CHECK LIST

X OR V MEANS FUNCTION EXPECTED
O MEANS DEFECTIVE
(REFER TO INSTRUMENT REPAIR LIST)

MONTH   YEAR

1 2 3 4 5 6 7 8 9 10 11 12 13 14 15 16 17 18 19 20 21 22 23 24 25 26 27 28 29 30 31

CRYOSTAT
HOODS
TISSUE PROCESSOR
COLDIN REFRIDGE
FOSTER REFRIDGE
CO2 INCUBATOR

FOSTER WALK IN
DEMINERALIZED H20

GLENCO REFRIDGE
FUME HOODS

BG II
STAT/LYTE
GEMINI I
GEMINI II
VOLTAGE
GILFORD

FIBROMETER
COLEMAN I
COLEMAN II

ZBI
COLDIN REFRIDGE
DILLON REFRIDGE

BB REFRIDGE I
BB REFRIDGE II
BB REFRIDGE III
RC3 CENTRIFUGE
FOSTER FREEZER

FIGURE 16

CATHOLIC MEDICAL CENTER

PIPETTORS: MONTHLY CALIBRATION CHECK   MONTH   YEAR

PIPETTOR LOCATION		NET WEIGHT OF WATER	TOLERENCES
FIBROMETER	0.1 ml.	_____	0.0997 gm ± 0.0003
	0.2 ml.	_____	0.1994 gm ± 0.0006
Gemini I	1.0 ml.	_____	0.9970 gm ± 0.016
Gemini II	1.0 ml.	_____	0.9970 gm ± 0.016
Osmometer	2.0 ml.	_____	1.9940 gm ± 0.032
Pregnancy MLA	50 ul.	_____	0.0498 gm ± 0.0003
MLA	100 ul.	_____	0.0997 gm ± 0.0003
Water Analysis	20 ul.	_____	0.0199 gm ± 0.0003
Oxford (urinalysis)	5.0 ml. sal.	_____	4.9850 gm ± 0.08
	5.0 ml. sulfo	_____	4.9850 gm ± 0.08

NOTE: 1.0 ml water at 25⁰C. weighs 0.9970 gm.

NOTE: Pipettors falling outside the indicated tolerances must be
readjusted to meet specifications or serviced to insure proper
volume uptake. Report out of spec. instruments to supervisor.

Tolerances: less than 1.0 ml = 0.3%
1.0 ml. or greater = 1.6%

FIGURE 17

MONTH:
YEAR:

DAILY	1	2	3	4	5	6	7	8	9	10	11	12	13	14	15	16	17	18	19	20	21	22	23	24	25	26	27	28	29	30	31
CHECK DRIFT																															
CHECK FOR SHORTS																															
PHOTOCELL RESPONSE																															

WEEKLY	FIRST	SECOND	THIRD	FOURTH	REMARKS
WAVELENGTH					
MONOCHROMATOR					
CLEAN CUVETTE WELL					
CLEAN EXICITER LAMP					

MONTHLY

NICKLE SULFATE TRAY LT. 670	OUR%	EXPT %	OUR O.D.	EXPT
70–420 1.0		15–25		0.824 / 0.602
0.75		25–35		0.602 / 0.456
ANDPASS 0.50		39–49		0.409 / 0.310
520 0.25		61–71		0.215 / 0.149

COBALT AMMONIUM SULFATE 520	OUR %	EXPT %	OUR O.D.	EXPT
1.0		15–25		0.824 / 0.602
0.75		25–35		0.602 / 0.456
0.50		39–49		0.409 / 0.310
0.25		61–71		0.215 / 0.149

CHROMIC PERCHLORATE 420	OUR %	EXPT %	OUR O.D.	EXPT
1.0		15–25		0.824 / 0.602
0.75		25–35		0.602 / 0.456
0.50		39–49		0.409 / 0.310
0.25		61–71		0.215 / 0.149

FIGURE 18

FIRE EXTINGUISHER CHECK

EXTINGUISHER NUMBER	LOCATION	PRESSURE √-IN GREEN 0-NOT FUNCT.	TECH	DATE
1	BLOOD BANK			
2	HEMATOLOGY			
3	CHEMISTRY			
4	BACTERIOLOGY			
5	HALL NEAR HISTOLOGY			
6	CONFERENCE ROOM			
7	OUTSIDE VOLATILE LIQUIDS			

COMMENTS:

EYEWASH CHECK

EYEWASH NUMBER	LOCATION	FUNCTIONING	√-IF OK 0-NOT FUNCT.	TECH	DATE
1	CHEMISTRY				
2	SPECIAL CHEMISTRY				
3	HISTOLOGY				
4	STAT LAB				

COMMENTS

FIGURE 19

VOLTAGE MONITORING   CMC LABORATORY

RECORD THE VOLTAGE READING OF THE VOLT METER DAILY
ESTIMATE THE INTERMEDIATE READING SINCE EACH DIVISION EQUALS 5 VOLTS.

DATE/TECH	VOLTAGE	DATE/TECH	VOLTAGE	DATE/TECH	VOLTAGE	DATE/TECH	VOLTAGE	DATE/TECH	VOLTAGE

it again, when an inspector says to you "show me", you must be able to produce written proof or else a negative action on the part of your laboratory will automatically be assumed.

Every accrediting agency such as College of American Pathologists, Joint Commission on Accreditation of Hospitals, CDC, American Association of Blood Banks and various state laboratory licensing agencies require instrument and equipment maintenance programs. If nothing else, this should be an incentive to set one up in your own respective health facility and be ready for your next inspector.

Purchasing of Quality Supplies and Inventory

Probably the most vital part of laboratory "quality" begins here. The purchasing of reagents is very crucial. If the person doing the purchasing knows nothing about the laboratory and is just out to get the most for his/her money, the laboratory will find itself quite often unable to do the work because the substitution reagent unfortunately will not do the same job. This tactic will often result in waste-- waste of time and waste of money. I'm not saying here that substitute reagents are bad, what I'm saying is if there is contemplation to purchase a substitute reagent other than the one recommended by the vendor of the instrument it should be evaluated first and after investigative procedures prove results are the same, then and only then should substitution be made. This therefore means involvement of not only the purchasing person but of section supervisors. Section supervisors should have a very definite say in the type of reagents and the type of glassware purchased for their areas. They know best what their needs are and should be listened to.

The purchase of glassware is another area that is critical. All volumetric glassware should be Class A and meet tolerance limits set by National Bureau of Standards, however, they should be rechecked by the laboratory before being put into use.

Procedure for calibration of volumetric glassware is as follows:

1. Weigh a clean flask to the fourth decimal place

2. Take pipet to be calibrated and carefully pipet water and transfer to flask

3. Weigh flask plus water

4. Subtract 1 from 3 = weight of water

5. Note temperature of the water

6. Density of water at 25°C is 0.9970

7. Calculate volume of water delivered as follows:

$$\text{Volume} = \frac{\text{Weight of Water} \quad (\#4)}{\text{Density at given temperature} \quad (\#6)}$$

8. Look to Tables 20 and 21 to see if error is within tolerable limits.

Inventory is also an integral part of a total quality control program. This is a personal decision as to how often it should be done in your laboratory. In our clinical setting we do it weekly. The following Laboratory Supply Inventory Sheet was designed by Miss Germaine Clement, BA, MT (ASCP), Assistant Chief Technologist

FIGURE 20

TOLERANCE LIMITS FOR VOLUMETRIC GLASSWARE

CAPACITY (ml)	TOLERANCE LIMITS (ml)				
	VOLUMETRIC PIPETTES	MEASURING PIPETTES	BURETTES	VOLUMETRIC FLASKS	GRADUATED CYLINDER
1/2	0.006	–	–	–	–
1	0.006	0.01	–	0.01	–
2	0.006	0.01	–	0.015	–
3	0.01	–	–	0.015	–
4	0.01	–	–	0.02	–
5	0.01	0.02	0.01	0.02	0.05
10	0.02	0.03	0.02	0.02	0.08
15	0.03	–	–	–	–
20	0.03	–	–	–	–
25	0.03	0.05	0.03	0.03	0.14
50	0.05	–	0.05	0.05	0.20
100	0.08	–	0.10	0.08	0.35
200	0.10	–	–	0.10	–
250	–	–	–	0.12	0.65
500	–	–	–	0.20	1.10
1,000	–	–	–	0.30	2.0
2,000	–	–	–	0.50	3.5

FIGURE 21

TOLERANCE LIMITS FOR PIPETTES
AS SPECIFIED BY THE NATIONAL BUREAU OF STANDARDS

CAPACITY (ml)	VOLUMETRIC PIPETTES		MEASURING PIPETTES MEASURING PIPETTES
	DELIVERY TIME (SECONDS)	LIMIT OF ERROR IN DELIVERY TIME (SECONDS)	DELIVERY TIME (SECONDS)
1/2	10	3	–
1	10	3	35
2	10	3	35
5	15	3	40
10	15	4	40
20	25	4	–
25	25	6	50
50	30	8	–
100	40	15	–
200	50	20	–

at Catholic Medical Center. It is simple, easy to use and has proven quite adequate for our setting (see Figure 22).

Error Detection—Charts

The basic item used for detecting errors occurring in any clinical analysis is the quality control chart. The object of the Levy-Jenning chart is to obtain the mean, standard deviations and coefficient of variation for laboratory determinations.

To use the chart (Fig. 4) control material must be used. It is a management decision as to which control material will be analyzed. There are three kinds of control sera to be considered:

1. Homemade pooled sera

2. Assayed commercial control sera

3. Unassayed commercial control sera

Homemade Pooled Sera

Homemade pooled sera appears to be the most reasonable cost-wise, but the time factor involved, as well as uncertainty as to results of material produced, could convert it to being more costly. I will briefly describe the method to produce it, but it would not be my method of choice.

1. Save left-over sera from patients (daily). Freeze at about 20°C. Plastic bottles could be kept in the freezer and the sera just poured into them daily. Make enough to last about 4 or 5 months. Sera kept frozen for more than 6 months is certain to give you problems.

2. About 3 weeks before your present pool runs out, thaw out all that you have accumulated. Mix with glass rod or magnetic stirrer. Do not shake.

3. Centrifuge at 3000 rmp for 15 minutes. (Do not expose to much light).

4. Pour into tubes equal to the amount of sera to be used daily. Use rubber caps (vacutainers) whenever possible.

5. Label containers with date of preparation, initials of technologist or technician, the expiration date and anything else you might feel is necessary.

6. Deep freeze at 20°C.

Often homemade pools do not have ranges for enzymes or the ranges for the constituents might not be satisfactory. If this occurs, compounds may be added. After addition of these chemicals the pool should be stirred for about 2 hours with a magnetic stirrer. After ascertaining that everything is dissolved, the mixture is filtered with Millipore filters, aliquoted then refrozen.

Please note, pools should not be frozen more than twice. If so, the constituents will start to degrade and the whole batch will be worthless. There are some advantages to the preparation of homemade pool:

1. It is inexpensive.

FIGURE 22
LAB. SUPPLY INVENTORY

DATE

ITEM

| ON HAND | ORDER | ON HAND | ORDER | ON HAND | ORDER | ON HAND | ORDER | ON HAND | ORDER | ON HAND | ORDER | ON HAND | ORDER | ON HAND | ORDER | ON HAND | ORDER | ON HAND | ORDER | ON HAND | ORDER | ON HAND | ORDER | ON HAND |

2.   It is the same as human sera.

3.   There is no change in value because of lyophilization.

Assayed Commercial Control Sera

For many reasons, smaller laboratories may find the use of assayed material more advantageous:

1.   Shelf life is longer (1-2 years).

2.   Mean and standard deviations have already been determined (if unable to attain mean for a particular assay it might be advisable to set your own mean, however you should check your procedure by perhaps sending an assay to another laboratory to be analyzed then you could procede with confidence).

In larger hospitals, assayed commercial control sera is a must. Its use may not be routine quality control, but may be used for trouble shooting or as a control for those assays not done frequently.

Unassayed Commercial Control Sera

Most large laboratories make use of unassayed control sera. The reasons are many, but some of the few most important ones are:

1.   Already prepared, no fuss in making own pool.

2.   Shelf life is long--1-2 years.

3.   When buying unassayed pool, you can belong to a group containing 100 or more laboratories all using the same material. This permits interlaboratory comparisons which can be very helpful.

Like everything in life there is always two sides to every story. There are disadvantages of unassayed commercial controls. If you are aware of the pitfalls then there is no problem. These include:

1.   Reconstitution--there is bound to be some degree of variation when adding water to the lyophilized sample.

2.   There will be some variation in filling by the vendor, even under the most perfect conditions.

3.   The base for the sera is animal in origin, again introducing some variation.

What this means is that the Levy-Jenning charts may not look as perfect with unassayed commercial control sera as they might with homemade pools. But the advantages far outweigh the very slight aberrations that the disadvantages might reveal and these are not significant enough to deter large laboratories from using commercial unassayed pools. The use of the monthly interlaboratory summary sheets alone gives the supervisor a tool to manage his section that certainly tips the balance in its favor.

Levy-Jenning Chart

To use the chart as a management tool in quality control, your manual must contain an outline for decision making. Your quality control program must have two pools, normal and abnormal. The manual should contain a section on:

1. Daily decisions

2. Monthly decisions

3. Annual decisions

4. Periodic decisions

The daily decision section should have items such as the following--items should be specific to your situation:

1. Accept run if both normal and abnormal controls are within ± 2 SD.

2. Reject run if 1 control is outside ± 2 SD. (At this point add any other reasons you feel a run should be rejected.)

3. When run is rejected the following procedures should take place: start run over using new vials of normal and abnormal pools. (This is just one of many rules you may wish your laboratory to follow; it is important for the management team to make the decisions, and communicate these to the laboratory personnel.)

4. Check points of 2 or 3 previous days for possible clues to problem.

MONTHLY DECISIONS

1. Pathologists and supervisors should meet to review quality control for the month.

    a. Levy-Jenning charts
    b. Youden plots
    c. CAP surveys
    d. Manuals
    e. New procedures

ANNUAL DECISIONS

1. Pathologists and supervisors should meet to review the following:

    a. Summary of a year's quality control monthly reviews
    b. Comprehensive surveys
    c. Procedure manuals

PERIODIC DECISIONS

1. Pathologists and supervisors should meet to discuss methodology changes, new procedures or new equipment to be purchased.

PREPARATION OF LEVY-JENNING CHART

Using commercially prepared unassayed control sera let us set up a chart. Step 1: determine acceptable range. As an example let us use BUN. To establish this, the determination must be run at least 20 times by as many technicians as possible. The accumulated data is then analyzed in the following manner. Using Figure 3, do the following:

FIGURE 23

MONTHLY QUALITY CONTROL REPORT

| Procedure BUN |
| Date 8-28-80 |
| Pool # 646 |

| 1. Average X = 40 |
| 2. ± Std. Dev. = 4.0 / 1 SD = 4.0 |
| # out of control 2 - #10 & #17 |

Evaluation:

Procedure for Calculating Average and Standard Deviation:

1. Record control analyses in column one.
2. Add column one.
3. Calculate average - line A.
4. Calculate and record in column two individual differences from average.
5. Square each individual difference, and record in column three.
6. Add column three.
7. Calculate standard deviation (SD) - line B.
8. Control limits: ± 3 x SD = 3 x _____ =

Calculations:

A. x = each individual measurement
   n = number of measurements =

Average = $\dfrac{\text{sum of x}}{n}$ or $\dfrac{\Sigma x}{n}$

Average = 40 =

(Record average in box 1 and 3.)

	Average: (3) 40	Diff. from Average:	Squared diff from Averag
1	40	0	0
2	40	0	0
3	43	3	9
4	39	1	1
5	40	0	0
6	41	1	1
7	45	5	25
8	41	1	1
9	38	2	4
10	29	11	121
11	42	2	4
12	43	3	9
13	43	3	9
14	39	1	1
15	38	2	4
16	39	1	1
17	49	9	81
18	43	3	9
19	40	0	0
20	42	2	4
21	38	2	4
22	34	6	36
23	37	3	9
24	38	2	4
25	43	3	9
26			

FIGURE 23 (continued)

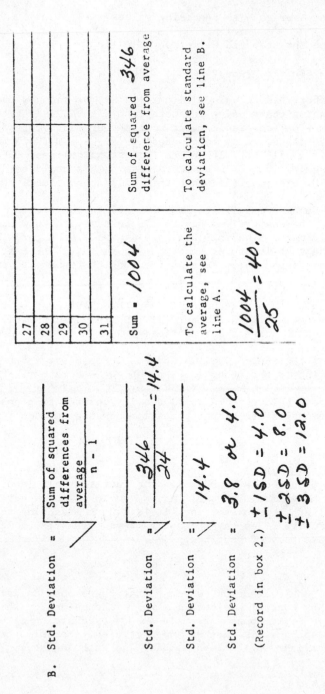

27		
28		
29		
30		
31		

Sum = 1004 | | Sum of squared differerce from average *346*

To calculate the average, see line A.

$$\frac{1004}{25} = 40.1$$

To calculate standard deviation, see line B.

B. Std. Deviation = $\sqrt{\dfrac{\text{Sum of squared differences from average}}{n-1}}$

Std. Deviation = $\sqrt{\dfrac{346}{24}} = 14.4$

Std. Deviation = $\sqrt{14.4}$

Std. Deviation = 3.8 or 4.0

(Record in box 2.) ± 1 SD = 4.0
± 2 SD = 8.0
± 3 SD = 12.0

1. Determine the average

2. Determine the standard deviation (Figure 23)

3. Eliminate values outside $\pm$ 3 SD

4. Re-determine average with remaining values

5. Re-determine the standard deviation

6. Assign acceptable range--average $\pm$ 2 SD

Since our BUN chart had no values beyond $\pm$ 3 SD, we can now proceed to setting up the actual Levy-Jenning chart using the data from Figure 23. At this time we must use $\pm$ 2 SD as upper limit of acceptable range unless your laboratory decides otherwise. Your chart Figure 24 is now ready to be used at the bench. This particular chart has a CV of 10% which is really not within the Federal guidelines. What you have to do now is work on narrowing your CV's to 5% or less. This could be done by accepting no values beyond $\pm$ 1 SD. You may find that this will automatically happen.

A chart must be examined daily to look for shifts and trends. (These were defined at the beginning of the chapter). This is the best way to know exactly what is happening in your department. The following are examples of a curve showing normal distribution and one that is out of control (Figure 25). The next example will be of a shift and a trend (Figure 26). Reasons for such charts are given under the definitions.

The important point to stress here is that the chart must be reviewed daily and notations must be made if and when abnormalities are seen, as well as what sort of action is being taken to correct any problem.

We have stressed the use of Quality Control in Chemistry, but most of these procedures can be applied to the other sections of the laboratory.

Many hospitals now belong to regional quality control programs and the SD's and CV's as well as the charts are computerized monthly saving much time for the busy supervisor.

External Survey Programs

At this point, we cannot stress enough the fact that all laboratories participate in external survey programs. This will allow you to compare your method with values obtained by several other laboratories. It is also a licensing requirement that laboratories show active files on external surveys. This is really one of the best ways to check the accuracy of your tests.

Quality Evaluation

When we speak about evaluation, we mean that there must be documentation to the fact that the quality control has been checked. The method by which it is done need not be complicated. Daily rounds are made and every chart, whether it be for instrumentation or Levy-Jennings, is checked and initialed. Monthly, the work is reviewed by the Section Supervisor, Chief Technologist and Pathologist and so documented.

FIGURE 24

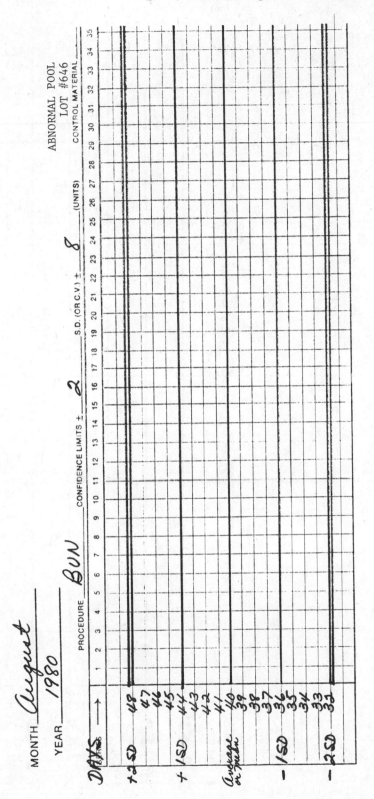

FIGURE 25

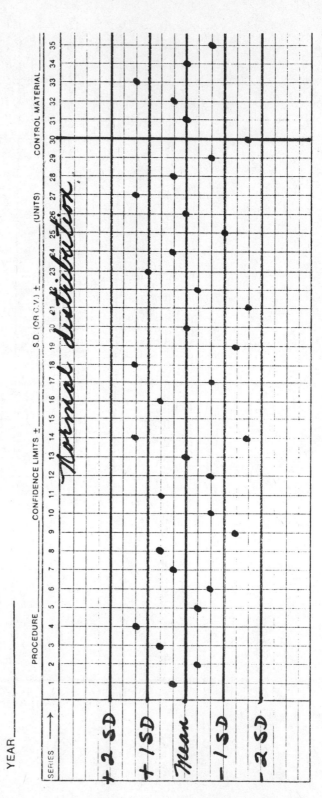

FIGURE 25 (continued)

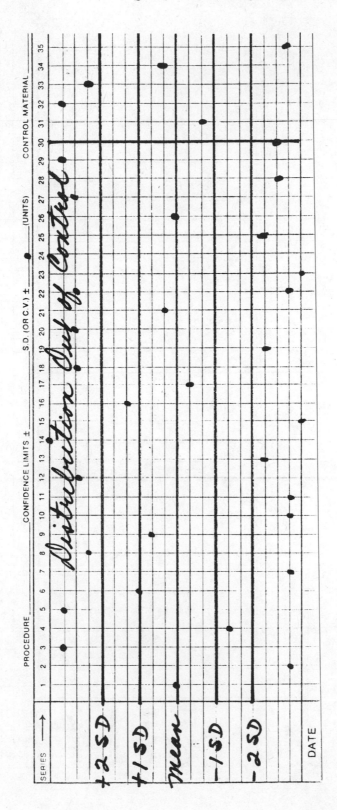
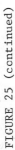

FIGURE 26

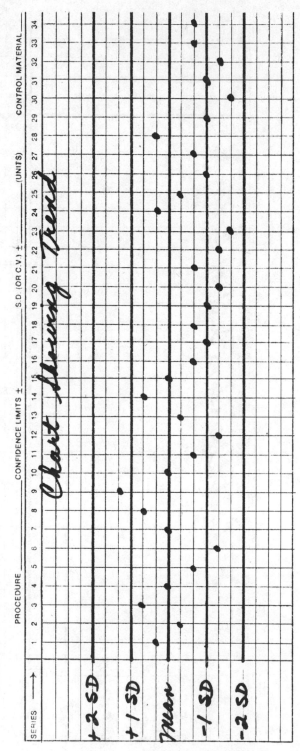

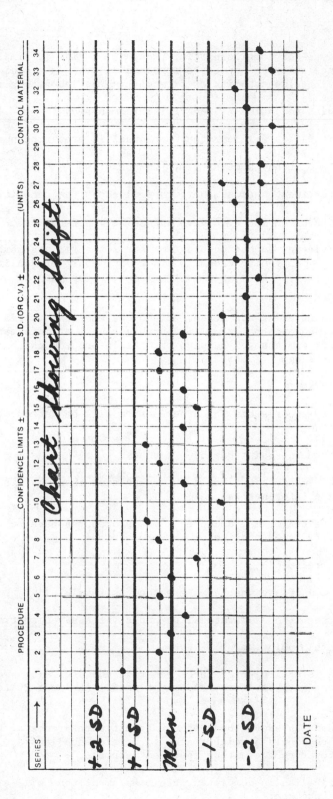

FIGURE 26 (continued)

Continuing Education

There are many types of continuing education. To define it simply, it means any educational experience that has no degree attached to it. This could be a seminar, or workshop given by outside agencies or from within the laboratory itself.

In-house continuing education is beneficial in many ways:

1. Active participation by laboratory personnel in preparation and presentation.

2. More people can attend because it is in-house.

3. Topics are pertinent because they are decided by the technicians.

4. Time limit can be set so work does not suffer.

The ASCP has continuing education programs for its affiliate members. No matter who the individual is, continuing education is a vital part of quality work in the laboratory. The only way to keep up with the latest techniques is to go out and find out about them.

Another form of continuing education that no one mentions is reading and more reading. The latest journals have an immeasurable source of information, and will serve as reference for any change you wish to make in procedures that are currently being used in your setting.

Method Evaluation and Selection

There are probably two reasons why a new method will be introduced into a clinical setting:

1. A revenue producing point has been reached.

2. Patient care demands a quicker turn around time than what is currently available through a reference lab.

Before a method is officially accepted a few procedures have to be undertaken. The following is a very brief outline of the procedures:

1. Seek out the reference.

2. Follow protocol to see whether the method is feasible.

3. Make a few runs with calibrators, or pools, or assayed control material.

4. Evaluate at this point.

5. If technique is not rejected check accuracy and precision. Run low and high controls along with patients randomly picked. At least 20 to 30 runs should be done.

6. These same samples should be checked against a reference method. Probably 2 or 3 samples should be either sent to a reference laboratory or checked in your own laboratory against an approved method.

7. Once the evaluation is completed, the management team will either accept or reject the procedure.

Supervision

For a quality control program to meet the objectives set forth, there must be constant surveillance. This means that the program will only give you what you put into it. Surveillance means daily, weekly, monthly and yearly checks, and everyone in the laboratory has to be interested and must want it to work.

BIBLIOGRAPHY AND RECOMMENDED READINGS

"College of American Pathologists Instruction Manual". Quality Assurance Service. 1973. Traverse City, MI.

Copeland, Bradley E., MD, Clare Shrukan C(ASCP), Kathleen Day, MT (ASCP), "A Decision Making Tool The Average Difference Test". 1974. American Society of Clinical Pathologists. Chicago, Illinois.

Dharan, Murali. "Total Quality Control in the Clinical Laboratory". 1977. C. V. Mosby Company. St. Louis, MO.

Feinstein, Alvan, R. "Clinical Biostatistics". 1977. C. V. Mosby Company. St. Louis, MO.

Galen, Robert S., MD, and S. Raymond Gambino, MD. 1975. "Beyond Normality". John Wiley and Sons. New York, NY.

Hirsch, Charles S., Morris, R. Crawford, Alan R. Moritz. *HANDBOOK OF LEGAL MEDICINE.* 1979. Fifth Edition. C. V. Mosby Company. St. Louis.

Inhorn, Stanley L., MD, Editor. "Quality Assurance Practices for Health Laboratories". 1978. American Public Health Association. Washington, DC.

Lundberg, George D., MD. *MANAGING THE PATIENT-FOCUSED LABORATORY.* 1975. Medical Economics Company. Oradell, NJ.

Medical Laboratory Observer. "A Management Primer for the Clinical Laboratory". July 1975. Medical Economics Company. Oradell, NJ.

Schuffstall, RM, MD, Brecharr Hemmaphardk, PhD, MBA. *THE HOSPITAL LABORATORY, MODERN CONCEPTS OF MANAGEMENT, OPERATIONS AND FINANCE.* 1979. C. V. Mosby Company. St. Louis, MO.

Vinson, Laurie T., Puliver, Edward and David Plaut. "Quality Control in the Blood Gas Laboratory". *Clinical Laboratory Products. April 1980.*

ACCURACY IN CLINICAL CHEMISTRY. Dade Publishers. Miami, FL.

Index